Crock Pot Cookbook for Beginners

1001 Best Crock Pot

Slow Cooker Recipes

(Latest Edition)

William Slinkard

CONTENTS

DESSERT RECIPES..47

POULTRY RECIPES **59**

BEEF, PORK & LAMB RECIPES 71

FISH & SEAFOOD RECIPES 82

SOUPS & STEWS RECIPES

SIDE DISH RECIPES 106

SNACK RECIPES 118

APPETIZERS RECIPES **129**

VEGETABLE & VEGETARIAN RECIPES **140**

Introduction

Slow cookers are cheap to buy, economical to use and they're great for making the most of budget ingredients. They offer a healthier, low-fat method of cooking and require the minimum amount of effort. Really, what's not to love?

10 top tips for using a slow cooker

1. Cut down your prep time

One of the main attractions for many people is the ease of a slow cooker, so when you're looking for recipes, avoid those that suggest a lot of pre-preparation. For many dishes, particularly soups and stews, you really can just throw all the ingredients in. It can be nice to cook the onions beforehand, as the flavour is different to when you put them in raw, but experiment both ways as you may find you prefer one. It can also be good to brown meat to give it some colour, but again, this is not essential.

2. Prepare for slow cooking the night before

If you're short on time in the morning, prepare everything you need for your slow-cooked meal the night before, put it into the slow-cooker dish, cover and store in the fridge overnight. Ideally the dish should be as close to room temperature as possible, so get it out of the fridge when you wake up and leave it for 20 minutes before turning the cooker on. If you need to heat your dish beforehand, then put the ingredients in a different container and transfer them in the morning.

3. Choose cheap cuts

Slow cookers are great for cooking cheaper cuts like beef brisket, pork shoulder, lamb shoulder and chicken thighs. You can also use less meat, as slow cooking really extracts a meaty flavour that permeates the whole dish. Bulk up with vegetables instead.

4. Trim fat from meat before slow cooking

You don't need to add oil to a slow cooker – the contents won't catch as long as there's enough moisture in there. You don't need a lot of fat on your meat either. Normally when you fry meat, a lot of the fat drains away, but this won't happen in a slow cooker so trim it off – otherwise you might find you have pools of oil in your stew. Removing the fat will give you a healthier result, and it'll still be tasty.

5. Reduce liquid when using a slow cooker

Because your slow cooker will have a tightly sealed lid, the liquid won't evaporate so if you're adapting a standard recipe, it's best to reduce the liquid by roughly a third. It should just cover the meat and vegetables. Don't overfill your slow cooker, or it may start leaking out the top, and the food won't cook so well. Half to two-thirds full is ideal – certainly no more than three-quarters.

6. Use flour to thicken sauces

Just as the the liquid doesn't reduce, it also doesn't thicken. You can roll meat in a small amount of seasoned flour before adding it to the slow cooker or use a little cornflour at the end. If you want to do the latter, take a tsp. or two of cornflour and mix it to a paste with a little cold water. Stir into your simmering slow cooker contents, then replace the lid.

7. Use the slow cooker low setting

Use the 'Low' setting as much as you can, finding that most dishes really benefit from a slow, gentle heat to really bring out the flavours. This also means you won't need to worry if you're heading out for the day – it'll take care of itself.

8. Leave your slow cooker recipe alone

Slow cookers are designed to do their own thing, so you don't need to keep checking the contents. Every time you take the lid off it will release some of the heat, so if you keep doing this you'll have to increase the cooking time.

9. Add all ingredients at the start (most of the time)

Ideally you want to choose recipes where most, if not all, of the ingredients can be added at the beginning, leaving you free to do other things. However, in most cases, pasta, rice and fresh herbs will need to be added towards the end.

10. How long should I cook a slow cooker recipe?

If a dish usually takes:

15-30 mins, cook it for 1-2 hours on High or 4-6 hours on Low

30 mins – 1 hour, cook it for 2-3 hours on High or 5-7 hours on Low

1-2 hours, cook it for 3-4 hours on High or 6-8 hours on Low

2-4 hours, cook it for 4-6 hours on High or 8-12 hours on Low

Root vegetables can take longer than meat and other vegetables so put these near the heat source, at the bottom of the pot.

BREAKFAST RECIPES

Quinoa And Chia Pudding

Ingredients: Servings: 2   Cooking Time: 6 Hours

1 C. coconut cream
2 tbsp. chia seeds
½ C. almond milk

1 tbsp. sugar
½ C. quinoa, rinsed
½ tsp. vanilla extract

Directions:
In your Crock Pot, mix the cream with the chia seeds and the other ingredients, toss, put the lid on and cook on Low for 6 hours.   Divide into 2 bowls and serve for breakfast.

Cranberry Quinoa

Ingredients: Servings: 4   Cooking Time: 2 Hours

3 C. coconut water
1 tsp. vanilla extract
1 C. quinoa
1/8 C. almonds, sliced

3 tsp. honey
1/8 C. coconut flakes
¼ C. cranberries, dried

Directions:
In your Crock Pot, mix coconut water with vanilla, quinoa, honey, almonds, coconut flakes and cranberries, toss, cover and cook on High for 2 hours.   Divide quinoa mix into bowls and serve.

Tomato Eggs

Ingredients: Servings: 4   Cooking Time: 2.5 Hours

2 C. tomatoes, chopped
¼ C. tomato juice
1 onion, diced

1 tsp. olive oil
½ tsp. ground black pepper
4 eggs

Directions:
Pour olive oil in the Crock Pot.   Add onion, tomato juice, and tomatoes.   Close the lid and cook the mixture on High for 1 hour. Then mix the tomato mixture and crack the eggs inside.   Close the lid and cook them on High for 1.5 hours more.

Apple And Chia Mix

Ingredients: Servings: 2   Cooking Time: 8 Hours

¼ C. chia seeds
2 apples, cored and roughly cubed
1 C. almond milk
2 tbsp. maple syrup

1 tsp. vanilla extract
½ tbsp. cinnamon powder
Cooking spray

Directions:
Grease your Crock Pot with the cooking spray, add the chia seeds, milk and the other ingredients, toss, put the lid on and cook on Low for 8 hours.   Divide the mix into bowls and serve for breakfast.

Breakfast Monkey Bread

Ingredients: Servings: 6   Cooking Time: 6 Hours

10 oz. biscuit rolls
1 tbsp. ground cardamom
1 tbsp. sugar

2 tbsp. coconut oil
1 egg, beaten

Directions:
Chop the biscuit roll roughly.   Mix sugar with ground cardamom.   Melt the coconut oil.   Put the ½ part of chopped biscuit rolls in the Crock Pot in one layer and sprinkle with melted coconut oil and ½ part of all ground cinnamon mixture. Then top it with remaining biscuit roll chops and sprinkle with cardamom mixture and coconut oil.   Then brush the bread with a beaten egg and close the lid.   Cook the meal on High for 6 hours.   Cook the cooked bread well.

Potato Omelet

Ingredients: Servings: 4   Cooking Time: 6 Hours

1 C. potatoes, sliced
1 onion, sliced
2 tbsp. olive oil

6 eggs, beaten
1 tsp. salt
½ tsp. ground black pepper

Directions:
Mix potatoes with ground black pepper and salt.   Transfer them in the Crock Pot, add olive oil and cook on high for 30 minutes. Then mix the potatoes and add onion and eggs.   Stir the mixture and cook the omelet on Low for 6 hours.

Apricot Butter

Ingredients: Servings: 4   Cooking Time: 7 Hours

1 C. apricots, pitted, chopped
1 tsp. ground cinnamon

3 tbsp. butter
1 tsp. brown sugar

Directions:
Put all ingredients in the Crock Pot and stir well   Close the lid and cook them on Low for 7 hours.   Then blend the mixture with the help of the immersion blender and cool until cold.

Ginger Apple Bowls

Ingredients: Servings: 2   Cooking Time: 6 Hours

2 apples, cored, peeled and cut into medium chunks
1 tbsp. sugar
1 tbsp. ginger, grated
1 C. heavy cream

¼ tsp. cinnamon powder
½ tsp. vanilla extract
¼ tsp. cardamom, ground

Directions:
In your Crock Pot, combine the apples with the sugar, ginger and the other ingredients, toss, put the lid on and cook on Low for 6 hours.   Divide into bowls and serve for breakfast.

Cinnamon Berries Oatmeal

Ingredients: Servings: 2   Cooking Time: 6 Hours

1 C. old fashioned oats
3 C. almond milk
1 C. blackberries
½ C. Greek yogurt
½ tsp. cinnamon powder
½ tsp. vanilla extract

Directions:

In your Crock Pot, mix the oats with the milk, berries and the other ingredients, toss, put the lid on and cook on Low for 6 hours. Divide into bowls and serve for breakfast.

Mayo Sausage Rolls

Ingredients: Servings: 11   Cooking Time: 3 Hours

1 lb. puff pastry
2 tbsp. flour
1 tbsp. mustard
1 egg, whisked
10 oz. breakfast sausages
1 tsp. paprika
1 tbsp. mayo

Directions:

Spread the puff pastry with a rolling pin and drizzle flour over it. Slice the puff pastry into long thick strips. Spread mustard, mayonnaise, and paprika on top of each pastry strip. Place one sausage piece at one end of each strip. Roll the puff pastry strip and brush the rolls with whisked egg. Cover the base of your Crock Pot with a parchment sheet. Place the puff pastry rolls in the cooker. Put the cooker's lid on and set the cooking time to 3 hours on High settings. Serve fresh.

Squash Bowls

Ingredients: Servings: 2   Cooking Time: 6 Hours

2 tbsp. walnuts, chopped
2 C. squash, peeled and cubed
½ C. coconut cream
½ tsp. cinnamon powder
½ tbsp. sugar

Directions:

In your Crock Pot, mix the squash with the nuts and the other ingredients, toss, put the lid on and cook on Low for 6 hours. Divide into bowls and serve.

Chicken- Pork Meatballs

Ingredients: Servings: 8   Cooking Time: 7 Hours

1 C. bread crumbs
2 tbsp. sour cream
9 oz. ground chicken
7 oz. ground pork
1 tsp. onion powder
1 onion, chopped
1 tsp. ketchup
¼ tsp. olive oil

Directions:

Thoroughly mix ground chicken, onion powder, sour cream, ground pork, ketchup, and onion in a large bowl. Add breadcrumbs to bind this mixture well. Make small meatballs out of this mixture and roll them in extra breadcrumbs. Brush the base of your Crock Pot with olive oil. Gently place the chicken-pork meatballs in the Crock Pot. Put the cooker's lid on and set the cooking time to 7 hours on Low settings. Serve warm.

Apple Oatmeal

Ingredients: Servings: 3   Cooking Time: 7 Hours 20 Minutes

¼ C. brown sugar
¼ tsp. salt
2 C. milk
2 tbsp. honey
2 tbsp. butter, melted
½ tsp. cinnamon
1 C. apple, peeled and chopped
½ C. walnuts, chopped
1 C. steel cut oats
½ C. dates, chopped

Directions:

Grease a crock pot and add milk, honey, brown sugar, melted butter, cinnamon and salt. Mix well and stir in the oats, apples, walnuts and dates. Cover and cook on LOW for about 7 hours. Dish out and stir well before serving.

Breakfast Meatballs

Ingredients: Servings: 8   Cooking Time: 7 Hours

2 C. ground pork
1 egg, beaten
1 tsp. garlic powder
1 tbsp. semolina
½ C. heavy cream
1 tsp. cayenne pepper

Directions:

Mix ground pork with egg, garlic powder, and semolina, Then make the meatballs and put them in the Crock Pot. Sprinkle them with cayenne pepper. After this, add heavy cream and close the lid. Cook the meatballs on low for 7 hours.

Kale Cups

Ingredients: Servings: 4   Cooking Time: 2.5 Hours

1 C. kale, chopped
4 eggs, beaten
1 tsp. chili powder
1 tsp. olive oil
½ C. Cheddar cheese, shredded

Directions:

Mix kale with eggs, olive oil, and chili powder. Transfer the mixture in the ramekins and top with Cheddar cheese. Place the ramekins in the Crock Pot. Close the lid and cook the meal on high for 2.5 hours.

Spinach Frittata

Ingredients: Servings: 6   Cooking Time: 2 Hours

2 C. spinach, chopped
1 tsp. smoked paprika
1 tsp. sesame oil
7 eggs, beaten
2 tbsp. coconut oil
¼ C. heavy cream

Directions:

Mix eggs with heavy cream. Then grease the Crock Pot with coconut oil and pour the egg mixture inside. Add smoked paprika, sesame oil, and spinach. Carefully mix the ingredients and close the lid. Cook the frittata on High for 2 hours.

Squash Butter

Ingredients: Servings: 4   Cooking Time: 2 Hours

1 C. butternut squash puree
4 tbsp. applesauce
1 tsp. allspices
2 tbsp. butter
1 tsp. cornflour

Directions:

Put all ingredients in the Crock Pot and mix until homogenous. Then close the lid and cook the butter on High for 2 hours. Transfer the cooked squash butter in the plastic vessel and cool it well.

Turkey Breakfast Casserole

Ingredients: Servings: 8   Cooking Time: 8 Hours 30 Minutes

1-lb. turkey sausages, cooked and drained
1 dozen eggs
1 (30 oz) package shredded hash browns, thawed
1 yellow onion, chopped
2 C. Colby Jack cheese, shredded
1 C. milk
1 tsp. salt
½ tsp. red pepper flakes, crushed
4 tbsp. flour
½ tsp. black pepper

Directions:

Grease a crockpot and layer with 1/3 of the hash browns, onions, sausages and cheese. Repeat these layers twice ending with the layer of cheese. Whisk together the rest of the ingredients in a large mixing bowl. Transfer this mixture into the crockpot and cover the lid. Cover and cook on LOW for about 8 hours. Dish out to serve the delicious breakfast.

Cilantro Shrimp Bake

Ingredients: Servings: 4   Cooking Time: 2.5 Hours

1 C. potato, mashed, cooked
¼ C. fresh cilantro, chopped
¼ C. cream
1 tsp. butter, melted
6 oz. shrimps, peeled, chopped
4 eggs, beaten

Directions:

Mix mashed potatoes with cream and eggs. Add butter and transfer the mixture in the Crock Pot. Then add cilantro and shrimps. Close the lid and cook the meal on High for 2.5 hours. Cool the cooked meal well and then cut into servings.

Apricot Oatmeal

Ingredients: Servings: 4   Cooking Time: 4 Hours

1 ½ C. oatmeal
1 C. of water
3 C. of milk
1 C. apricots, pitted, sliced
1 tsp. butter

Directions:

Put oatmeal in the Crock Pot. Add water, milk, and butter. Close the lid and cook the mixture on high for 1 hour. Then add apricots, carefully mix the oatmeal and close the lid. Cook the meal on Low for 3 hours.

Artichoke Pepper Frittata

Ingredients: Servings: 4   Cooking Time: 3 Hours

14 oz. canned artichokes hearts, drained and chopped
12 oz. roasted red peppers, chopped
8 eggs, whisked
¼ C. green onions, chopped
4 oz. feta cheese, crumbled
Cooking spray

Directions:

Coat the base of your Crock Pot with cooking spray. Add green onions, roasted peppers, and artichokes to the Crock Pot. Pour whisked eggs over the veggies and drizzle cheese on top. Put the cooker's lid on and set the cooking time to 3 hours on Low settings. Slice and serve.

Pork And Eggplant Casserole

Ingredients: Servings: 2   Cooking Time: 6 Hours

1 red onion, chopped
1 eggplant, cubed
½ lb. pork stew meat, ground
½ tsp. chili powder
3 eggs, whisked
½ tsp. garam masala
1 tbsp. sweet paprika
1 tsp. olive oil

Directions:

In a bowl, mix the eggs with the meat, onion, eggplant and the other ingredients except the oil and stir well. Grease your Crock Pot with oil, add the pork and eggplant mix, spread into the pot, put the lid on and cook on Low for 6 hours. Divide the mix between plates and serve for breakfast.

Cranberry Maple Oatmeal

Ingredients: Servings: 2   Cooking Time: 6 Hours

1 C. almond milk
½ C. steel cut oats
½ tsp. vanilla extract
½ C. cranberries
1 tbsp. maple syrup
1 tbsp. sugar

Directions:

In your Crock Pot, mix the oats with the berries, milk and the other ingredients, toss, put the lid on and cook on Low for 6 hours. Divide into bowls and serve for breakfast.

Carrots Casserole

Ingredients: Servings: 2   Cooking Time: 3 Hours

1 tsp. ginger, ground
½ lb. carrots, peeled and grated
2 eggs, whisked
½ tsp. garlic powder
½ tsp. rosemary, dried
Salt and black pepper to the taste
1 red onion, chopped
1 tbsp. parsley, chopped
2 garlic cloves, minced
½ tbsp. olive oil

Directions:

Grease your Crock Pot with the oil and mix the carrots with the eggs, ginger and the other ingredients inside. Toss, put the lid on, cook High for 3 hours, divide between plates and serve.

Creamy Strawberries Oatmeal

Ingredients: Servings: 8   Cooking Time: 8 Hours

6 C. water
2 C. milk
2 C. steel cut oats
1 tsp. cinnamon powder

1 C. Greek yogurt
2 C. strawberries, halved
1 tsp. vanilla extract

Directions:
In your Crock Pot, mix water with milk, oats, yogurt, cinnamon, strawberries and vanilla, toss, cover and cook on Low for 8 hours. Divide into bowls and serve for breakfast.

Chocolate Oatmeal

Ingredients: Servings: 5   Cooking Time: 4 Hours

1 oz. dark chocolate, chopped
1 tsp. vanilla extract
2 C. oatmeal

2 C. of coconut milk
½ tsp. ground cardamom

Directions:
Put all ingredients in the Crock Pot and stir carefully with the help of the spoon. Close the lid and cook the meal for 4 hours on Low.

Morning Ham Muffins

Ingredients: Servings: 4   Cooking Time: 2.5 Hours

4 eggs, beaten
3 oz. Mozzarella, shredded
3 oz. ham, chopped

1 tsp. olive oil
1 tsp. dried parsley
½ tsp. salt

Directions:
Mix eggs with dried parsley, salt, and ham. Add mozzarella and stir the muffin mixture carefully. Sprinkle the silicone muffin molds with olive oil. After this, pour the egg and ham mixture in the muffin molds and transfer in the Crock Pot. Cook the muffins on High for 2.5 hours.

Cranberry Almond Quinoa

Ingredients: Servings: 4   Cooking Time: 2 Hours

3 C. of coconut water
1 tsp. vanilla extract
1 C. quinoa
1/8 C. almonds, sliced

3 tsp. honey
1/8 C. coconut flakes
¼ C. cranberries, dried

Directions:
Add coconut water, honey, vanilla, quinoa, almonds, cranberries, and coconut flakes to the Crock Pot. Put the cooker's lid on and set the cooking time to 2 hours on High settings. Dish out and serve.

Beans Breakfast Bowls

Ingredients: Servings: 2   Cooking Time: 3 Hours And 10 Minutes

2 spring onions, chopped
½ green bell pepper, chopped
½ red bell pepper, chopped

5 oz. canned pinto beans, drained
½ C. corn
½ tsp. turmeric powder

½ yellow onion, chopped
5 oz. canned black beans, drained
5 oz. canned red kidney beans, drained

1 tsp. chili powder
½ tsp. hot sauce
A pinch of salt and black pepper
1 tbsp. olive oil

Directions:
Heat up a pan with the oil over medium-high heat, add the spring onions, bell peppers and the onion, sauté for 10 minutes and transfer to the Crock Pot. Add the beans and the other ingredients, toss, put the lid on and cook on High for 3 hours. Divide the mix into bowls and serve for breakfast.

Hash Browns And Sausage Casserole

Ingredients: Servings: 12   Cooking Time: 4 Hours

30 oz. hash browns
1 lb. sausage, browned and sliced
8 oz. mozzarella cheese, shredded
8 oz. cheddar cheese, shredded

6 green onions, chopped
½ C. milk
12 eggs
Cooking spray
Salt and black pepper to the taste

Directions:
Grease your Crock Pot with cooking spray and add half of the hash browns, half of the sausage, half of the mozzarella, cheddar and green onions. In a bowl, mix the eggs with salt, pepper and milk and whisk well. Add half of the eggs mix into the Crock Pot, then layer the remaining hash browns, sausages, mozzarella, cheddar and green onions. Top with the rest of the eggs, cover the Crock Pot and cook on High for 4 hours. Divide between plates and serve hot.

Saucy Beef Meatloaf

Ingredients: Servings: 8   Cooking Time: 7 Hours

12 oz. ground beef
1 tsp. salt
1 tsp. ground coriander
1 tbsp. ground mustard
¼ tsp. ground chili pepper

6 oz. white bread, chopped
½ C. milk
1 tsp. ground black pepper
3 tbsp. tomato sauce

Directions:
Soak the white bread cubes in the milk and keep them aside for 3 minutes. Whisk ground beef with chili pepper, mustard, black pepper, salt, and ground coriander in a bowl. Now add the bread-milk mixture into the beef and mix well. Cover the base of your Crock Pot with aluminum foil. Spread the beef-bread mixture in the foil. Top the meatloaf with tomato sauce. Put the cooker's lid on and set the cooking time to 7 hours on Low settings. Slice and serve.

Biscuit Roll Bread

Ingredients: Servings: 6   Cooking Time: 2 Hours

12 oz. biscuit rolls, diced

1 tsp. vanilla extract
4 tbsp. butter, melted

1 tbsp. ground
cinnamon
3 oz. white sugar

1 egg white
4 tbsp. brown sugar

Directions:

Whisk sugar with melted butter, cinnamon in a bowl. Split the biscuit roll cubes into 2 parts and place on half of all the cubes in the Crock Pot. Top this layer with the cinnamon butter mixture evenly. Place the remaining parts of the biscuit roll cubes on top. Put the cooker's lid on and set the cooking time to 2 hours on Low settings. Now beat egg white with brown sugar until it is fluffy. Top the cooked bread with the egg white icing. Serve.

Cinnamon Quinoa

Ingredients: Servings: 4   Cooking Time: 4 Hours

1 C. quinoa
2 C. milk
2 C. water
¼ C. stevia

1 tsp. cinnamon
powder
1 tsp. vanilla extract

Directions:

In your Crock Pot, mix quinoa with milk, water, stevia, cinnamon and vanilla, stir, cover, cook on Low for 3 hours and 30 minutes, stir, cook for 30 minutes more, divide into bowls and serve for breakfast.

Sausage Frittata

Ingredients: Servings: 5   Cooking Time: 4 Hours

½ onion, diced
8 oz. sausages,
chopped
1 tsp. coconut oil

1 C. Mozzarella,
shredded
6 eggs, beaten
½ tsp. cayenne
pepper

Directions:

Put sausages in the Crock Pot. Add onion and coconut oil. Close the lid and cook the ingredients on high for 2 hours. Then stir them well. Add eggs, cayenne pepper, and shredded mozzarella. Carefully stir the meal and close the lid. Cook it on high for 2 hours.

Breakfast Meat Rolls

Ingredients: Servings: 12   Cooking Time: 4.5 Hours

1-lb. puff pastry
1 C. ground pork
1 tbsp. garlic, diced

1 egg, beaten
1 tbsp. sesame oil

Directions:

Roll up the puff pastry. Then mix ground pork with garlic and egg. Then spread the puff pastry with ground meat mixture and roll. Cut the puff pastry rolls on small rolls. Then sprinkle the rolls with sesame oil. Arrange the meat rolls in the Crock Pot and close the lid. Cook breakfast on High for 4.5 hours.

Brussels Sprouts Omelet

Ingredients: Servings: 4   Cooking Time: 4 Hours

4 eggs, whisked
Salt and black pepper
to the taste

2 garlic cloves,
minced
12 oz. Brussels

1 tbsp. olive oil
2 green onions,
minced

sprouts, sliced
2 oz. bacon, chopped

Directions:

Drizzle the oil on the bottom of your Crock Pot and spread Brussels sprouts, garlic, bacon, green onions, eggs, salt and pepper, toss, cover and cook on Low for 4 hours. Divide between plates and serve right away for breakfast.

Quinoa Cauliflower Medley

Ingredients: Servings: 7   Cooking Time: 9 Hours

8 oz. potato, peeled
and cubed
7 oz. cauliflower, cut
in florets
7 oz. chickpea,
canned
1 C. tomatoes,
chopped

1 C. onion, chopped
13 oz. almond milk
3 C. chicken stock
8 tbsp. quinoa
1/3 tbsp. miso
1 tsp. minced garlic
2 tsp. curry paste

Directions:

Spread the chopped potatoes, tomatoes, and onion in the Crock Pot. Whisk curry paste with chicken stock and miso in a separate bowl. Pour this mixture over the layer of the veggies. Now top this mixture with chickpeas, cauliflower florets, quinoa, garlic, and almond milk. Put the cooker's lid on and set the cooking time to 9 hours on Low settings. Serve.

Broccoli Omelet

Ingredients: Servings: 4   Cooking Time: 2 Hours

1 tbsp. cream cheese
3 oz. broccoli,
chopped

5 eggs, beaten
1 tomato, chopped
1 tsp. avocado oil

Directions:

Mix eggs with cream cheese and transfer in the Crock Pot. Add avocado oil, broccoli, and tomato. Close the lid and cook the omelet on High for 2 hours.

Greek Breakfast Casserole

Ingredients: Servings: 4   Cooking Time: 4 Hours

12 eggs, whisked
Salt and black pepper
to the taste
½ C. milk
1 red onion, chopped
1 C. baby bell
mushrooms, sliced

½ C. sun-dried
tomatoes
1 tsp. garlic, minced
2 C. spinach
½ C. feta cheese,
crumbled

Directions:

In a bowl, mix the eggs with salt, pepper and milk and whisk well. Add garlic, onion, mushrooms, spinach and tomatoes, toss well, pour this into your Crock Pot, sprinkle cheese all over, cover and cook on Low for 4 hours. Slice, divide between plates and serve for breakfast.

Apple Crumble

Ingredients: Servings: 2   Cooking Time: 5 Hours

1 tbsp. liquid honey 1 tbsp. almond butter
2 Granny Smith 1 tsp. vanilla extract
apples
4 oz. granola
4 tbsp. water

Directions:

Cut the apple into small wedges. Remove the seeds from the apples and chop them into small pieces. Put them in the Crock Pot. Add water, almond butter, vanilla extract, and honey. Cook the apples for 5 hours on Low. Then stir them carefully. Put the cooked apples and granola one-by-one in the serving glasses.

Baby Carrots In Syrup

Ingredients: Servings: 5   Cooking Time: 7 Hours

3 C. baby carrots 1 C. apple juice
2 tbsp. brown sugar 1 tsp. vanilla extract

Directions:

Mix apple juice, brown sugar, and vanilla extract. Pour the liquid in the Crock Pot. Add baby carrots and close the lid. Cook the meal on Low for 7 hours.

Boiled Bacon Eggs

Ingredients: Servings: 6   Cooking Time: 2 Hours

7 oz. bacon, sliced 1 tbsp. minced garlic
1 tsp. salt 1 tsp. ground black
6 eggs, hard-boiled, pepper
peeled 4 oz. Parmesan
½ C. cream cheese, shredded
3 tbsp. mayonnaise 1 tsp. dried dill

Directions:

Place a non-skillet over medium heat and add bacon slices. Drizzle salt and black pepper on top, then cook for 1 minute per side. Transfer the bacon slices to a plate and keep them aside. Whisk mayonnaise with minced garlic, dried dill, and cream in a bowl. Spread this creamy mixture into the base of your Crock Pot. Take the peeled eggs and wrap then with cooked bacon slices. Place the wrapped eggs in the creamy mixture. Drizzle shredded cheese over the wrapped eggs. Put the cooker's lid on and set the cooking time to 2 hours on High settings. Serve and devour.

Bacon And Egg Casserole

Ingredients: Servings: 8   Cooking Time: 5 Hours

20 oz. hash browns Cooking spray
8 oz. cheddar cheese, ½ C. milk
shredded 12 eggs
8 bacon slices, Salt and black pepper
cooked and chopped to the taste
6 green onions, Salsa for serving
chopped

Directions:

Grease your Crock Pot with cooking spray, spread hash browns, cheese, bacon and green onions and toss. In a bowl, mix the eggs with salt, pepper and milk and whisk really well. Pour this over hash browns, cover and cook on Low for 5 hours. Divide between plates and serve with salsa on top.

Ham Omelet

Ingredients: Servings: 2   Cooking Time: 3 Hours

Cooking spray ½ C. ham, chopped
4 eggs, whisked ½ C. cheddar cheese,
1 tbsp. sour cream shredded
2 spring onions, 1 tbsp. chives,
chopped chopped
1 small yellow onion, A pinch of salt and
chopped black pepper

Directions:

Grease your Crock Pot with the cooking spray and mix the eggs with the sour cream, spring onions and the other ingredients inside. Toss the mix, spread into the pot, put the lid on and cook on High for 3 hours. Divide the mix between plates and serve for breakfast right away.

Chorizo Eggs

Ingredients: Servings: 4   Cooking Time: 1.5 Hours

5 oz. chorizo, sliced 1 tsp. butter, softened
4 eggs, beaten
2 oz. Parmesan,
grated

Directions:

Grease the Crock Pot bottom with butter. Add chorizo and cook them on high for 30 minutes. Then flip the sliced chorizo and add eggs and Parmesan. Close the lid and cook the meal on High for 1 hour more.

Chia Seeds And Chicken Breakfast

Ingredients: Servings: 4   Cooking Time: 3 Hours

1 lb. chicken breasts, ¼ C. chia seeds
skinless, boneless
and cubed ½ tsp. oregano,
½ tsp. basil, dried chopped
¾ C. flaxseed, Salt and black pepper
ground to the taste
¼ C. parmesan, 2 eggs
grated 2 garlic cloves,
minced

Directions:

In a bowl, mix flaxseed with chia seeds, parmesan, salt, pepper, oregano, garlic and basil and stir. Put the eggs in a second bowl and whisk them well. Dip chicken in eggs mix, then in chia seeds mix, put them in your Crock Pot after you've greased it with cooking spray, cover and cook on High for 3 hours. Serve them right away for a Sunday breakfast.

Sweet Eggs

Ingredients: Servings: 4   Cooking Time: 4 Hours

4 oz. white bread, 1 tsp. vanilla extract
chopped 1 tsp. avocado oil
2 tbsp. sugar
6 eggs, beaten
¼ C. milk

Directions:

Mix eggs with sugar and milk. Add vanilla extract and bread. Then brush the Crock Pot bottom with avocado oil. Pour the egg mixture inside and close the lid. Cook the meal on Low for 4 hours.

Turkey Omelet

Ingredients: Servings: 4   Cooking Time: 5 Hours

½ tsp. garlic powder
6 oz. ground turkey
4 eggs, beaten

1 tbsp. coconut oil
½ tsp. salt
¼ C. milk

Directions:

Mix milk with salt, eggs, and garlic powder. Then add ground turkey. Grease the Crock Pot bowl bottom with coconut oil. Put the egg mixture in the Crock Pot, flatten it, and close the lid. Cook the omelet on Low for 5 hours.

Green Muffins

Ingredients: Servings: 8   Cooking Time: 2 ½   hrs

1 C. spinach, washed
5 tbsp. butter
1 C. flour
1 tsp. salt

½ tsp. baking soda
1 tbsp. lemon juice
1 tbsp. sugar
3 eggs

Directions:

Add the spinach leaves to a blender jug and blend until smooth. Whisk the eggs in a bowl and add the spinach mixture. Stir in baking soda, salt, sugar, flour, and lemon juice. Mix well to form a smooth spinach batter. Divide the dough into a muffin tray lined with muffin cups. Place this muffin tray in the Crock Pot. Put the cooker's lid on and set the cooking time to 2 hours 30 minutes on High settings. Serve.

Tender Granola

Ingredients: Servings: 4   Cooking Time: 30 Minutes

4 oz. rolled oats
1 tbsp. coconut oil
1 tbsp. liquid honey
3 oz. almonds,
chopped

½ tsp. ground
cinnamon
2 tbsp. dried
cranberries
Cooking spray

Directions:

In the mixing bowl mix rolled oats, coconut oil, almonds, ground cinnamon, and dried cranberries. Then make the tiny balls from the mixture. Spray the Crock Pot with the cooking spray and put the oat balls inside. Close the lid and cook the granola for 30 minutes on High.

Breakfast Muffins

Ingredients: Servings: 4   Cooking Time: 3 Hours

7 eggs, beaten
1 bell pepper, diced
½ tsp. salt
½ tsp. cayenne
pepper

2 tbsp. almond meal
1 tsp. avocado oil

Directions:

Brush the muffin molds with avocado oil. In the mixing bowl, mix eggs, bell pepper, salt, cayenne pepper, and almond meal. Pour the muffin mixture in the muffin molds and transfer in the Crock Pot. Cook the muffins on high for 3 hours.

Cheddar Eggs

Ingredients: Servings: 4   Cooking Time: 2 Hours

1 tsp. butter, softened
4 eggs

½ tsp. salt
1/3 C. Cheddar
cheese, shredded

Directions:

Grease the Crock Pot bowl with butter and crack the eggs inside. Sprinkle the eggs with salt and shredded cheese. Close the lid and cook on High for 2 hours.

Cauliflower Rice Pudding

Ingredients: Servings: 2   Cooking Time: 2 Hours

¼ C. maple syrup
1 C. cauliflower rice

3 C. almond milk
2 tbsp. vanilla extract

Directions:

Put cauliflower rice in your Crock Pot, add maple syrup, almond milk and vanilla extract, stir, cover and cook on High for 2 hours. Stir your pudding again, divide into bowls and serve for breakfast.

Breakfast Stuffed Peppers

Ingredients: Servings: 3   Cooking Time: 4 Hours

3 bell peppers, halved
and deseeded
Salt and black pepper
to the taste
4 eggs
2 tbsp. green onions,
chopped

½ C. milk
½ C. ham, chopped
¼ C. spinach,
chopped
¾ C. cheddar cheese,
shredded

Directions:

In a bowl, mix the eggs with salt, pepper, green onion, milk, spinach, ham and half of the cheese and stir well. Line your Crock Pot with tin foil, divide eggs mix in each bell pepper half, arrange them all in the Crock Pot, sprinkle the rest of the cheese all over them, cover and cook on Low for 4 hours. Divide peppers between plates and serve for breakfast.

Blueberry Quinoa Oatmeal

Ingredients: Servings: 4   Cooking Time: 8 Hours

½ C. quinoa
1 C. steel cut oats
1 tsp. vanilla extract
Zest of 1 lemon,
grated
1 tsp. vanilla extract

5 C. water
2 tbsp. flaxseed
1 tbsp. butter, melted
3 tbsp. maple syrup
1 C. blueberries

Directions:

In your Crock Pot, mix butter with quinoa, water, oats, vanilla, lemon zest, flaxseed, maple syrup and blueberries, stir, cover and cook on Low for 8 hours. Divide into bowls and serve for breakfast.

Bacon Eggs

Ingredients: Servings: 2   Cooking Time: 2 Hours

2 eggs, hard-boiled, peeled	2 bacon slices
¼ tsp. ground black pepper	1 tsp. olive oil
	½ tsp. dried thyme

Directions:

Sprinkle the bacon with ground black pepper and dried thyme. Then wrap the eggs in the bacon and sprinkle with olive oil. Put the eggs in the Crock Pot and cook on High for 2 hours.

Cheesy Eggs

Ingredients: Servings: 2   Cooking Time: 3 Hours

4 eggs, whisked	2 oz. feta cheese, crumbled
¼ C. spring onions, chopped	A pinch of salt and black pepper
1 tbsp. oregano, chopped	Cooking spray
1 C. milk	

Directions:

In a bowl, combine the eggs with the spring onions and the other ingredients except the cooking spray and whisk. Grease your Crock Pot with cooking spray, add eggs mix, stir , put the lid on and cook on Low for 3 hours. Divide between plates and serve for breakfast.

Mexican Eggs

Ingredients: Servings: 8   Cooking Time: 2 Hours And 15 Minutes

Cooking spray	1 C. half and half
10 eggs	A pinch of salt and black pepper
12 oz. Monterey jack, shredded	10 oz. taco sauce
½ tsp. chili powder	4 oz. canned green chilies, chopped
1 garlic clove, minced	8 corn tortillas

Directions:

In a bowl, mix the eggs with half and half, 8 oz. of cheese, salt, pepper, chili powder, green chilies and garlic and whisk everything. Grease your Crock Pot with cooking spray, add eggs mix, cover and cook on Low for 2 hours. Spread taco sauce and the rest of the cheese all over, cover and cook on Low for 15 minutes more. Divide eggs on tortillas, wrap and serve for breakfast.

Stuffed Baguette

Ingredients: Servings: 4   Cooking Time: 5 Hours

6 oz. baguette	4 oz. ham, cooked and shredded
7 oz. breakfast sausages, chopped	6 oz. Parmesan, shredded
3 tbsp. whipped cream	3 tbsp. ketchup
1 tsp. minced garlic	2 oz. green olives
1 tsp. onion powder	

Directions:

Slice the baguette in half and remove the flesh from the center of these halves. Toss chopped sausages with cheese shreds, onion powder, minced garlic, cream, shredded ham and ketchup in a large bowl. Divide this cheese-sausage mixture into the baguette halves. Place these stuffed baguette halves in the Crock Pot. Put the cooker's lid on and set the cooking time to 5 hours on Low settings. Slice the stuffed baguettes and serve.

Spinach Tomato Frittata

Ingredients: Servings: 6   Cooking Time: 2 Hours

1 tbsp. olive oil	3 eggs
1 yellow onion, chopped	2 tbsp. milk
1 C. mozzarella cheese, shredded	Salt and black pepper to the taste
3 egg whites	1 C. baby spinach
	1 tomato, chopped

Directions:

Grease your Crock Pot with theoil and spread onion, spinach, and tomatoes on the bottom. In a bowl, mix the eggs with egg whites, milk, salt, and pepper, whisk well and pour over the veggies from the pot. Sprinkle mozzarella all over, cover the Crock Pot, cook on Low for 2 hrs; slice, divide between plates, and serve for breakfast.

"baked" Creamy Brussels Sprouts

Ingredients: Servings: 2 (serving Size Is ½ Of Recipe—6.3 Ounces)   Cooking Time: 2 Hours And 25 Minutes

14 Brussels sprouts	½ C. cream cheese
¼ C. Parmesan cheese, grated	1 tsp. balsamic vinegar
2 garlic cloves	Salt and pepper to taste
2 tbsp. extra virgin olive oil	

Directions:

Rinse the Brussels sprouts in cold water to remove dirt and dust. Discard the first leaves. Pour oil into Crock-Pot and add Brussels sprouts. Add in the remaining ingredients and stir. Cover and cook for 3-4 hours on low or 1-2 hours on HIGH. Before serving, sprinkle with Parmesan or feta cheese. Let cheese melt for 2 or 3 minutes.

Oats Granola

Ingredients: Servings: 8   Cooking Time: 2 Hours

5 C. old-fashioned rolled oats	½ C. peanut butter
1/3 C. coconut oil	1 tbsp. vanilla
2/3 C. honey	2 tsp. cinnamon powder
½ C. almonds, chopped	1 C. craisins
	Cooking spray

Directions:

Grease your Crock Pot with cooking spray, add oats, oil, honey, almonds, peanut butter, vanilla, craisins and cinnamon, toss just a bit, cover and cook on High for 2 hours, stirring every 30 minutes. Divide into bowls and serve for breakfast.

Hot Eggs Mix

Ingredients: Servings: 2   Cooking Time: 2 Hours

Cooking spray
4 eggs, whisked
¼ C. sour cream
A pinch of salt and black pepper
½ tsp. chili powder
½ tsp. hot paprika

½ red bell pepper, chopped
½ yellow onion, chopped
2 cherry tomatoes, cubed
1 tbsp. parsley, chopped

Directions:

In a bowl, mix the eggs with the cream, salt, pepper and the other ingredients except the cooking spray and whisk well.   Grease your Crock Pot with cooking spray, pour the eggs mix inside, spread, stir, put the lid on and cook on High for 2 hours.   Divide the mix between plates and serve.

Huevos Rancheros

Ingredients: Servings: 2   Cooking Time: 3 Hours 15 Minutes

1 tbsp. butter
½ C. black beans
2 tbsp. guacamole
¼ tsp. cumin powder
¼ C. light cream

½ red onion, thinly sliced
2 eggs
½ oz. Mexican blend cheese, shredded
2 tbsp. red enchilada sauce

Directions:

Put all the ingredients in a large bowl except guacamole and butter and mix thoroughly.   Put butter in the crockpot and stir in the mixed ingredients.   Cover and cook on LOW for about 3 hours.   Dish out and top with guacamole to serve.

Orange Pudding

Ingredients: Servings: 4   Cooking Time: 4 Hours

1 C. carrot, grated
2 C. of milk
1 tbsp. cornstarch

1 tsp. vanilla extract
½ tsp. ground nutmeg

Directions:

Put the carrot in the Crock Pot.   Add milk, vanilla extract, and ground nutmeg.   Then add cornstarch and stir the ingredients until cornstarch is dissolved.   Cook the pudding on low for 4 hours.

Walnut And Cheese Balls

Ingredients: Servings: 5   Cooking Time: 1.5 Hours

1 C. walnuts, grinded
2 eggs, beaten
3 oz. Parmesan, grated

¼ C. breadcrumbs
2 tbsp. coconut oil, melted

Directions:

Mix grinded walnuts and breadcrumbs.   Then add eggs and Parmesan.   Carefully mix the mixture and make the medium size balls from them.   Then pour melted coconut oil in the Crock Pot.   Add walnuts balls. Arrange them in one layer and close the lid.   Cook the balls on high for 1 hour.   Then flip them on another side and cook for 30 minutes more.

Egg Quiche

Ingredients: Servings: 4   Cooking Time: 7 Hours

4 eggs, beaten
1 bell pepper, diced
1 onion, diced
1 tsp. chili flakes

½ tsp. ground paprika
2 tbsp. flax meal

Directions:

Mix eggs with flax meal.   Add bell pepper, chili flakes, onion, and ground paprika.   Pour the quiche mixture in the Crock Pot and close the lid.   Cook the meal on low for 7 hours.

Worcestershire Asparagus Casserole

Ingredients: Servings: 4   Cooking Time: 5 Hours

2 lb. asparagus spears, cut into 1-inch pieces
1 C. mushrooms, sliced
1 tsp. olive oil

Salt and black pepper to the taste
2 C. coconut milk
1 tsp. Worcestershire sauce
5 eggs, whisked

Directions:

Grease your Crock Pot with the oil and spread asparagus and mushrooms on the bottom.   In a bowl, mix the eggs with milk, salt, pepper and Worcestershire sauce, whisk, pour into the Crock Pot, toss everything, cover and cook on Low for 6 hours. Divide between plates and serve right away for breakfast.

Herbed Egg Scramble

Ingredients: Servings: 2   Cooking Time: 6 Hours

4 eggs, whisked
¼ C. mozzarella, shredded
1 tbsp. chives, chopped
1 tbsp. oregano, chopped

¼ C. heavy cream
1 tbsp. rosemary, chopped
A pinch of salt and black pepper
Cooking spray

Directions:

Grease your Crock Pot with the cooking spray, and mix the eggs with the cream, herbs and the other ingredients inside.   Stir well, put the lid on, cook for 6 hours on Low, stir once again, divide between plates and serve.

Cheesy Sausage Casserole

Ingredients: Servings: 6-8   Cooking Time: 4-5 Hours

1 ½ C. cheddar cheese, shredded
½ C. mayonnaise
2 C. green cabbage, shredded
2 C. zucchini, diced
½ C. onion, diced
8 large eggs
1 lb. pork sausage

1 tsp. sage, ground, dried
2 tsp. prepared yellow mustard
Cayenne pepper to taste
¼ tsp. sea salt
¼ tsp. black pepper

26

Directions:

Using cooking spray, grease the inside of the Crock-Pot. In a mixing bowl, whisk together eggs, mayonnaise, cheese, mustard, dried ground sage, cayenne pepper, salt, and black pepper. Layer half of the sausage, cabbage, zucchini, and onions into the Crock-Pot. Repeat with the remaining ingredients of zucchini, onion, sausage and cabbage. Pour the egg mixture onto the layered ingredients. Cook for 4-5 hours on LOW, until it is golden brown on the edges and set. Serve warm.

Sausage Pie(2)

Ingredients: Servings: 4   Cooking Time: 3 Hours

½ C. flour
¼ C. skim milk
1 tsp. baking powder
1 tsp. salt

½ tsp. chili flakes
4 sausages, chopped
1 egg, beaten
Cooking spray

Directions:

Mix flour with skin milk and baking powder. Then add salt, chili flakes, and egg. Stir the mixture until smooth. You will get the batter. Spray the Crock Pot with cooking spray from inside. Then pour the batter in the Crock Pot. Add chopped sausages and close the lid. Cook the pie on High for 3 hours.

Peachy Cinnamon Butter

Ingredients: Servings: 8   Cooking Time: 8 Hours

15 oz. peach, pitted, peeled and cubed
2 C. of sugar
1 tbsp. ground cinnamon

¼ tsp. salt
1 tsp. fresh ginger, peeled and grated
5 tbsp. lemon juice

Directions:

Take a blender jug and add peach cubes into the jug. Blender until peaches are pureed. Pour this peach puree into the Crock Pot. Stir in salt, sugar, grated ginger, and cinnamon. Put the cooker's lid on and set the cooking time to 8 hours on Low settings. Stir in lemon juice and mix well. Add the peach butter to glass jars. Allow the jars to cool and serve with bread.

Egg Casserole

Ingredients: Servings: 4   Cooking Time: 6 Hours 30 Minutes

¾ C. milk
½ tsp. salt
8 large eggs
½ tsp. dry mustard
¼ tsp. black pepper
4 C. hash brown potatoes, partially thawed

½ C. green bell pepper, chopped
4 green onions, chopped
12 oz. ham, diced
½ C. red bell pepper, chopped
1½ C. cheddar cheese, shredded

Directions:

Whisk together eggs, dry mustard, milk, salt and black pepper in a large bowl. Grease the crockpot and put 1/3 of the hash brown potatoes, salt and black pepper. Layer with 1/3 of the diced ham, red bell peppers, green bell peppers, green onions and cheese. Repeat the layers twice, ending with the cheese and top

with the egg mixture. Cover and cook on LOW for about 6 hours. Serve this delicious casserole for breakfast.

Breakfast Salad

Ingredients: Servings: 4   Cooking Time: 2.5 Hours

1 C. ground beef
1 tsp. chili powder
1 tbsp. olive oil

1 onion, diced
2 C. arugula, chopped
1 C. tomatoes, chopped

Directions:

Mix ground beef with chili powder, diced onion, and olive oil. Put the mixture in the Crock Pot and close the lid. Cook it on High for 2.5 hours. Then transfer the mixture in the salad bowl, cool gently. Add tomatoes and arugula. Mix the salad.

Green Buttered Eggs

Ingredients: Servings: 2   Cooking Time: 3 Hours

2 tbsp. organic grass-fed butter
1 tbsp. coconut oil
2 cloves of garlic, chopped
½ C. cilantro, chopped

1 tsp. thyme leaves
4 organic eggs, beaten
¼ tsp. cayenne pepper
Salt and pepper to taste

Directions:

Place butter and coconut oil in a skillet heated over medium flame. Add in the garlic and sauté until fragrant. Add in the cilantro and thyme leaves. Continue stirring until crisp. Pour into the CrockPot and add in the beaten eggs. Season with cayenne pepper, salt and black pepper to taste. Close the lid and cook on high for 2 hours and on low for 3 hours.

Goat Cheese Frittata

Ingredients: Servings: 4   Cooking Time: 2.5 Hours

2 oz. goat cheese, crumbled
5 eggs, beaten
2 oz. bell pepper, chopped

1 tbsp. flour
1 tsp. butter, softened
1 oz. cilantro, chopped

Directions:

Mix flour with eggs and bell pepper. Then grease the Crock Pot bottom with butter and pour the egg mixture inside. Then top the mixture with crumbled goat cheese and cilantro. Close the lid and cook the meal on High for 2.5 hours.

Basil Sausage And Broccoli Mix

Ingredients: Servings: 2   Cooking Time: 8 Hours And 10 Minutes

1 yellow onion, chopped
2 spring onions, chopped
1 C. pork sausage, chopped
1 C. broccoli florets

4 eggs, whisked
2 tsp. basil, dried
A pinch of salt and black pepper
A drizzle of olive oil

Directions:

Heat up a pan with the oil over medium-high heat, add the yellow onion and the sausage, toss, cook for 10 minutes and transfer to the Crock Pot.   Add the eggs and the other ingredients, toss, put the lid on and cook on Low for 8 hours.   Divide between plates and serve for breakfast.

Shredded Chicken Muffins

Ingredients: Servings: 4   Cooking Time: 2.5 Hours

6 oz. chicken fillet, boiled	1 tsp. ground black pepper
4 eggs, beaten	1 tsp. olive oil
1 tsp. salt	

Directions:

Shred the chicken fillet with the help of the fork and mix with eggs, salt, and ground black pepper.   Then brush the muffin molds with olive oil and transfer the shredded chicken mixture inside.   Put the muffins in the Crock Pot.   Close the lid and cook them on High for 2.5 hours.

Chai Breakfast Quinoa

Ingredients: Servings: 2   Cooking Time: 6 Hours

1 C. quinoa	2 C. milk
1 egg white	¼ tsp. cinnamon powder
¼ tsp. vanilla extract	
1 and ½ tbsp. brown sugar	¼ tsp. vanilla extract
¼ tsp. cardamom, ground	¼ tsp. nutmeg, ground
¼ tsp. ginger, grated	1 tbsp. coconut flakes

Directions:

In your Crock Pot, mix quinoa with egg white, milk, vanilla, sugar, cardamom, ginger, cinnamon, vanilla and nutmeg, stir a bit, cover and cook on Low for 6 hours.   Stir, divide into bowls and serve for breakfast with coconut flakes on top.

Peach, Vanilla And Oats Mix

Ingredients: Servings: 2   Cooking Time: 8 Hours

½ C. steel cut oats	½ tsp. vanilla extract
2 C. almond milk	1 tsp. cinnamon powder
½ C. peaches, pitted and roughly chopped	

Directions:

In your Crock Pot, mix the oats with the almond milk, peaches and the other ingredients, toss, put the lid on and cook on Low for 8 hours.   Divide into bowls and serve for breakfast right away.

Mushroom Chicken Casserole

Ingredients: Servings: 5   Cooking Time: 8 Hours

8 oz. mushrooms, sliced	7 oz. chicken fillet, sliced
1 C. cream	1 tsp. butter
1 carrot, peeled and grated	1 tsp. fresh rosemary
6 oz. Cheddar cheese, shredded	1 tsp. salt
	½ tsp. coriander

Directions:

Add the mushroom slices, grated carrot in the Crock Pot. Season the chicken strips with coriander and rosemary.   Place these chicken slices in the cooker and top it with cream, butter, salt, and cheese.   Put the cooker's lid on and set the cooking time to 8 hours on Low settings.   Serve.

Veggies Casserole

Ingredients: Servings: 8   Cooking Time: 4 Hours

8 eggs	¾ C. almond milk
4 egg whites	1 tsp. sweet paprika
2 tsp. mustard	4 bacon strips, chopped
A pinch of salt and black pepper	6 oz. cheddar cheese, shredded
2 red bell peppers, chopped	Cooking spray
1 yellow onion, chopped	

Directions:

In a bowl, mix the eggs with egg whites, mustard, milk, salt, pepper and sweet paprika and whisk well.   Grease your Crock Pot with cooking spray and spread bell peppers, bacon and onion on the bottom.   Add mixed eggs, sprinkle cheddar all over, cover and cook on Low for 4 hours.   Divide between plates and serve for breakfast.

Salami Eggs

Ingredients: Servings: 4   Cooking Time: 2.5 Hours

4 oz. salami, sliced	4 eggs
1 tsp. butter, melted	1 tbsp. chives, chopped

Directions:

Pour the melted butter in the Crock Pot.   Crack the eggs inside. Then top the eggs with salami and chives.   Close the lid and cook them on High for 2.5 hours.

Buttery Oatmeal

Ingredients: Servings: 2   Cooking Time: 3 Hours

Cooking spray	1 apple, cored and cubed
2 C. coconut milk	
1 C. old fashioned oats	2 tbsp. butter, melted
1 pear, cubed	

Directions:

Grease your Crock Pot with the cooking spray, add the milk, oats and the other ingredients, toss, put the lid on and cook on High for 3 hours.   Divide the mix into bowls and serve for breakfast.

Eggs And Sweet Potato Mix

Ingredients: Servings: 2   Cooking Time: 6 Hours

½ red onion, chopped	½ tsp. olive oil
½ green bell pepper, chopped	4 eggs, whisked
2 sweet potatoes, peeled and grated	1 tbsp. chives, chopped
	A pinch of red pepper, crushed

½ red bell pepper, chopped
1 garlic clove, minced
A pinch of salt and black pepper

Directions:
In a bowl, mix the eggs with the onion, bell peppers and the other ingredients except the oil and whisk well. Grease your Crock Pot with the oil, add the eggs and potato mix, spread, put the lid on and cook on Low for 6 hours. Divide everything between plates and serve.

Lentils And Quinoa Mix

Ingredients: Servings: 6   Cooking Time: 8 Hours

3 garlic cloves, minced	4 C. veggie stock
1 yellow onion, chopped	1 C. lentils
1 celery stalk, chopped	14 oz. pinto beans
2 red bell peppers, chopped	2 tbsp. chili powder
12 oz. canned tomatoes, chopped	½ C. quinoa
	1 tbsp. oregano, chopped
	2 tsp. cumin, ground

Directions:
In your Crock Pot, mix garlic with the onion, celery, bell peppers, tomatoes, stock, lentils, pinto beans, chili powder, quinoa, oregano and cumin, stir, cover, cook on Low for 8 hours, divide between plates and serve for breakfast

Radish Bowl

Ingredients: Servings: 4   Cooking Time: 1.5 Hours

1 tbsp. dried dill	2 C. radish, halved
1 tbsp. olive oil	4 eggs, beaten
	¼ tsp. salt
	¼ C. milk

Directions:
Mix radish with dried dill, olive oil, salt, and milk and transfer in the Crock Pot. Cook the radish on High for 30 minutes. Then shake the vegetables well and add eggs. Mix the mixture gently and close the lid. Cook the meal on High for 1 hour.

Cowboy Breakfast Casserole

Ingredients: Servings: 6   Cooking Time: 3 Hours

1-lb. ground beef	5 eggs, beaten
1 C. grass-fed Monterey Jack cheese, shredded	1 avocado, peeled and diced
Salt and pepper to taste	A handful of cilantro, chopped
	A dash of hot sauce

Directions:
In a skillet over medium flame, sauté the beef for three minutes until slightly golden. Pour into the CrockPot and pour in eggs. Sprinkle with cheese on top and season with salt and pepper to taste. Close the lid and cook on high for 4 hours or on low for 6 hours. Serve with avocado, cilantro and hot sauce.

Chocolate Toast

Ingredients: Servings: 4   Cooking Time: 40 Minutes

4 white bread slices	1 banana, mashed
1 tbsp. vanilla extract	1 tbsp. coconut oil
2 tbsp. Nutella	¼ C. full-fat milk

Directions:
Mix vanilla extract, Nutella, mashed banana, coconut oil, and milk. Pour the mixture in the Crock Pot and cook on High for 40 minutes. Make a quick pressure release and cool the chocolate mixture. Spread the toasts with cooked mixture.

Ginger Raisins Oatmeal

Ingredients: Servings: 2   Cooking Time: 8 Hours

1 C. almond milk	¼ C. raisins
½ C. steel cut oats	
½ tsp. ginger, ground	1 tbsp. orange juice
1 tbsp. orange zest, grated	½ tsp. vanilla extract
	½ tbsp. honey

Directions:
In your Crock Pot, combine the milk with the oats, raisins and the other ingredients, toss, put the lid on and cook on Low for 8 hours. Divide into 2 bowls and serve for breakfast.

Quinoa And Banana Mix

Ingredients: Servings: 8   Cooking Time: 6 Hours

2 C. quinoa	2 tbsp. maple syrup
2 bananas, mashed	1 tsp. cinnamon powder
4 C. water	Cooking spray
2 C. blueberries	
2 tsp. vanilla extract	

Directions:
Grease your Crock Pot with cooking spray, add quinoa, bananas, water, blueberries, vanilla, maple syrup and cinnamon, stir, cover and cook on Low for 6 hours. Stir again, divide into bowls and serve for breakfast.

Sweet Vegetable Rice Pudding

Ingredients: Servings: 4   Cooking Time: 1 Hour

2 C. cauliflower, shredded	3 C. of milk
1 tbsp. potato starch	2 tbsp. maple syrup

Directions:
Mix potato starch with milk and pour in the Crock Pot. Add maple syrup and cauliflower shred. Cook the mixture on High for 1 hour.

Eggs And Vegetables Omelet

Ingredients: Servings: 4   Cooking Time: 3 Hours

2 tbsp. coconut oil	½ C. broccoli, chopped
4 eggs, beaten	
1 C. spinach, chopped	1 C. grass-fed sharp cheddar cheese, shredded
½ C. cauliflower, chopped	

Salt and pepper to taste

Directions:

Grease the inside of the CrockPot with coconut oil. Pour in eggs, spinach, cauliflower, and broccoli. Stir to combine. Add in the cheese and season with salt and pepper to taste. Close the lid and cook on high for 2 hours or on low for 3 hours.

Quinoa Breakfast Bars

Ingredients: Servings: 8   Cooking Time: 4 Hours

2 tbsp. maple syrup
2 tbsp. almond butter, melted
Cooking spray
½ tsp. cinnamon powder
1 C. almond milk
2 eggs

½ C. raisins
1/3 C. quinoa
1/3 C. almonds, roasted and chopped
1/3 C. dried apples, chopped
2 tbsp. chia seeds

Directions:

In a bowl, mix almond butter with maple syrup, cinnamon, milk, eggs, quinoa, raisins, almonds, apples and chia seeds and stir really well. Grease your Crock Pot with the spray, line it with parchment paper, spread quinoa mix, cover and cook on Low for 4 hours. Leave mix aside to cool down, slice and serve for breakfast.

Basil Sausages

Ingredients: Servings: 5   Cooking Time: 4 Hours

1-lb. Italian sausages, chopped
1 tsp. dried basil
¼ C. of water

1 tbsp. olive oil
1 tsp. ground coriander

Directions:

Sprinkle the chopped sausages with ground coriander and dried basil and transfer in the Crock Pot. Add olive oil and water. Close the lid and cook the sausages on high for 4 hours.

Eggs With Spinach And Yogurt

Ingredients: Servings: 4   Cooking Time: 3 Hours

1 clove of garlic, minced
2/3 C. plain Greek yogurt
2 tbsp. grass-fed butter, unsalted
4 large eggs, beaten
1 tsp. fresh oregano, chopped

Salt and pepper to taste
2 tbsp. olive oil
10 C. fresh spinach, chopped
¼ tsp. red pepper flakes, crushed
2 tbsp. scallions, chopped

Directions:

In a mixing bowl, combine garlic, yogurt, butter, and eggs. Stir in oregano and season with salt and pepper to taste. Grease the bottom of the CrockPot with olive oil. Arrange the spinach and pour over the egg mixture. Sprinkle with pepper flakes and scallions on top. Close the lid and cook on high for 2 hours or on low for 3 hours.

Chicken Cabbage Medley

Ingredients: Servings: 5   Cooking Time: 4.5 Hours

6 oz. ground chicken
10 oz. cabbage, chopped
1 white onion, sliced
½ C. tomato juice
1 tsp. sugar

½ tsp. salt
1 tsp. ground black pepper
4 tbsp. chicken stock
2 garlic cloves

Directions:

Whisk tomato juice with black pepper, salt, sugar, and chicken stock in a bowl. Spread the onion slices, chicken, and cabbage in the Crock Pot. Pour the tomato-stock mixture over the veggies and top with garlic cloves. Put the cooker's lid on and set the cooking time to 4 hours 30 minutes on High settings. Serve.

Granola Bowls

Ingredients: Servings: 2   Cooking Time: 4 Hours

½ C. granola
2 tbsp. brown sugar
2 tbsp. cashew butter

¼ C. coconut cream
1 tsp. cinnamon powder
½ tsp. nutmeg, ground

Directions:

In your Crock Pot, mix the granola with the cream, sugar and the other ingredients, toss, put the lid on and cook on Low for 4 hours. Divide into bowls and serve for breakfast.

Berry-berry Jam

Ingredients: Servings: 6   Cooking Time: 4 Hours

1 C. white sugar
1 C. strawberries
1 tbsp. gelatin
3 tbsp. water

1 tbsp. lemon zest
1 tsp. lemon juice
½ C. blueberries

Directions:

Take a blender jug and add berries, sugar, lemon juice, and lemon zest to puree. Blend this blueberry-strawberry mixture for 3 minutes until smooth. Pour this berry mixture into the base of your Crock Pot. Put the cooker's lid on and set the cooking time to 1 hour on High settings. Mix gelatin with 3 tbsp. water in a bowl and pour it into the berry mixture. Again, put the cooker's lid on and set the cooking time to 3 hours on High settings. Allow the jam to cool down. Serve.

Baby Spinach Rice Mix

Ingredients: Servings: 4   Cooking Time: 6 Hours

¼ C. mozzarella, shredded
½ C. baby spinach
½ C. wild rice
1 and ½ C. chicken stock
½ tsp. turmeric powder

½ tsp. oregano, dried
A pinch of salt and black pepper
3 scallions, minced
¾ C. goat cheese, crumbled

Directions:

In your Crock Pot, mix the rice with the stock, turmeric and the other ingredients, toss, put the lid on and cook on Low for 6 hours. Divide the mix into bowls and serve for breakfast.

Corn Casserole

Ingredients: Servings: 6   Cooking Time: 8 Hours

1 C. sweet corn kernels	2 tbsp. cream cheese
1 chili pepper, chopped	5 oz. ham, chopped
1 tomato, chopped	1 tsp. garlic powder
1 C. Mozzarella, shredded	2 eggs, beaten

Directions:
Mix sweet corn kernels, with chili pepper, tomato, and ham. Add minced garlic and stir the ingredients. Transfer it in the Crock Pot and flatten gently. Top the casserole with eggs, cream cheese, and Mozzarella. Cook the casserole on LOW for 8 hours.

Morning Pie

Ingredients: Servings: 6   Cooking Time: 3 Hours

½ C. oatmeal	1 C. full-fat milk
1 C. butternut squash, diced	½ tsp. ground cinnamon
1 tsp. vanilla extract	1 tsp. sesame oil
	4 pecans, crushed

Directions:
Mix oatmeal and milk in the Crock Pot. Add diced butternut squash, vanilla extract, and ground cinnamon. Then add sesame oil and pecans. Carefully mix the ingredients and close the lid. Cook the pie on Low for 3 hours. Then cool the pie and cut it into servings.

Quinoa Bars

Ingredients: Servings: 8   Cooking Time: 4 Hours

2 tbsp. maple syrup	½ C. raisins
2 tbsp. almond butter, melted	1/3 C. quinoa
Cooking spray	1/3 C. almonds, toasted and chopped
½ tsp. cinnamon powder	1/3 C. dried apples, chopped
1 C. almond milk	2 tbsp. chia seeds
2 eggs	

Directions:
Mix quinoa with almond butter, cinnamon, milk, maple syrup, eggs, apples, chia seeds, almonds, and raisins in a suitable bowl. Coat the base of your Crock Pot with cooking spray and parchment paper. Now evenly spread the quinoa-oats mixture over the parchment paper. Put the cooker's lid on and set the cooking time to 4 hours on Low settings. Slice and serve.

Broccoli Omelette

Ingredients: Servings: 4   Cooking Time: 2 Hours

½ C. milk	1 C. broccoli florets
6 eggs	1 yellow onion,

Salt and black pepper to the taste	chopped
A pinch of chili powder	1 garlic clove, minced
A pinch of garlic powder	1 tbsp. cheddar cheese, shredded
1 red bell pepper, chopped	Cooking spray

Directions:
Start by cracking eggs in a large bowl and beat them well. Stir in all the veggies, cheese, and spices then mix well. Pour the eggs-veggie mixture into the Crock Pot. Put the cooker's lid on and set the cooking time to 2 hours on High settings. Slice and serve warm.

Creamy Quinoa With Nuts

Ingredients: Servings: 5   Cooking Time: 3 Hours

1 oz. nuts, crushed	1 tsp. salt
2 C. quinoa	¼ tsp. chili flakes
1 C. heavy cream	1 oz. Parmesan, grated
1 C. of water	

Directions:
Put quinoa, heavy cream, water, salt, and chili flakes in the Crock Pot. Cook the ingredients on High for 3 hours. Then add grated cheese and crushed nuts. Stir the meal well and transfer in the serving plates.

Bacon Muffins

Ingredients: Servings: 5   Cooking Time: 4 Hours

½ C. flour	2 eggs, beaten
2 tbsp. coconut oil	2 oz. bacon, chopped, cooked
1 tsp. baking powder	¼ C. milk

Directions:
Mix flour, milk, and eggs. Add coconut oil, baking powder, and bacon. Stir the mixture carefully. Then pour the batter in the muffin molds. Transfer them in the Crock Pot and close the lid. Cook the muffins on High for 4 hours.

Baguette Boats

Ingredients: Servings: 4   Cooking Time: 3 Hours

6 oz. baguette (2 baguettes)	½ C. Mozzarella, shredded
4 ham slices	1 tsp. olive oil
1 tsp. minced garlic	1 egg, beaten

Directions:
Cut the baguettes into the halves and remove the flesh from the bread. Chop the ham and mix it with egg, Mozzarella, and minced garlic. Fill the baguettes with ham mixture. Then brush the Crock Pot bowl with olive oil from inside. Put the baguette boats in the Crock Pot and close the lid. Cook them for 3 hours on High.

Cheese And Turkey Casserole

Ingredients: Servings: 4   Cooking Time: 6 Hours

8 oz. ground turkey
5 oz. Monterey jack cheese, shredded
1 tbsp. dried parsley

1 tsp. butter
1 tsp. chili powder
1 red onion, diced
¼ C. of water

Directions:

Put all ingredients in the Crock Pot and mix carefully.   Close the lid and cook the casserole on low for 6 hours.

Banana And Coconut Oatmeal

Ingredients: Servings: 6   Cooking Time: 7 Hours

Cooking spray
2 bananas, sliced
1 C. steel cut oats
28 oz. canned coconut milk
½ C. water
1 tbsp. butter
2 tbsp. brown sugar

¼ tsp. nutmeg, ground
½ tsp. cinnamon powder
½ tsp. vanilla extract
1 tbsp. flaxseed, ground

Directions:

Grease your Crock Pot with cooking spray, add banana slices, oats, coconut milk, water, butter, sugar, cinnamon, butter, vanilla and flaxseed, toss a bit, cover and cook on Low for 7 hours. Divide into bowls and serve for breakfast.

Kale & Feta Breakfast Frittata

Ingredients: Servings: 6 (4.8 oz. Per Serving)   Cooking Time: 3 Hours And 5 Minutes

2 C. kale, chopped
½ C. feta, crumbled
2 tsp. olive oil
Salt and pepper to taste

3 green onions, chopped
1 large green pepper, diced
8 eggs

Directions:

Heat the olive oil in Crock-Pot and sauté the kale, diced pepper, and chopped green onion for about 2-3 minutes. Beat the eggs in a mixing bowl, pour over other ingredients, and stir. Add salt and pepper and sprinkle crumbled feta cheese on top. Cover and cook on LOW for 2-3 hours, or until the cheese has melted. Serve hot.

LUNCH & DINNER RECIPES

Vegetarian Gumbo

Ingredients: Servings: 6   Cooking Time: 8 1/2 Hours

2 tbsp. olive oil
1 sweet onion, chopped
1 celery stalk, sliced
2 garlic cloves, chopped
1 red bell pepper, cored and diced
2 tbsp. all-purpose flour
2 C. vegetable stock

1 C. diced tomatoes
1 can (15 oz.) kidney beans, drained
2 C. sliced mushrooms
1 summer squash, cubed
1 C. chopped okra
1 tsp. Cajun seasoning
1/2 C. coconut milk

Salt and pepper to taste

Directions:

Heat the oil in a skillet and add the onion, celery, garlic and bell pepper and cook for 5 minutes until softened. Add the flour and cook for 1 additional minute then transfer the mixture in your Crock Pot.   Add the remaining ingredients and season with salt and pepper.   Cook on low settings for 8 hours.   Serve the gumbo warm.

Pork Soup

Ingredients: Servings: 2   Cooking Time: 6 Hours

½ C. canned black beans, drained and rinsed
1 lb. pork stew meat, cubed
3 C. beef stock
1 small red bell pepper, chopped
1 yellow onion, chopped

1 tsp. Italian seasoning
½ tbsp. olive oil
Salt and black pepper to the taste
½ C. canned tomatoes, crushed
1 tbsp. basil, chopped

Directions:

In your Crock Pot, mix the pork with the beans, stock and the other ingredients, toss, put the lid on and cook on Low for 6 hours.   Divide into bowls and serve.

Summer Lasagna

Ingredients: Servings: 8   Cooking Time: 6 1/2 Hours

1 large zucchini
1 large eggplant
1 can diced tomatoes
1 C. white rice
1/2 tsp. dried oregano
2 tbsp. chopped parsley

1 celery stalk, diced
2 C. vegetable stock
Salt and pepper to taste
1 1/2 C. shredded mozzarella

Directions:

Cut the zucchini and eggplant into thin ribbons using a vegetable peeler.   Mix the tomatoes, white rice, celery, oregano, parsley, salt and pepper.   Layer the zucchini, eggplant and rice mixture in your Crock Pot.   Add the stock and top with cheese.   Cook on low settings for 6 hours.   Serve the lasagna warm.

Savory Chowder

Ingredients: Servings: 6   Cooking Time: 6 Hours 20 Minutes

¼ C. red onions, chopped
2 C. cauliflower, chopped
¼ tsp. thyme
2 tsp. parsley
1 C. organic chicken broth

1 can clams
1 pint half-and-half
2 slices bacon, cooked
1 tsp. salt
1 garlic clove, minced
1/8 tsp. pepper

Directions:

Put all the ingredients in a crock pot and stir well. Cover and cook on LOW for about 6 hours. Ladle out in a bowl and serve hot.

Tofu Korma

Ingredients: Servings: 6   Cooking Time: 8 1/4 Hours

8 oz. firm tofu, cubed	1/2 tsp. grated ginger
2 tbsp. olive oil	1/2 tsp. turmeric
2 red bell peppers, cored and diced	powder
	1/4 tsp. chili powder
1 carrot, diced	1/2 tsp. curry powder
1/2 celery stalk, diced	1 C. vegetable stock
2 C. cauliflower florets	1/2 C. coconut milk
1 C. diced tomatoes	Salt and pepper to taste

Directions:

Heat the oil in a skillet and add the tofu. Cook on all sides until golden brown then transfer in your Crock Pot. Add the remaining ingredients in your crock pot and season with salt and pepper. Cook on low settings for 8 hours. Serve the korma warm and fresh.

Bavarian Beef Roast

Ingredients: Servings: 6   Cooking Time: 10 1/4 Hours

2 tbsp. all-purpose flour	2 lb. beef roast
	1 C. apple juice
2 tbsp. mustard seeds	1/2 C. beef stock
1 tsp. prepared horseradish	Salt and pepper to taste

Directions:

Season the beef with salt and pepper and sprinkle with flour. Combine the beef roast and the rest of the ingredients in your crock pot. Add salt and pepper as needed and cook on low settings for 10 hours. Serve the roast while still warm.

Slow Cooked Thyme Chicken

Ingredients: Servings: 2   Cooking Time: 7 Hours

1 lb. chicken legs	1 carrot, chopped
1 tbsp. thyme, chopped	½ yellow onion, chopped
2 garlic cloves, minced	A pinch of salt and white pepper
½ C. chicken stock	Juice of ½ lemon

Directions:

In your Crock Pot, mix the chicken legs with the thyme, garlic and the other ingredients, toss, put the lid on and cook on Low for 7 hours. Divide between plates and serve.

Thai Chicken Vegetable Medley

Ingredients: Servings: 6   Cooking Time: 4 1/4 Hours

2 chicken breasts, cut into strips	2 zucchinis, sliced
	1 leek, sliced
2 red bell peppers, cored and sliced	1 tbsp. red Thai curry paste
2 heirloom tomatoes, peeled and diced	1 C. coconut milk
	1/2 C. vegetable stock

2 C. button mushrooms	Salt and pepper to taste
4 garlic cloves, minced	

Directions:

Combine all the ingredients in your crock pot. Add salt and pepper to taste and cover with a lid. Cook on low settings for 4 hours. Serve the dish warm or chilled.

Beef Cabbage Rolls

Ingredients: Servings: 8   Cooking Time: 6 1/2 Hours

16 green cabbage leaves	2 tbsp. chopped parsley
1 1/2 lb. ground beef	1 egg
1/2 C. white rice	1 tbsp. all-purpose flour
2 onions, finely chopped	Salt and pepper to taste
2 garlic cloves, minced	1 1/2 C. beef stock
	2 lemons, juiced

Directions:

Bring a pot of water to a boil. Add the cabbage leaves and cook for 2 minutes just to soften them. Drain well and allow to cool. Mix the beef, rice, onions, garlic, parsley, egg and flour. Season with salt and pepper and mix well. Place the cabbage leaves on your working board and place a few spoonfuls of beef mixture at one end of each leaf. Roll the leaves tightly, hiding the ends in. Place the cabbage rolls in your crock pot. Add the stock and lemon juice and cook on low settings for 6 hours. Serve the rolls warm.

African Inspired Chicken Stew

Ingredients: Servings: 8   Cooking Time: 5 1/4 Hours

1 1/2 C. red lentils	1/2 tsp. chili powder
2 lb. skinless chicken drumsticks	1 tsp. coriander powder
1 tbsp. butter	1/4 tsp. all-spice powder
2 large red onions, chopped	1/4 tsp. ground cloves
4 garlic cloves, minced	1 C. coconut milk
	1 C. vegetable stock
1 tsp. grated ginger	

Directions:

Combine the lentils, chicken, butter, spices, coconut milk and stock in your Crock Pot. Add enough salt and pepper and cook on low settings for 5 hours. Serve the stew warm and fresh.

Green Lentils Salad

Ingredients: Servings: 2   Cooking Time: 4 Hours

¼ C. green lentils	2 C. lettuce, chopped
1 C. chicken stock	¼ C. Greek Yogurt
½ tsp. ground cumin	

Directions:

Mix green lentils with chicken stock and transfer in the Crock Pot. Cook the ingredients on High for 4 hours. Then cool the lentils and transfer them in the salad bowl. Add ground cumin, lettuce, and Greek yogurt. Mix the salad carefully.

Smoky Pork Chili

Ingredients: Servings: 8   Cooking Time: 6 1/4 Hours

1 tbsp. canola oil	1 C. dark beer
6 bacon slices, chopped	1 tsp. cumin powder
1 lb. ground pork	1 lb. dried black beans, rinsed
2 onions, chopped	2 1/2 C. vegetable stock
4 garlic cloves, chopped	1 C. diced tomatoes
2 tbsp. tomato paste	2 bay leaves
1 1/2 tsp. smoked paprika	1 thyme sprig
	Salt and pepper to taste

Directions:

Heat the oil in a skillet and add the bacon. Cook until crisp then stir in the pork. Sauté for a few additional minutes then transfer in your Crock Pot. Add the rest of the ingredients and adjust the taste with salt and pepper. Cook on low settings for 6 hours. Serve the chili warm and fresh.

Soy Braised Chicken

Ingredients: Servings: 6   Cooking Time: 3 1/4 Hours

6 chicken thighs	1 bay leaf
2 shallots, sliced	1/2 tsp. cayenne pepper
2 garlic cloves, chopped	Salt and pepper to taste
1/4 C. apple cider	Cooked white rice for serving
1/4 C. soy sauce	
1 tbsp. brown sugar	

Directions:

Combine the chicken, shallots, garlic cloves, apple cider, soy sauce, leaf, brown sugar and cayenne pepper in your crock pot. Adjust the taste with salt and pepper if needed and cook on high settings for 3 hours. Serve the chicken warm.

Chickpea Curry

Ingredients: Servings: 6   Cooking Time: 4 1/4 Hours

2 tbsp. coconut oil	1/2 tsp. turmeric powder
1 sweet onion, chopped	1/4 tsp. curry powder
2 garlic cloves, chopped	4 C. cooked chickpeas, drained
1/2 tsp. grated ginger	1 can diced tomatoes
1/2 tsp. cumin powder	1/2 C. vegetable stock
1/4 tsp. ground coriander	1/2 C. coconut milk
	Salt and pepper to taste

Directions:

Heat the coconut oil in a skillet and add the onion and garlic. Cook for 2 minutes until softened then add the spices and cook for 30 seconds just to release flavor. Transfer in your Crock Pot and add the remaining ingredients. Adjust the taste with salt and pepper and cook on low settings for 4 hours. Serve the curry warm.

Sweet Farro

Ingredients: Servings: 3   Cooking Time: 6 Hours

1/2 C. farro	2 tbsp. dried cranberries
2 C. of water	
1/2 C. heavy cream	2 tbsp. sugar

Directions:

Chop the cranberries and put in the Crock Pot. Add water, heavy cream, sugar, and farro. Mix the ingredients with the help of the spoon and close the lid. Cook the farro on low for 6 hours.

Hominy Beef Chili

Ingredients: Servings: 6   Cooking Time: 3 1/4 Hours

1 lb. ground beef	2 jalapeno peppers, chopped
1 large onion, chopped	1/2 tsp. cumin powder
4 garlic cloves, chopped	1 tsp. chili powder
2 carrots, diced	2 C. frozen corn
2 red bell peppers, cored and diced	Salt and pepper to taste
1 can (15 oz.) hominy, drained	1 bay leaf
1 can fire roasted tomatoes	Grated Cheddar for serving

Directions:

Mix the ground beef, onion, garlic, carrots, bell peppers, hominy, tomatoes, jalapeno peppers, cumin powder, chili powder and corn in your crock pot. Add the bay leaf, salt and pepper to taste and cook on high settings for 3 hours. Serve the chili warm, topped with grated Cheddar.

Sour Cream Pork Chops

Ingredients: Servings: 6   Cooking Time: 6 1/4 Hours

6 pork chops, bone in	2 tbsp. chopped parsley
1 C. sour cream	Salt and pepper to taste
1/2 C. chicken stock	
2 green onions, chopped	

Directions:

Combine the pork chops, sour cream, stock, onions and parsley in your crock pot. Add salt and pepper to taste and cook on low settings for 6 hours. Serve the pork chops warm and fresh, topped with plenty of sauce.

Asparagus Barley Stew

Ingredients: Servings: 6   Cooking Time: 6 1/4 Hours

1 bunch asparagus, trimmed and chopped	1 C. pearl barley
	2 C. vegetable stock
1 shallot, chopped	Salt and pepper to taste
1 garlic clove, chopped	1/2 C. grated Parmesan
1/2 tsp. fennel seeds	

Directions:

10.   Combine the asparagus, shallot, garlic, fennel seeds, pearl barley and stock in your Crock Pot. 1Add salt and pepper to taste and cook on low settings for 6 hours. 1When done, stir in the Parmesan and serve the stew warm and fresh.

Gruyere Flank Steaks

Ingredients: Servings: 4   Cooking Time: 3 1/4 Hours

4 flank steaks
Salt and pepper to taste
1 C. crumbled gruyere cheese
1 tsp. Worcestershire sauce

1/2 C. white wine
1/2 C. cream cheese
1 tsp. Dijon mustard
Salt and pepper to taste

Directions:

Season the steaks with salt and pepper. Place them in your Crock Pot.   Mix the rest of the ingredients in a bowl then spoon the mixture over the steaks.   Cover the pot and cook on high settings for 3 hours.   Serve the steaks warm with your favorite side dish.

Chickpeas Stew(2)

Ingredients: Servings: 2   Cooking Time: 6 Hours

½ tbsp. olive oil
2 garlic cloves, minced
1 red chili pepper, chopped
¼ C. carrots, chopped
6 oz. canned tomatoes, chopped
6 oz. canned chickpeas, drained

1 red onion, chopped
½ C. chicken stock
1 bay leaf
½ tsp. coriander, ground
A pinch of red pepper flakes
½ tbsp. parsley, chopped
Salt and black pepper to the taste

Directions:

In your Crock Pot, mix the chickpeas with the onion, garlic and the other ingredients, toss, put the lid on and cook on Low for 6 hours.   Divide into bowls and serve.

Sweet And Spicy Pulled Pork

Ingredients: Servings: 8   Cooking Time: 9 1/4 Hours

4 lb. pork shoulder
1 tbsp. cumin powder
1 tsp. chili powder
1/4 C. brown sugar
1 tsp. dry mustard

2 chipotle peppers, chopped
6 garlic cloves, minced
1/4 tsp. ground cloves
1 1/2 tsp. salt
1 C. pineapple juice
1 C. chickens tock

Directions:

Mix the brown sugar, cumin powder, chili powder, dry mustard, chipotle peppers, garlic and ground cloves, as well as salt in a bowl.   Spread this mix over the meat and rub it well.   Place the meat in your Crock Pot and add the pineapple juice and stock. Cover and cook on low settings for 9 hours.   When done, shred the meat into fine threads using 2 forks.   It's best served warm.

Beans And Rice

Ingredients: Servings: 6   Cooking Time: 3 Hours

1 lb. pinto beans, dried
1/3 C. hot sauce
Salt and black pepper to the taste
1 tbsp. garlic, minced
1 tsp. garlic powder

½ tsp. cumin, ground
1 tbsp. chili powder
3 bay leaves
½ tsp. oregano, dried
1 C. white rice, cooked

Directions:

In your Crock Pot, mix pinto beans with hot sauce, salt, pepper, garlic, garlic powder, cumin, chili powder, bay leaves and oregano, stir, cover and cook on High for 3 hours.   Divide rice between plates, add pinto beans on top and serve for lunch

Spiced Chicken Over Wild Rice

Ingredients: Servings: 6   Cooking Time: 7 1/4 Hours

6 chicken thighs
1 tsp. cumin powder
1/2 tsp. chili powder
Salt and pepper to taste

1 C. wild rice
2 celery stalk, diced
1 carrot, diced
2 C. sliced mushrooms
2 C. vegetable stock

Directions:

Season the chicken with cumin powder, chili, salt and pepper. Combine the rice, celery, carrot, mushrooms, stock, salt and pepper in your crock pot.   Place the chicken on top and cook on low settings for 7 hours.   Serve the chicken and rice warm or chilled.

Bacon Wrapped Beef Tenderloin

Ingredients: Servings: 6   Cooking Time: 8 1/4 Hours

2 lb. beef tenderloin
1 tsp. cumin powder
1 tsp. smoked paprika
8 slices bacon

1 tsp. dried thyme
2 tbsp. olive oil
1 C. beef stock
Salt and pepper to taste

Directions:

Season the beef tenderloin with salt, pepper, cumin powder, paprika and thyme. Drizzle with olive oil and rub the meat well. Wrap the beef in bacon slices and place in your crock pot.   Add the stock and cover the pot with its lid.   Cook on low settings for 8 hours.   When done, slice and serve the tenderloin warm with your favorite side dish.

Beef Salsa Chili

Ingredients: Servings: 8   Cooking Time: 7 1/2 Hours

2 lb. beef roast, cubed
2 tbsp. canola oil
2 red onions, chopped
2 garlic cloves, chopped
2 carrots, diced
2 red bell peppers, cored and diced
1 leek, sliced
1 1/2 C. red salsa

1 bay leaf
1 tsp. cumin seeds
1 tsp. chili powder
2 C. dried black bean
4 C. chicken stock or water
Salt and pepper to taste

Directions:

Heat the oil in a skillet or frying pan and add the beef. Cook for a few minutes until golden brown then transfer in your crock pot. Add the rest of the ingredients and season with salt and pepper. Cook on low settings for 7 hours. The chili is best served warm, but it can also be re-heated.

Caribbean Sticky Pork Ribs

Ingredients: Servings: 8   Cooking Time: 7 1/4 Hours

6 lb. pork ribs
1 can crushed pineapple
2 tbsp. honey
1 tsp. Worcestershire sauce
1/2 tsp. all spice powder

1 tsp. hot sauce
1/4 tsp. chili powder
2 onions, sliced
2 garlic cloves, chopped
Salt and pepper to taste

Directions:

Mix the pineapple, honey, hot sauce, Worcestershire sauce, all spice and chili powder, salt and pepper, as well as onions and garlic in your Crock Pot. Place the pork ribs on top and drizzle them with the sauce found in the pot. Cover and cook on low settings for 7 hours. Serve the pork ribs warm and fresh.

Layered Sweet Potatoes

Ingredients: Servings: 8   Cooking Time: 6 1/2 Hours

2 tbsp. olive oil
2 large sweet potatoes, peeled and finely sliced
2 onions, finely sliced
1 pinch nutmeg

2 C. whole milk
1/2 C. cream cheese
2 eggs, beaten
1/2 tsp. garlic powder
Salt and pepper to taste

Directions:

Grease your Crock Pot then layer the potatoes and onions in your Crock Pot. Mix the nutmeg, milk, eggs and garlic powder in a bowl. Add salt and pepper to taste then pour over the veggies. Cook on low settings for 6 hours. Serve the dish warm.

Spicy Vegetarian Chili

Ingredients: Servings: 8   Cooking Time: 6 1/2 Hours

2 tbsp. olive oil
2 shallots, chopped
4 garlic cloves, chopped
2 C. cauliflower florets
1 can (15 oz.) chickpeas, drained
1 can (15 oz.) black beans, drained
1 can fire toasted tomatoes
1 C. canned corn, drained

1 zucchini, cubed
2 red bell peppers, cored and diced
1 celery stalk, diced
1 tsp. chili powder
1 C. tomato sauce
2 C. vegetable stock
1 bay leaf
Salt and pepper to taste
Sour cream for serving

Directions:

Heat the oil in a skillet and add the shallots and garlic. Cook for a few minutes until softened then transfer in your Crock Pot. Add the remaining ingredients and adjust the taste with salt and

pepper. Cook on low settings for 6 hours. Serve the chili warm, topped with sour cream.

Root Vegetable Beef Stew

Ingredients: Servings: 8   Cooking Time: 8 1/2 Hours

3 lb. beef sirloin roast, cubed
4 carrots, sliced
2 parsnips, sliced
1 celery root, peeled and cubed
4 garlic cloves, chopped
4 large potatoes, peeled and cubed

1 turnip, peeled and cubed
1 bay leaf
1 lemon, juiced
1 tsp. Worcestershire sauce
1 C. beef stock
Salt and pepper to taste

Directions:

Combine the beef, carrots, parsnips, celery root, garlic, potatoes, turnip, bay leaf, lemon juice, Worcestershire sauce and stock in your crock pot. Add salt and pepper to taste and cover with its lid. Cook on low settings for 8 hours. Serve the roast and vegetables warm.

Cinnamon Pork Ribs

Ingredients: Servings: 2   Cooking Time: 8 Hours

2 lb. baby back pork ribs
1 tbsp. cinnamon powder
2 tbsp. olive oil
1/2 tsp. allspice, ground
1/2 C. beef stock

A pinch of salt and black pepper
1/2 tsp. garlic powder
1 tbsp. balsamic vinegar
1 tbsp. tomato paste

Directions:

In your Crock Pot, mix the pork ribs with the cinnamon, the oil and the other ingredients, toss, put the lid on and cook on Low for 8 hours. Divide ribs between plates and serve for lunch with a side salad.

Lunch Roast

Ingredients: Servings: 8   Cooking Time: 8 Hours

2 lb. beef chuck roast
Salt and black pepper to the taste
1 yellow onion, chopped
2 tsp. olive oil
8 oz. tomato sauce
1/4 C. lemon juice
1/4 C. water

1/4 C. ketchup
1/4 C. apple cider vinegar
1 tbsp. Worcestershire sauce
2 tbsp. brown sugar
1/2 tsp. mustard powder
1/2 tsp. paprika

Directions:

In your Crock Pot, mix beef with salt, pepper, onion oil, tomato sauce, lemon juice, water, ketchup, vinegar, Worcestershire sauce, sugar, mustard and paprika, toss well, cover and cook on Low for 8 hours. Slice roast, divide between plates, drizzle cooking sauce all over and serve for lunch.

Mustard Baked Potatoes

Ingredients: Servings: 6   Cooking Time: 4 1/4 Hours

3 lb. potatoes, peeled and cubed
1 tbsp. Dijon mustard
1/4 C. vegetable stock
1/2 tsp. cumin seeds
4 garlic cloves, minced
1/2 tsp. salt

Directions:
Combine all the ingredients in your Crock Pot. Mix well until evenly coated. Cover with a lid and cook on low settings for 4 hours. Serve the potatoes warm.

Pork Stew

Ingredients: Servings: 8   Cooking Time: 5 Hours

2 pork tenderloins, cubed
Salt and black pepper to the taste
2 carrots, sliced
1 yellow onion, chopped
2 celery ribs, chopped
2 tbsp. tomato paste
3 C. beef stock
1/3 C. plums, dried, pitted and chopped
1 rosemary spring
1 thyme spring
2 bay leaves
4 garlic cloves, minced
1/3 C. green olives, pitted and sliced
1 tbsp. parsley, chopped

Directions:
In your Crock Pot, mix pork with salt, pepper, carrots, onion, celery, tomato paste, stock, plums, rosemary, thyme, bay leaves, garlic, olives and parsley, cover and cook on Low for 5 hours. Discard thyme, rosemary and bay leaves, divide stew into bowls and serve for lunch.

Balsamic Vegetable Sauce

Ingredients: Servings: 8   Cooking Time: 6 1/2 Hours

1 large onion, chopped
4 garlic cloves, chopped
2 red bell peppers, cored and diced
2 cans (15 oz. each) diced tomatoes
2 C. vegetable stock
10 oz. soy crumbles
2 tbsp. balsamic vinegar
1/2 tsp. dried basil
1/2 tsp. dried oregano
Salt and pepper to taste

Directions:
Combine all the ingredients in your crock pot. Season with salt and pepper as needed and cook on low settings for 6 hours. Serve the sauce warm and fresh or freeze it into individual portions for later.

Bean And Spinach Enchilada Sauce

Ingredients: Servings: 8   Cooking Time: 6 1/4 Hours

1 can (15 oz.) black beans, drained
10 oz. frozen spinach, thawed and drained
1 C. frozen corn
1/2 tsp. chili powder
1 C. tomato sauce
1 can fire roasted tomatoes
1/2 lime, juiced
1/2 tsp. cumin powder
Salt and pepper to taste

Directions:
Combine all the ingredients in your crock pot, adding salt and pepper as needed. Cook on low settings for 6 hours. Serve the enchilada sauce warm or keep cooking it after wrapping it in flour tortillas. The sauce can also be frozen into individual portions to serve later.

Green Pea Chicken With Biscuit Topping

Ingredients: Servings: 6   Cooking Time: 6 1/2 Hours

1 shallot, chopped
1 leek, sliced
2 garlic cloves, chopped
2 chicken breasts, cubed
1 1/2 C. green peas
1/2 lb. baby carrots
1 tbsp. cornstarch
1 C. vegetables tock
1/4 C. white wine
1 C. all-purpose flour
1/2 C. butter, chilled and cubed
1/2 C. buttermilk, chilled
Salt and pepper to taste

Directions:
Combine the shallot, leek, garlic, chicken, green peas, baby carrots, cornstarch, stock and wine in your crock pot. Season with salt and pepper. For the topping, mix the flour, butter, buttermilk, salt and pepper in your food processor. Pulse just until mixed then spoon the mixture over the vegetables in the crock pot. Cover and cook on low settings for 6 hours. Serve the dish warm.

Mexican Lunch Mix

Ingredients: Servings: 12   Cooking Time: 7 Hours

12 oz. beer
1/4 C. flour
2 tbsp. tomato paste
1 jalapeno pepper, chopped
4 tsp. Worcestershire sauce
2 tsp. red pepper flakes, crushed
1 and 1/2 tsp. cumin, ground
2 tsp. chili powder
1 bay leaf
Salt and black pepper to the taste
2 garlic cloves, minced
1/2 tsp. sweet paprika
1/2 tsp. red vinegar
3 lb. pork shoulder butter, cubed
2 potatoes, chopped
1 yellow onion, chopped

Directions:
In your Crock Pot, mix pork with potatoes, onion, beef, flour, tomato paste, jalapeno, bay leaf, Worcestershire sauce, pepper flakes, cumin, chili powder, garlic, paprika and vinegar, toss, cover and cook on Low for 7 hours. Divide between plates and serve for lunch.

Autumnal Stew

Ingredients: Servings: 6   Cooking Time: 6 1/4 Hours

4 C. butternut squash cubes
1 shallot, chopped
2 garlic cloves, chopped
2 ripe tomatoes, peeled and diced
1/4 tsp. cumin powder
1 pinch chili powder

2 red apples, peeled and diced
1 celery stalk, sliced
1 carrot, sliced

1/2 C. tomato sauce
1/2 C. vegetable stock
Salt and pepper to taste

Directions:

Combine all the ingredients in your Crock Pot. Add salt and pepper to taste and cook on low settings for 6 hours. Serve the stew warm and fresh.

Mustard Short Ribs

Ingredients: Servings: 2   Cooking Time: 8 Hours

2 beef short ribs, bone in and cut into individual ribs
Salt and black pepper to the taste

½ C. BBQ sauce
1 tbsp. mustard
1 tbsp. green onions, chopped

Directions:

In your Crock Pot, mix the ribs with the sauce and the other ingredients, toss, put the lid on and cook on Low for 8 hours. Divide the mix between plates and serve.

Caramelized Onion Beef Pot Roast

Ingredients: Servings: 8   Cooking Time: 8 1/2 Hours

4 lb. beef roast
4 large onions, sliced
3 tbsp. canola oil
4 garlic cloves, chopped
2 carrots, sliced

1 celery root, peeled and cubed
2 large potatoes, peeled and cubed
1 C. beef stock
1/2 C. water
Salt and pepper to taste

Directions:

Heat the oil in a frying pan and add the onions. Cook for 10 minutes until golden brown, slightly caramelized. Transfer in your Crock Pot and add the rest of the ingredients. Season with enough salt and pepper and cook on low settings for 8 hours. Serve the pot roast warm.

Honey Garlic Chicken Thighs With Snap Peas

Ingredients: Servings: 6   Cooking Time: 6 1/4 Hours

6 chicken thighs
1/2 tsp. cumin powder
1/2 tsp. smoked paprika
1/2 tsp. fennel seeds

3 tbsp. honey
2 tbsp. soy sauce
1 lb. snap peas
1/4 C. vegetable stock

Directions:

Combine the chicken, honey, cumin powder, paprika, fennel seeds and soy sauce in a bowl and mix well until evenly coated. Mix the snap peas and stock in your crock pot. Place the chicken over the snap peas and cover with a lid. Cook on low settings for 6 hours. Serve the chicken and snap peas warm.

Ravioli Stew

Ingredients: Servings: 6   Cooking Time: 6 1/4 Hours

1 celery stalk, sliced
2 carrots, sliced
2 garlic cloves, chopped
1 can (15 oz.) cannellini beans, drained
1/2 tsp. dried basil

1 shallot, chopped
1 C. diced tomatoes
10 oz. spinach ravioli
1 C. vegetable stock
Salt and pepper to taste
Grated Parmesan for serving

Directions:

Combine all the ingredients in your Crock Pot and season with salt and pepper. Cook the stew on low settings for 6 hours. Serve the stew warm, topped with grated Parmesan cheese.

Bacon Baked Beans

Ingredients: Servings: 6   Cooking Time: 8 1/4 Hours

6 bacon slices, chopped
1 tbsp. olive oil
1 lb. black beans, rinsed
1 large onion, chopped
1 celery stalk, diced
1 carrot, diced

1 C. tomato sauce
1 C. fire roasted tomatoes
1/4 tsp. cumin seeds
1/4 tsp. chili powder
Salt and pepper to taste

Directions:

Heat the oil in a skillet and add the bacon. Cook until crisp then transfer in your Crock Pot. Add the remaining ingredients and adjust the taste with salt and pepper. Cook on low settings for 8 hours. Serve the beans warm.

Sweet And Spicy Vegetable Curry

Ingredients: Servings: 6   Cooking Time: 3 1/4 Hours

2 tbsp. olive oil
2 shallots, chopped
4 garlic cloves, chopped
2 carrots, sliced
1 red bell pepper, cored and diced
2 celery stalks, sliced
1/2 head green cabbage, shredded
1 green apple, peeled and diced
1 C. canned chickpeas, drained

1 parsnip, diced
2 C. cauliflower florets
1 C. tomato sauce
1 C. vegetable stock
1/2 tsp. chili powder
1/2 tsp. cumin powder
1 tsp. curry powder
1 tbsp. brown sugar
1/2 C. coconut milk
Salt and pepper to taste

Directions:

Heat the oil in your Crock Pot and add the shallots, garlic, carrots, parsnip, bell pepper and celery. Cook for 5 minutes until softened then transfer in your Crock Pot. Add the remaining ingredients and season with salt and pepper. Cook on high settings for 3 hours. The curry is best served warm.

Red Lentil Dal

Ingredients: Servings: 10   Cooking Time: 6 1/4 Hours

2 C. red lentils, rinsed
4 C. water
1 can diced tomatoes

1/2 tsp. cumin powder
1/2 tsp. fenugreek

1 sweet onion,
chopped
2 garlic cloves,
chopped
1 tsp. grated ginger
1 tsp. turmeric
powder
1/4 tsp. ground
cardamom
1 bay leaf

seeds
1/2 tsp. mustard
seeds
1 tsp. fennel seeds
Salt and pepper to
taste
1 lemon, juiced for
serving
Cooked rice for
serving

Directions:
Combine the seeds in a skillet and cook for 1 minute just until their flavor is released. Place aside.   Combine the rest of the ingredients in your Crock Pot.   Add the seeds as well and cook on low settings for 6 hours.   To serve, spoon the dal over cooked rice and finish with a drizzle of lemon juice.

French Style Braised Beef Sirloin

Ingredients: Servings: 8   Cooking Time: 8 1/4 Hours

4 lb. beef sirloin
1 C. dry white wine
4 large onions, sliced
6 garlic cloves,
chopped
1/2 lb. button
mushrooms

2 carrots, sliced
1 celery stalk, sliced
1 C. beef stock
1 thyme sprig
1 rosemary sprig
Salt and pepper to
taste

Directions:
Combine the wine, onions, garlic, mushrooms, carrots, celery stalk, beef stock, thyme and rosemary sprig in your crock pot. Season the beef with salt and pepper and place in the pot.   Cover with its lid and cook on low settings for 8 hours.   When done, slice the beef and serve it warm.

Italian Style Pork Shoulder

Ingredients: Servings: 6   Cooking Time: 7 1/4 Hours

2 lb. pork shoulder
1 large onion, sliced
4 garlic cloves,
chopped
2 celery stalks, sliced
2 ripe tomatoes,
peeled and diced

1/4 C. white wine
1 tsp. dried thyme
1 tsp. dried basil
1 thyme sprig
Salt and pepper to
taste

Directions:
Combine all the ingredients in your crock pot, adjusting the taste with enough salt and pepper.   Cover with a lid and cook on low settings for 7 hours.   Serve the pork shoulder warm and fresh with your favorite side dish.

Maple Chicken Mix

Ingredients: Servings: 2   Cooking Time: 6 Hours

2 spring onions,
chopped
1 lb. chicken breast,
skinless and boneless
2 garlic cloves,
minced
1 tbsp. maple syrup

A pinch of salt and
black pepper
½ C. chicken stock
½ C. tomato sauce
1 tbsp. chives,
chopped
1 tsp. basil, dried

Directions:
In your Crock Pot mix the chicken with the garlic, maple syrup and the other ingredients, toss, put the lid on and cook on Low for 6 hours.   Divide the mix between plates and serve for lunch.

Balsamic Roasted Root Vegetables

Ingredients: Servings: 4   Cooking Time: 3 1/4 Hours

1/2 lb. baby carrots
2 sweet potatoes,
peeled and cubed
1 turnip, peeled and
sliced
1 large red onion,
sliced
2 tbsp. olive oil

2 parsnips, sliced
1 tbsp. brown sugar
2 tbsp. balsamic
vinegar
1/4 C. vegetable stock
Salt and pepper to
taste

Directions:
Combine all the ingredients in your crock pot.   Add salt and pepper to taste and cook on high settings for 3 hours.   Serve the vegetables warm and fresh.

Adobo Chicken With Bok Choy

Ingredients: Servings: 4   Cooking Time: 6 1/2 Hours

4 chicken breasts
4 garlic cloves,
minced
1 sweet onion,
chopped
2 tbsp. soy sauce

1 tbsp. brown sugar
1 tsp. paprika
1 C. chicken stock
1 head bok choy,
shredded

Directions:
Mix the chicken, garlic, onion, soy sauce, brown sugar, paprika and stock in your crock pot.   Cook on low settings for 4 hours then add the bok choy and continue cooking for 2 additional hours.   Serve the chicken and bok choy warm.

Creamy Chicken Soup

Ingredients: Servings: 6   Cooking Time: 6 Hours

2 chicken breasts,
skinless and boneless
1 C. yellow corn
1 C. peas
1 celery stalk,
chopped
1 C. carrots, chopped
2 gold potatoes,
cubed

4 oz. cream cheese,
soft
1 yellow onion,
chopped
4 C. chicken stock
2 tsp. garlic powder
3 C. heavy cream
Salt and black pepper
to the taste

Directions:
In your Crock Pot, mix chicken with corn, peas, carrots, potatoes, celery, cream cheese, onion, garlic powder, stock, heavy cream, salt and pepper, stir, cover and cook on Low for 6 hours. Transfer chicken to a cutting board, shred meat using 2 forks, return to the Crock Pot, stir, ladle soup into bowls and serve for lunch.

Lentils Soup(2)

Ingredients: Servings: 6   Cooking Time: 6 Hours

1 yellow onion, chopped
6 carrots, sliced
1 yellow bell pepper, chopped
4 garlic cloves, minced
A pinch of cayenne pepper
3 C. red lentils
4 C. chicken stock
Salt and black pepper to the taste
2 C. water
1 tsp. lemon zest, grated
1 tsp. lemon juice
1 tbsp. rosemary, chopped

Directions:

In your Crock Pot, mix onion with carrots, bell pepper, garlic, cayenne, lentils, stock, salt, pepper and water, stir, cover and cook on Low for 6 hours. Add lemon zest, lemon juice and rosemary, stir, ladle into bowls and serve for lunch.

Button Mushroom Beef Stew

Ingredients: Servings: 6   Cooking Time: 6 1/2 Hours

2 lb. beef roast, cubed
1 tbsp. all-purpose flour
2 tbsp. canola oil
2 carrots, diced
1 celery root, peeled and diced
1 can fire roasted tomatoes
1 lb. button mushrooms
1 C. beef stock
2 bay leaves
1 red chili, chopped
Salt and pepper to taste

Directions:

Season the beef with salt and pepper and sprinkle it with flour. Heat the oil in a frying pan and add the beef. Cook for a few minutes until golden then transfer in your Crock Pot. Add the rest of the ingredients and adjust the taste with salt and pepper. Cover and cook on low settings for 6 hours. Serve the stew warm or chilled.

Beef Stew(2)

Ingredients: Servings: 2   Cooking Time: 6 Hours And 10 Minutes

1 tbsp. olive oil
1 red onion, chopped
1 carrot, peeled and sliced
1 lb. beef meat, cubed
1/2 C. canned tomatoes, chopped
2 tbsp. tomato sauce
1/2 C. beef stock
2 tbsp. balsamic vinegar
2 garlic cloves, minced
1/2 C. black olives, pitted and sliced
1 tbsp. rosemary, chopped
Salt and black pepper to the taste

Directions:

Heat up a pan with the oil over medium-high heat, add the meat, brown for 10 minutes and transfer to your Crock Pot. Add the rest of the ingredients, toss, put the lid on and cook on High for 6 hours. Divide between plates and serve right away!

Sweet Peppers With Rice

Ingredients: Servings: 6   Cooking Time: 6 Hours

6 sweet peppers
1/2 C. white rice, half-cooked
1/2 onion, minced
1 tsp. ground black pepper
1 tsp. ground coriander
1/2 C. tomato juice
1 tbsp. cream cheese

Directions:

In the mixing bowl mix rice, onion, ground black pepper, and ground coriander. Then remove the seeds from the sweet peppers. Fill the sweet peppers with rice mixture ad transfer in the Crock Pot one-by-one. Pour the tomato juice over the Crock Pot. Add cream cheese. Close the lid and cook the meal on Low for 6 hours.

Bbq Beef Brisket

Ingredients: Servings: 8   Cooking Time: 6 1/4 Hours

2 tbsp. brown sugar
1 tsp. cumin powder
1 tsp. smoked paprika
1 tsp. chili powder
1 tsp. celery seeds
4 lb. beef brisket
1 tsp. salt
1/4 C. apple cider vinegar
1/2 C. beef stock
1 C. ketchup
1 tbsp. Worcestershire sauce
2 tbsp. soy sauce

Directions:

Mix the sugar, cumin powder, paprika, chili powder, celery seeds and salt in a bowl. Spread the mix over the brisket and rub it well into the meat. Combine the vinegar, stock, ketchup, Worcestershire sauce and soy sauce in your crock pot. Add the beef and cook on low settings for 6 hours. Serve the beef brisket sliced and warm.

Kitchen Sink Stew

Ingredients: Servings: 8   Cooking Time: 7 1/2 Hours

1 onion, chopped
2 garlic cloves, chopped
1/2 tsp. smoked paprika
1 C. canned corn, drained
2 C. sliced mushrooms
1 C. frozen green peas
2 C. chopped okra
1 zucchini, cubed
2 tbsp. tomato paste
1 C. diced tomatoes
1 can (15 oz.) black beans, drained
1/2 tsp. dried oregano
Salt and pepper to taste

Directions:

Combine all the ingredients in your crock pot. Add salt and pepper to taste and cook on low settings for 7 hours. The stew is best served warm, but you can also re-heat it or freeze it into individual portions for later.

Coffee Beef Roast

Ingredients: Servings: 6   Cooking Time: 4 1/4 Hours

2 lb. beef sirloin
2 tbsp. olive oil
4 garlic cloves, minced
1 C. strong brewed coffee
1/2 C. beef stock
Salt and pepper to taste

Directions:

Combine all the ingredients in your crock pot, adding salt and pepper to taste. Cover with a lid and cook on high settings for 4 hours. Serve the roast warm and fresh with your favorite side dish.

Mexican Tortilla Chip Casserole

Ingredients: Servings: 6   Cooking Time: 2 1/2 Hours

1 1/2 C. frozen corn	2 potatoes, peeled
1 can fire roasted tomatoes	and cubed
	1 C. water
1 C. red salsa	Salt and pepper to
1/2 tsp. cumin powder	taste
	6 oz. tortilla chips
1/2 tsp. chili powder	1 1/2 C. grated Cheddar

Directions:

Combine the corn with tomatoes, red salsa, cumin powder, chili powder, potatoes, salt and pepper in your crock pot. Add the water and mix then top with tortilla chips and cheese. Cook on high settings for 2 hours. Serve the casserole warm and fresh.

Pineapple Slow Cooked Tofu

Ingredients: Servings: 6   Cooking Time: 6 1/4 Hours

18 oz. firm tofu, cubed	1 chipotle pepper, chopped
1 can crushed pineapple	2 tbsp. soy sauce
1 shallot, chopped	2 tbsp. tomato paste
4 garlic cloves, minced	1 lime, juiced
	1/2 tsp. sesame oil
1 tsp. grated ginger	Salt and pepper to taste
1 tbsp. date syrup	

Directions:

Combine all the ingredients in your crock pot. Add salt and pepper as needed and cook on low settings for 6 hours. Serve the dish fresh or chilled.

Pinto Bean Chili With Butternut Squash

Ingredients: Servings: 8   Cooking Time: 6 1/4 Hours

3 C. butternut squash cubes	2 tbsp. tomato paste
	1 C. vegetable stock
2 cans (15 oz.) pinto beans, drained	1/2 tsp. chili powder
	1 bay leaf
1 C. canned corn, drained	1 thyme sprig
	Salt and pepper to
1 large onion, chopped	taste
	1 lime, sliced
2 garlic cloves, chopped	
1/2 C. tomato sauce	

Directions:

Combine the butternut squash, pinto beans, canned corn, onion, garlic and tomato paste in your Crock Pot. Add the remaining ingredients and season with salt and pepper. Cook on low settings for 6 hours. Serve the chili warm, drizzled with lime juice.

Spicy Chickpea Stew

Ingredients: Servings: 6   Cooking Time: 8 1/4 Hours

1 1/2 C. dried chickpeas, rinsed	1 celery stalk, diced
	1 bay leaf
2 shallots, chopped	1/2 tsp. garlic powder
1 can fire roasted tomatoes	1/4 tsp. chili powder
	Salt and pepper to
1 tsp. dried oregano	taste
2 C. vegetable stock	

Directions:

Combine the chickpeas, shallots, celery, tomatoes, oregano, stock and spices in your crock pot. Add salt and pepper as needed and cook on low settings for 7 hours. Serve the chickpea chili warm and fresh or store it in individual containers in the freezer.

Salsa Chicken(1)

Ingredients: Servings: 2   Cooking Time: 8 Hours

7 oz. mild salsa	1 green bell pepper, chopped
1 lb. chicken breast, skinless, boneless and cubed	Cooking spray
	1 tbsp. cilantro, chopped
1 small yellow onion, chopped	1 red bell pepper, chopped
½ tsp. coriander, ground	1 tbsp. chili powder
½ tsp. rosemary, dried	

Directions:

Grease the Crock Pot with the cooking spray and mix the chicken with the salsa, onion and the other ingredients inside. Put the lid on, cook on Low for 8 hours, divide into bowls and serve for lunch.

Spiced Beef Tenderloin

Ingredients: Servings: 8   Cooking Time: 7 1/4 Hours

4 lb. beef tenderloin	2 tbsp. honey
1 tbsp. cumin powder	2 tbsp. olive oil
1 tsp. chili powder	1/2 tsp. ground cloves
1 tsp. smoked paprika	1/4 tsp. nutmeg
1 tsp. ground ginger	1 tsp. ground coriander
	1 C. beef stock
	1 1/2 tsp. salt

Directions:

Mix the cumin powder, chili, paprika, ginger, honey, olive oil, cloves, nutmeg, salt and ground coriander in a bowl. Spread this mixture over the beef and rub it well into the meat with your fingertips. Place the beef in your crock pot and add the stock. Cover the pot and cook on low settings for 7 hours.

Red Chile Pulled Pork

Ingredients: Servings: 8   Cooking Time: 7 1/4 Hours

4 lb. pork roast	1 C. tomato sauce
2 red chilis, seeded and chopped	1 C. red salsa

1 large onion,
chopped

Salt and pepper to
taste

Directions:

Combine all the ingredients in your Crock Pot. Add salt and pepper to fit your taste and cook under the lid on low settings for 7 hours. When done, shred the pork into fine threads using two forks. Serve the pork warm and fresh or re-heat it later.

Mediterranean Crock Pot Stew

Ingredients: Servings: 6   Cooking Time: 6 1/2 Hours

2 tbsp. olive oil
1 large onion,
chopped
2 carrots, sliced
2 red bell peppers,
cored and diced
2 ripe tomatoes,
peeled and diced
4 sun-dried tomatoes,
chopped
2 zucchinis, cubed

1/2 C. pitted black
olives
2 tbsp. tomato paste
1 tbsp. lemon juice
1 1/2 C. vegetable
stock
Salt and pepper to
taste
2 tbsp. pesto sauce
for serving

Directions:

Heat the oil in a skillet and stir in the onion, carrots and bell peppers and cook for 5 minutes. Transfer in your Crock Pot and add the remaining ingredients, seasoning with salt and pepper to taste. Cook on low settings for 6 hours. Serve the stew warm and fresh.

Sweet Potato Shepherd's Pie

Ingredients: Servings: 6   Cooking Time: 6 3/4 Hours

1 lb. ground beef
2 tbsp. canola oil
1 large onion, finely
chopped
2 carrots, grated
2 celery stalks,
chopped
4 garlic cloves,
chopped

1 C. diced tomatoes
1/2 tsp. chili powder
Salt and pepper to
taste
2 lb. sweet potatoes,
peeled and cubed
1/2 C. grated
Parmesan

Directions:

Heat the oil in a skillet and add the beef. Cook for a few minutes, stirring often, then add then transfer in your crock pot. Add the onion, carrots, celery stalks, garlic and tomatoes, as well as chili powder, salt and pepper. Cook the sweet potatoes in a steamer for 15 minutes then mash them finely. Add salt and pepper to taste then spoon the sweet potatoes over the beef mixture. Top with grated cheese and cook on low settings for 6 hours. Serve the pie warm.

Crock Pot Jambalaya

Ingredients: Servings: 8   Cooking Time: 6 1/2 Hours

2 tbsp. olive oil
8 oz. firm tofu, cubed
1 large onion,
chopped
2 red bell peppers,
cored and diced
2 garlic cloves,

2 ripe tomatoes,
peeled and diced
1/2 head cauliflower,
cut into florets
1 large sweet potato,
peeled and cubed
1 tbsp. tomato paste

chopped
1/2 tsp. Cajun
seasoning

1 1/4 C. vegetable
stock
Salt and pepper to
taste

Directions:

Heat the oil in a skillet and add the tofu. Cook on low settings for a few minutes until golden brown. Transfer in your Crock Pot and add the rest of the ingredients, adjusting the taste with salt and pepper. Cook on low settings for 6 hours. Serve the jambalaya warm and fresh.

Basmati Rice With Artichoke Hearts

Ingredients: Servings: 5   Cooking Time: 6 Hours

4 artichoke hearts,
canned, chopped
1 C. Arborio rice
1 tbsp. apple cider
vinegar
2 C. of water

½ C. of coconut milk
1 tsp. coconut oil
1 onion, sliced
1 oz. Parmesan,
grated

Directions:

Put rice in the Crock Pot. Add coconut milk and water. Close the lid and cook the mixture on low for 6 hours. Meanwhile, melt the coconut oil. Add onion and roast it for 2 minutes. Then stir it well, add apple cider vinegar, and artichoke hearts. Roast the ingredients for 3 minutes. When the rice is cooked, transfer it in the plates and top with roasted artichoke mixture and Parmesan.

Quinoa Chili(1)

Ingredients: Servings: 6   Cooking Time: 6 Hours

2 C. veggie stock
30 oz. canned black
beans, drained
28 oz. canned
tomatoes, chopped
1 green bell pepper,
chopped
1 yellow onion,
chopped
2 sweet potatoes,
cubed

½ C. quinoa
1 tbsp. chili powder
2 tbsp. cocoa powder
2 tsp. cumin, ground
Salt and black pepper
to the taste
¼ tsp. smoked
paprika

Directions:

In your Crock Pot, mix stock with quinoa, black beans, tomatoes, bell pepper, onion, sweet potatoes, chili powder, cocoa, cumin, paprika, salt and pepper, stir, cover and cook on High for 6 hours. Divide into bowls and serve for lunch.

Chicken And Eggplant Stew

Ingredients: Servings: 2   Cooking Time: 8 Hours

1 C. tomato paste
½ C. chicken stock
1 lb. chicken breast,
skinless, boneless
and cubed
1 small red onion,
chopped
1 red bell pepper,
chopped

2 eggplants, cubed
½ tbsp. smoked
paprika
1 tsp. cumin, ground
Cooking spray
Salt and black pepper
to the taste
Juice of ½ lemon

½ tsp. rosemary, dried

½ tbsp. parsley, chopped

Directions:
In your Crock Pot, mix the chicken with the stock, tomato paste and the other ingredients, toss, put the lid on and cook on Low for 8 hours. Divide into bowls and serve for lunch.

Veggie Medley Roasted Pork Tenderloin

Ingredients: Servings: 6   Cooking Time: 7 1/4 Hours

2 1/2 lb. pork tenderloin
2 ripe heirloom tomatoes, peeled
2 carrots, sliced
1 shallot

4 garlic cloves
1 C. cauliflower florets
1 C. chicken stock
Salt and pepper to taste

Directions:
Combine the tomatoes, carrots, shallot, garlic, cauliflower, stock, salt and pepper in your blender. Pulse until smooth then combine it with the pork tenderloin in your crock pot. Cover with a lid and cook on low settings for 7 hours. When done, slice and serve the pork tenderloin warm.

Brazilian Pork Stew

Ingredients: Servings: 6   Cooking Time: 7 1/4 Hours

1/2 lb. dried black beans
1 1/2 lb. pork shoulder, cubed
2 sweet onions, chopped
4 bacon slices, chopped
4 garlic cloves, chopped

1 tsp. cumin seeds
1/2 tsp. ground coriander
2 bay leaves
1 tsp. white wine vinegar
2 C. chicken stock
Salt and pepper to taste

Directions:
Combine the beans and pork with the rest of the ingredients in your crock pot. Add salt and pepper to taste and cover with a lid. Cook on low settings for 7 hours. Serve the stew warm and fresh.

Eggplant Parmigiana

Ingredients: Servings: 6   Cooking Time: 8 1/4 Hours

4 medium eggplants, peeled and finely sliced
1/4 C. all-purpose flour

4 C. marinara sauce
1 C. grated Parmesan
Salt and pepper to taste

Directions:
Season the eggplants with salt and pepper and sprinkle with flour. Layer the eggplant slices and marinara sauce in your crock pot. Top with the grated cheese and cook on low settings for 8 hours. Serve the parmigiana warm or chilled.

Chunky Pasta Sauce

Ingredients: Servings: 8   Cooking Time: 8 1/4 Hours

1 can (15 oz.) black beans, drained
1 can (15 oz.) kidney beans
2 C. tomato sauce
1 C. fire roasted tomatoes
1 C. frozen corn
1 C. green peas

1 celery stalk, sliced
1 tsp. cumin powder
1 tsp. dried oregano
1 C. vegetable stock
Salt and pepper to taste

Directions:
Combine all the ingredients in your crock pot. Add salt and pepper to taste and cook on low settings for 8 hours. Serve the sauce right away or freeze it into individual portions for later serving.

Herbed Barley Casserole

Ingredients: Servings: 8   Cooking Time: 7 1/4 Hours

1 C. pearl barley
1 large onion, finely chopped
4 garlic cloves, chopped
1 tsp. dried oregano
1 tsp. dried basil
1/2 tsp. dried thyme
1 C. diced tomatoes
2 red bell peppers, cored and diced

1 zucchini, diced
2 C. sliced mushrooms
2 C. vegetable stock
2 tbsp. pine nuts
2 tbsp. chopped parsley
1 tbsp. chopped cilantro
Salt and pepper to taste

Directions:
Combine the pearl barley and the remaining ingredients in your crock pot. Add salt and pepper to taste and cook on low settings for 7 hours. The casserole is best served warm.

Savory Sweet Potato Apple Casserole

Ingredients: Servings: 6   Cooking Time: 6 1/4 Hours

1 1/2 lb. sweet potatoes, peeled and cubed
4 red apples, peeled, cored and diced
2 garlic cloves, minced

2 shallots, chopped
1 tbsp. brown sugar
1 pinch nutmeg
1 C. vegetable stock
Salt and pepper to taste

Directions:
Combine all the ingredients in your crock pot and season with salt and pepper. Cook on low settings for 6 hours. Serve the casserole warm or chilled.

Coffee Sriracha Roasted Beef

Ingredients: Servings: 4   Cooking Time: 6 1/4 Hours

1 1/2 lb. beef roast
1 C. freshly brewed coffee
1 tsp. Worcestershire sauce
1/2 C. beef stock

1 tbsp. Sriracha sauce
2 garlic cloves, minced
Salt and pepper to taste

Directions:

Combine the beef roast, coffee, Worcestershire sauce, Sriracha sauce, garlic and stock in your crock pot. Season the dish with salt and pepper and cook on low settings for 6 hours. Serve the roasted beef warm with your favorite side dish.

Lemon Garlic Whole Roasted Chicken

Ingredients: Servings: 8   Cooking Time: 8 1/4 Hours

1 large whole chicken	1 thyme sprig
1 lemon, sliced	Salt and pepper to
8 garlic cloves,	taste
crushed	1/2 C. vegetable stock
1 rosemary sprig	

Directions:

Place half of the lemon slices and garlic in your crock pot. Season the chicken with salt and pepper and place it over the lemon. Top with the remaining lemon and rosemary and thyme sprig. Add the stock as well. Cover and cook on low settings for 8 hours. Serve the chicken warm or chilled.

Creamy Panade

Ingredients: Servings: 4   Cooking Time: 2.5 Hours

5 oz. bread, toasted, chopped	¼ C. Mozzarella, shredded
1 tsp. garlic powder	3 C. of water
½ C. red kidney beans, canned	6 oz. sausages, chopped

Directions:

Put chopped sausages in the Crock Pot. Add water, cheese, red kidney beans, garlic powder, and bread. Gently stir the mixture and close the lid. Cook the panade on high for 2.5 hours.

Cheesy Potato Casserole

Ingredients: Servings: 6   Cooking Time: 6 1/2 Hours

2 1/2 lb. potatoes, peeled and sliced	1/2 tsp. dried oregano
2 large onions, sliced	1/2 tsp. dried thyme
2 tomatoes, sliced	1/2 C. vegetable stock
4 garlic cloves, minced	Salt and pepper to taste
1 1/2 C. tomato sauce	1 1/2 C. grated Cheddar

Directions:

Layer the potatoes and onions in your crock pot. Finish the layering with tomatoes. Mix the garlic, tomato sauce, oregano, thyme and stock in a bowl. Add salt and pepper to taste then pour this mixture over the potatoes. Top with cheese and cook on low settings for 6 hours. Serve the casserole warm and fresh.

Fennel Braised Chicken

Ingredients: Servings: 4   Cooking Time: 6 1/4 Hours

4 chicken breasts	1 bay leaf
1 fennel bulb, sliced	1 1/2 C. chicken stock
1 sweet onion, sliced	Salt and pepper to
2 carrots, sliced	taste
2 oranges, juiced	

Directions:

Combine all the ingredients in your crock pot. Add salt and pepper to taste and cook on low settings for 6 hours. Serve the chicken warm.

Quick Zucchini Stew

Ingredients: Servings: 4   Cooking Time: 1 3/4 Hours

1 tbsp. olive oil	2 ripe tomatoes, diced
1 shallot, chopped	1 bay leaf
1 garlic clove, chopped	1/2 C. Vegetable stock
2 large zucchinis, cubed	Salt and pepper to taste

Directions:

Combine all the ingredients in your Crock Pot. Add salt and pepper to taste and cook on high settings for 1 1/2 hours. Serve the soup warm and fresh.

Three Pepper Roasted Pork Tenderloin

Ingredients: Servings: 8   Cooking Time: 8 1/4 Hours

3 lb. pork tenderloin	1/4 C. three pepper mix
2 tbsp. Dijon mustard	Salt and pepper to
1 C. chicken stock	taste

Directions:

Season the pork with salt and pepper. Brush the meat with mustard. Spread the pepper mix on your chopping board then roll the pork through this mixture, making sure to coat it well. Place carefully in your crock pot and pour in the stock. Cook on low settings for 8 hours. Serve the pork tenderloin sliced and warm with your favorite side dish.

Molasses Baked Beans

Ingredients: Servings: 6   Cooking Time: 6 1/4 Hours

1 lb. dried white beans, rinsed	2 tbsp. tomato paste
4 C. water	1 C. diced tomatoes
2 tbsp. molasses	1 tsp. mustard seeds
1 tbsp. brown sugar	Salt and pepper to taste

Directions:

Combine all the ingredients in your crock pot. Season with salt and pepper to taste. Cover with a lid and cook on low settings for 6 hours. Serve the beans warm and fresh.

Pork Cannellini Bean Stew

Ingredients: Servings: 6   Cooking Time: 3 3/4 Hours

1 lb. pork tenderloin, cubed	2 carrots, sliced
2 tbsp. canola oil	2 red bell peppers, cored and diced
2 celery stalks, sliced	1 1/2 C. dried cannellini beans, rinsed
1/2 tsp. dried basil	
1/2 tsp. dried oregano	3 C. chicken stock
	1 rosemary sprig
	Salt and pepper to taste

Directions:

Heat the oil in a skillet and add the pork. Cook for a few minutes until golden. Transfer the pork in your Crock Pot. Add the rest of the ingredients and season with salt and pepper as needed. Cook the stew on high settings for 3 1/2 hours. Serve the stew warm and fresh.

Chicken Layered Potato Casserole

Ingredients: Servings: 8   Cooking Time: 6 1/2 Hours

2 lb. potatoes, peeled and sliced	1/2 tsp. garlic powder
2 chicken breasts, cut into thin strips	1/4 tsp. onion powder
1/4 tsp. chili powder	1 C. heavy cream
1/4 tsp. cumin powder	1 1/2 C. whole milk
	Salt and pepper to taste

Directions:

Combine the cream, milk, chili powder, cumin powder, garlic powder and onion powder. Layer the potatoes and chicken in your Crock Pot. Pour the milk mix over the potatoes and chicken, seasoning with salt and pepper. Cook on low settings for 6 hours. Serve the casserole warm or chilled.

Chicken Sweet Potato Stew

Ingredients: Servings: 6   Cooking Time: 3 1/4 Hours

2 chicken breasts, cubed	1/2 tsp. garlic powder
2 tbsp. butter	1 pinch cinnamon powder
2 shallots, chopped	1 1/2 C. vegetable stock
2 lb. sweet potatoes, peeled and cubed	Salt and pepper to taste
1/2 tsp. cumin powder	

Directions:

Combine the chicken, butter and shallots in your crock pot. Cook for 5 minutes then transfer in your crock pot. Add the sweet potatoes, cumin powder, garlic and cinnamon, as well as stock, salt and pepper. Cook on high settings for 3 hours. Serve the stew warm or chilled.

Layered Eggplant Parmesan Bake

Ingredients: Servings: 6   Cooking Time: 4 1/4 Hours

2 large eggplants, peeled and sliced	2 C. tomato sauce
1/2 tsp. chili powder	2 C. grated Parmesan
1 tsp. dried basil	Salt and pepper to taste

Directions:

Mix the tomato sauce with chili powder and basil. Layer the eggplants, tomato sauce and Parmesan in your Crock Pot, adding salt and pepper as needed. Cover and cook on low settings for 4 hours. Serve the bake warm and fresh.

Stout Carrot Chicken Stew

Ingredients: Servings: 8   Cooking Time: 8 1/4 Hours

8 chicken thighs	1 lb. baby carrots
4 bacon slices,	1 C. tomato sauce
chopped	2 tbsp. tomato paste
2 tbsp. canola oil	1 1/2 C. stout beer
4 garlic cloves, chopped	1 tbsp. lemon juice
1 large onion, chopped	2 bay leaves
1/2 lb. button mushrooms	1 rosemary sprig
	Salt and pepper to taste

Directions:

Heat the canola oil in a crock pot and add the bacon. Cook until crisp then stir in the chicken. Cook on all sides until golden brown then transfer in your crock pot. Add the remaining ingredients and season well with salt and pepper. Cook on low settings for 8 hours. Serve the dish warm and fresh.

Spinach And Mushroom Soup

Ingredients: Servings: 6   Cooking Time: 3 Hours

2/3 C. yellow onion, chopped	1 and 1/2 C. half and half
16 oz. baby spinach	
3 tbsp. butter	1/4 tsp. thyme, dried
Salt and black pepper to the taste	16 oz. cheese tortellini
5 C. veggie stock	2 tsp. garlic powder
3 garlic cloves, minced	3 C. mushrooms, sliced
1/2 tsp. Italian seasoning	1/2 C. parmesan, grated

Directions:

Heat up a pan with the butter over medium-high heat, add onion, garlic, mushrooms and spinach, stir and cook for a few minutes. Transfer to your Crock Pot, add salt, pepper, stock, Italian seasoning, half and half, thyme, garlic powder and parmesan, cover and cook on High for 2 hours and 30 minutes. Add tortellini, stir, cover, cook on High for 30 minutes more, ladle into bowls and serve for lunch.

Mediterranean Chickpea Feta Stew

Ingredients: Servings: 8   Cooking Time: 8 1/4 Hours

2 C. dried chickpeas, rinsed	1 pinch chili powder
1 large onion, chopped	2 heirloom tomatoes, peeled and diced
2 carrots, diced	2 C. vegetable stock
1 celery stalk, diced	Salt and pepper to taste
1 tsp. dried oregano	8 oz. feta cheese for servings
1 tsp. dried basil	

Directions:

Combine the chickpeas, onion, carrots, celery, oregano, basil, chili powder, tomatoes, salt and pepper, as well as stock in your crock pot. Cover and cook on low settings for 8 hours. Serve the stew warm, topped with crumbled feta cheese.

Beef And Cabbage

Ingredients: Servings: 2   Cooking Time: 8 Hours

1 lb. beef stew meat, cubed	1 C. tomato paste
	1/2 tsp. sweet paprika

1 C. green cabbage,
shredded
1 C. red cabbage,
shredded
1 carrot, grated
½ C. water

1 tbsp. chives,
chopped
A pinch of salt and
black pepper

Directions:

In your Crock Pot, mix the beef with the cabbage, carrot and the other ingredients, toss, put the lid on and cook on Low for 8 hours.   Divide the mix between plates and serve for lunch.

Lemon Pepper Chicken

Ingredients: Servings: 6   Cooking Time: 3 1/4 Hours

2 lb. chicken
drumsticks
2 tbsp. butter
2 garlic cloves,
chopped

1 lemon, juiced
1 thyme sprig
1 C. vegetable stock
Salt and pepper to
taste

Directions:

Combine all the ingredients in your crock pot.   Add salt and pepper as needed and cook the chicken on high settings for 3 hours.   Serve the chicken warm with your favorite side dish.

Roasted Rosemary Pork And Potatoes

Ingredients: Servings: 6   Cooking Time: 6 1/2 Hours

2 lb. pork roast,
cubed
3 large carrots, sliced
1 1/2 lb. potatoes,
peeled and cubed

1 celery root, peeled
and cubed
2 rosemary sprigs
Salt and pepper to
taste
1 C. chicken stock

Directions:

Combine the pork roast, carrots, celery, potatoes, rosemary and stock in your crock pot.   Add salt and pepper and cook on low settings for 6 hours.   Serve the dish warm and fresh.

Hoisin Braised Tofu

Ingredients: Servings: 4   Cooking Time: 2 1/4 Hours

4 slices firm tofu
1 tbsp. soy sauce
1 tsp. grated ginger
1 tsp. rice vinegar

1/2 C. hoisin sauce
1/2 tsp. sesame oil
2 garlic cloves,
minced
1 tsp. molasses

Directions:

Mix the hoisin sauce, ginger, vinegar, sesame oil, garlic and molasses in your Crock Pot.   Add the tofu and coat it well then cover the pot with its lid and cook on high settings for 2 hours. Serve the tofu warm with your favorite side dish.

Mexican Vegetable Casserole

Ingredients: Servings: 6   Cooking Time: 6 1/4 Hours

1 can (15 oz.) black
beans, drained
1 can (10 oz.) sweet
corn, drained
2 jalapeno peppers,

1/2 C. all-purpose
flour
1/4 C. butter, chilled
and cubed
1/4 tsp. cumin

chopped
1 can fire roasted
tomatoes
Salt and pepper to
taste

powder
1/2 tsp. baking
powder
1/2 C. chilled
buttermilk

Directions:

Combine the beans, corn, jalapeno peppers and tomatoes in your Crock Pot. Add salt and pepper to taste.   In a bowl, mix the flour, cumin and butter and rub the mixture well until sandy.   Stir in the chilled buttermilk and mix quickly with a fork.   Drop spoonfuls of batter over the vegetables and cover the pot with its lid.   Cook on low settings for 6 hours.   Serve the casserole warm.

Beef Three Bean Casserole

Ingredients: Servings: 8   Cooking Time: 6 1/4 Hours

1 lb. ground beef
4 bacon slices,
chopped
2 tbsp. canola oil
1 can (15 oz.) black
beans, drained
1 can (15 oz.) red
beans, drained
1 can (15 oz.) kidney
beans, drained
2 carrots, diced

1 celery stalk, diced
4 garlic cloves,
chopped
1 tbsp. molasses
1/4 tsp. cayenne
pepper
1 C. beef stock
1/4 C. tomato paste
Salt and pepper to
taste
1 1/2 C. grated
Cheddar

Directions:

Heat the oil in a frying pan and add the beef and bacon. Cook for 5 minutes, stirring often then transfer the mixture in your Crock Pot.   Add the beans, carrots, celery, garlic, molasses, cayenne, stock and tomato paste, as well as salt and pepper.   Top with Cheddar and cook on low settings for 6 hours.   The casserole is best served warm.

3-grain Porridge

Ingredients: Servings: 6   Cooking Time: 8 Hours

½ C. of wheat berries
½ C. pearl barley
3 oz. goat cheese,
crumbled

¼ wild rice
2 tbsp. butter
1 tsp. salt
5 C. of water

Directions:

Pour water in the Crock Pot.   Add wheat berries, pearl barley, and wild rice.   Then add salt and cook the mixture on low for 8 hours.   When the grains are cooked, add goat cheese and butter. Carefully mix the meal and transfer in the serving plates.

Beef Stew(1)

Ingredients: Servings: 5   Cooking Time: 7 Hours And 30 Minutes

2 potatoes, peeled
and cubed
1 lb. beef stew meat,
cubed
11 oz. tomato juice
14 oz. beef stock

3 bay leaves
Salt and black pepper
to the taste
½ tsp. chili powder
½ tsp. thyme, dried

46

2 celery ribs, chopped
2 carrots, chopped
1 yellow onion, chopped

1 tbsp. water
2 tbsp. cornstarch
½ C. peas
½ C. corn

Directions:

In your Crock Pot, mix potatoes with beef, tomato juice, stock, ribs, carrots, bay leaves, onion, salt, pepper, chili powder and thyme, stir, cover and cook on Low for 7 hours. Add cornstarch mixed with water, peas and corn, stir, cover and cook on Low for 30 minutes more. Divide into bowls and serve for lunch.

DESSERT RECIPES

Classic Banana Foster

Ingredients: Servings: 3   Cooking Time: 3 Hours

3 bananas, peeled chopped
2 tbsp. sugar
2 tbsp. butter, melted

1 tsp. vanilla extract
1 tbsp. rum
3 ice cream balls

Directions:

Put the bananas in the Crock Pot in one layer. Then sprinkle them with sugar, butter, vanilla extract, and rum. Close the lid and cook on Low for 3 hours. Transfer the cooked bananas in the ramekins and top with ice cream balls.

Stuffed Apples

Ingredients: Servings: 5   Cooking Time: 1 Hour And 30 Minutes

5 apples, tops cut off and cored
5 figs
1/3 C. sugar
1 tsp. dried ginger
¼ C. pecans, chopped
2 tsp. lemon zest, grated

¼ tsp. nutmeg, ground
½ tsp. cinnamon powder
1 tbsp. lemon juice
1 tablespoon vegetable oil
½ C. water

Directions:

In a bowl, mix figs with sugar, ginger, pecans, lemon zest, nutmeg, cinnamon, oil and lemon juice, whisk really well, stuff your apples with this mix and put them in your Crock Pot. Add the water, cover, cook on High for 1 hour and 30 minutes, divide between dessert plates and serve.

Pineapple Coconut Tapioca Pudding

Ingredients: Servings: 8   Cooking Time: 6 1/4 Hours

1 1/2 C. tapioca pearls
1 C. sweetened condensed milk
1 can crushed pineapple

2 C. coconut milk
1/2 C. coconut flakes
1 tsp. vanilla extract

Directions:

Combine all the ingredients in your crock pot. Cover and cook for 6 hours on low settings. The pudding is best served chilled.

Gingerbread

Ingredients: Servings: 4   Cooking Time: 5 Hours

4 tbsp. coconut oil
½ C. flour

1 tbsp. gingerbread spices
¼ C. of sugar

Directions:

Mix all ingredients in the mixing bowl and knead the dough. Roll it up and cut into the cookies with help of the cookie cutter. Line the Crock Pot with baking paper. Put the cookies in the Crock Pot in one layer and bake them on High for 2.5 hours. Repeat the same steps with remaining cookies.

Berries Salad

Ingredients: Servings: 2   Cooking Time: 1 Hour

2 tbsp. brown sugar
1 tbsp. lime juice
1 tbsp. lime zest, grated

1 C. blueberries
½ C. cranberries
1 C. blackberries
1 C. strawberries
½ C. heavy cream

Directions:

In your Crock Pot, mix the berries with the sugar and the other ingredients, toss, put the lid on and cook on High for 1 hour. Divide the mix into bowls and serve.

Cardamom Apple Jam

Ingredients: Servings: 4   Cooking Time: 2.5 Hours

1 C. apples, chopped
1 tsp. ground cardamom

2 tbsp. brown sugar
1 tsp. agar

Directions:

Mix apples with brown sugar and transfer in the Crock Pot. Leave the apples until they get the juice. Then add ground cardamom and agar. Mix the mixture. Close the lid and cook the jam on High for 2.5 hours. Then blend the mixture until smooth and cool to room temperature.

Crustless Peach Pie

Ingredients: Servings: 8   Cooking Time: 4 1/4 Hours

4 large peaches, pitted and sliced
1 1/4 C. all-purpose flour
1/2 C. ground almonds

1/4 C. white sugar
1/2 tsp. cinnamon powder
1/2 tsp. ground ginger
1 C. butter, melted

Directions:

Mix the peaches, flour, almonds, sugar, cinnamon and ginger in your crock pot. Drizzle the butter over the pie and cook on low settings for 4 hours. Serve the pie chilled.

Milk Fondue

Ingredients: Servings: 3   Cooking Time: 4 Hours

5 oz. milk chocolate, chopped
1 tbsp. butter
1 tsp. vanilla extract
¼ C. milk

Directions:
Put the chocolate in the Crock Pot in one layer. Then top it with butter, vanilla extract, and milk. Close the lid and cook the dessert on Low for 4 hours. Gently stir the cooked fondue and transfer in the ramekins.

Mixed-berry Marmalade

Ingredients: Servings: 12   Cooking Time: 3 Hrs.

1 lb. cranberries
1 lb. strawberries
½ lb. blueberries
3.5 oz. black currant
2 lbs. sugar
Zest of 1 lemon
2 tbsp. water

Directions:
Toss all the berries with sugar, water, and lemon zest in the insert of Crock Pot. Put the cooker's lid on and set the cooking time to 3 hours on High settings. Divide the marmalade mixture into the jars and allow it to cool. Serve.

Soft Sable Cookies

Ingredients: Servings: 2   Cooking Time: 2 Hours

1 tsp. sesame seeds
2 tbsp. butter, softened
½ tsp. baking powder
1 egg yolk, whisked
2 tsp. brown sugar
1/3 C. flour
½ tsp. olive oil

Directions:
Mix butter with baking powder, brown sugar, and flour. Knead a soft dough and cut into 2 pieces. Then roll the balls from the dough and press them gently. Brush every ball with the help of the egg yolk and sprinkle with sesame seeds. Brush the Crock Pot bowl with olive oil and put the cookies inside. Cook them on High for 2 hours. Then cool the cookies well.

Mango Tapioca Pudding

Ingredients: Servings: 6   Cooking Time: 6 1/4 Hours

1 C. tapioca pearls
2 C. coconut milk
1 C. water
1 ripe mango, peeled and cubed
1/2 C. shredded coconut
1/4 C. white sugar
1 cinnamon stick

Directions:
Combine all the ingredients in your Crock Pot. Cover the pot and cook on low settings for 6 hours. Allow the pudding to cool completely before serving.

Fluffy Vegan Cream

Ingredients: Servings: 6   Cooking Time: 1.5 Hours

1 C. coconut cream
1 avocado, pitted, peeled, chopped
½ C. of soy milk
1 tbsp. corn starch

Directions:
Pour soy milk in the Crock Pot. Add corn starch and stir until smooth. Then close the lid and cook the liquid on high for 1.5

hours. Meanwhile, whip the coconut cream and blend the avocado. Mix the blended avocado with thick soy milk mixture and then carefully mix it with whipped coconut cream.

Chocolate Mango Mix

Ingredients: Servings: 2   Cooking Time: 1 Hour

¼ C. dark chocolate, cut into chunks
1 C. mango, peeled and chopped
1 C. crème fraiche
2 tbsp. sugar
½ tsp. almond extract

Directions:
In your Crock Pot, mix the crème fraiche with the chocolate and the other ingredients, toss, put the lid on and cook on Low for 1 hour. Blend using an immersion blender, divide into bowls and serve.

Maple Plums And Mango

Ingredients: Servings: 2   Cooking Time: 1 Hour

2 tsp. orange zest
1 tbsp. orange juice
1 C. plums, pitted and halved
1 C. mango, peeled and cubed
1 tbsp. maple syrup
3 tbsp. sugar

Directions:
In your Crock Pot, mix the plums with the mango and the other ingredients, toss, put the lid on and cook on High for 1 hour. Divide into bowls and serve cold

Banana Ice Cream

Ingredients: Servings: 2   Cooking Time: 5 Hours

½ C. cream
4 tbsp. sugar
4 bananas, chopped
2 egg yolks

Directions:
Mix sugar with egg yolks and blend until you get a lemon color mixture. After this, mix the cream with egg yolks and transfer in the Crock Pot. Cook the mixture on low for 5 hours. Stir the liquid from time to time. After this, mix the cream mixture with bananas and blend until smooth. Place the mixture in the plastic vessel and refrigerate until solid.

Pear Walnut Cake

Ingredients: Servings: 8   Cooking Time: 4 1/2 Hours

1 C. butter, softened
1 C. white sugar
3 eggs
1 C. all-purpose flour
1 C. ground walnuts
1/4 C. cocoa powder
1/4 tsp. salt
1 tsp. baking powder
1/2 tsp. cinnamon powder
4 ripe pears, peeled, cored and sliced

Directions:
Mix the butter and sugar in a bowl until creamy and pale. Add the eggs one by one and mix well. Fold in the flour, walnuts, cocoa powder, salt, baking powder and cinnamon with a spatula. Spoon the batter in your Crock Pot and top with pear slices. Bake in the crock pot for 4 hours on low settings. Allow the cake to cool in the pot before slicing.

S'mores Cake

Ingredients: Servings: 6   Cooking Time: 2 Hours

1 C. chocolate cake mix
¼ C. pudding mix
3 eggs, beaten
3 tbsp. butter, melted
¼ C. plain yogurt
3 oz. marshmallows
3 oz. graham crackers, crushed
Cooking spray

Directions:

Mix chocolate cake mix with pudding mix. Add eggs, plain yogurt, and butter. Stir it until homogenous. After this, add graham crackers and carefully mix them again. Spray the Crock Pot bottom with cooking spray and put the chocolate mixture inside. Cook it on high for 2 hours. Then add marshmallows and broil the mixture.

Lemon Poppy Seed Cake

Ingredients: Servings: 8   Cooking Time: 4 1/2 Hours

3/4 C. butter, softened
3/4 C. white sugar
1 large lemon, zested and juiced
2 eggs
1 C. all-purpose flour
1/2 C. fine cornmeal
1 tsp. baking soda
1/2 tsp. baking powder
1/2 tsp. salt
2 tbsp. poppy seeds
1 C. buttermilk

Directions:

Mix the flour, cornmeal, baking soda, baking powder, salt and poppy seeds in a bowl. Combine the butter, sugar and lemon zest in a bowl and mix well for 5 minutes. Add the eggs and lemon zest and mix well. Fold in the flour mixture, alternating it with the buttermilk. Spoon the batter in your crock pot and cook on low settings for 4 hours. Allow the cake to cool in the pot before slicing and serving.

Raspberry Biscuits

Ingredients: Servings: 8   Cooking Time: 6.5 Hours

4 eggs, beaten
1 C. of sugar
1 C. flour
1 tsp. ground cinnamon
1 tbsp. coconut flakes
1 C. raspberries
Cooking spray

Directions:

Blend the eggs with sugar until you get a smooth and fluffy mixture. Add flour, ground cinnamon, and coconut flakes. Mix the mixture until smooth. Spray the Crock Pot with cooking spray and pour the dough inside. Then sprinkle the dough with raspberries and close the lid. Cook the meal on Low for 6.5 hours. After this, remove the cooked dessert from the Crock Pot and cut into servings.

Cranberry Cookies

Ingredients: Servings: 6   Cooking Time: 2.5 Hours

2 oz. dried cranberries, chopped
3 tbsp. peanut butter
1 C. flour
1 tsp. baking powder
3 tbsp. sugar
1 tbsp. cream cheese

Directions:

Mix peanut butter with flour, baking powder, and sugar. Add cream cheese and cranberries and knead the dough. Make the small balls and press them gently to get the shape of the cookies. After this, line the Crock Pot bowl with baking paper. Put the cookies inside and close the lid. Cook the cookies on high for 2.5 hours.

Caramel Apple Crisp

Ingredients: Servings: 8   Cooking Time: 6 1/2 Hours

6 Granny Smith apples, peeled, cored and sliced
1 tbsp. cornstarch
1/2 tsp. cinnamon powder
1/2 C. caramel sauce
1 C. all-purpose flour
1/2 C. rolled oats
1/4 C. butter, chilled
1 pinch salt

Directions:

Mix the apples, caramel sauce, cinnamon and cornstarch in your Crock Pot. For the topping, mix the flour, oats, butter and salt in a bowl until grainy. Spread the topping over the apples and cook on low settings for 6 hours. Allow the crisp to cool in the pot before serving.

Hot Fudge Chocolate Cake

Ingredients: Servings: 10   Cooking Time: 2 1/2 Hours

1 C. cocoa powder
1 C. all-purpose flour
2 tsp. baking powder
1/2 tsp. salt
1 C. white sugar
1/4 C. butter, melted
2 eggs
1 tsp. vanilla extract
1 C. plain yogurt
3/4 C. whole milk

Directions:

Mix the dry ingredients in a bowl then add the wet ingredients and give it a quick mix just until combined. Pour the batter in your greased Crock Pot. Cover the pot and bake for 2 hours on high settings. Allow the cake to cool completely before slicing and serving.

Chocolate Cream

Ingredients: Servings: 4   Cooking Time: 2 Hours

1 C. chocolate chips
2 tbsp. butter
2/3 C. heavy cream
2 tsp. brandy
2 tbsp. sugar
¼ tsp. vanilla extract

Directions:

In your Crock Pot, mix chocolate chips with butter, cream, brandy, sugar and vanilla extract, cover and cook on Low for 2 hours. Divide into bowls and serve warm.

Berry Cobbler

Ingredients: Servings: 6   Cooking Time: 2 Hours

1 lb. fresh blackberries
1 lb. fresh blueberries
¾ C. water
¾ C. sugar+ 2 tablespoons
1 tsp. baking powder
2 tbsp. palm sugar
1/3 C. milk
1 egg, whisked
1 tsp. lemon zest,

¾ C. flour
¼ C. tapioca flour
½ C. arrowroot powder

grated
3 tbsp. vegetable oil

Directions:

Put blueberries, blackberries, ¾ C. sugar, water and tapioca in your Crock Pot, cover and cook on High for 1 hour. In a bowl, mix flour with arrowroot, the rest of the sugar and baking powder and stir well. In a second bowl, mix the egg with milk, oil and lemon zest. Combine egg mixture with flour mixture, stir well, drop tbsp. of this mix over the berries, cover and cook on High for 1 more hour. Leave cobbler to cool down, divide into dessert bowls and serve.

Orange Curd

Ingredients: Servings: 6   Cooking Time: 7 Hours

2 C. orange juice
1 tbsp. orange zest, grated
4 egg yolks
1 C. of sugar

1 tbsp. cornflour
1 tsp. vanilla extract

Directions:

Whisk the egg yolks with sugar until you get a lemon color mixture. Then add orange juice, vanilla extract, cornflour, and orange zest. Whisk the mixture until smooth. Pour the liquid in the Crock Pot and close the lid. Cook the curd on low for 7 hours. Stir the curd every 1 hour.

Yogurt Cheesecake

Ingredients: Servings: 2   Cooking Time: 3 Hours

For the crust:
1 tbsp. coconut oil, melted
½ C. graham cookies, crumbled
For the filling:
3 oz. cream cheese, soft

1 C. Greek yogurt
½ tbsp. cornstarch
3 tbsp. sugar
1 egg, whisked
1 tsp. almond extract
Cooking spray

Directions:

In a bowl mix the cookie crumbs with butter and stir well. Grease your Crock Pot with the cooking spray, line it with parchment paper and press the crumbs on the bottom. In a bowl, mix the cream cheese with the yogurt and the other ingredients, whisk well and spread over the crust. Put the lid on, cook on Low for 3 hours, cool down and keep in the fridge for 1 hour before serving.

Caramel Cream

Ingredients: Servings: 2   Cooking Time: 2 Hours

1 and ½ tsp. caramel extract
1 C. water
2 oz. cream cheese
2 eggs
1 and ½ tbsp. sugar

For the caramel sauce:
2 tbsp. sugar
2 tbsp. butter, melted
¼ tsp. caramel extract

Directions:

In your blender, mix cream cheese with water, 1 and ½ tbsp. sugar, 1 and ½ tsp. caramel extract and eggs and blend well. Pour this into your Crock Pot, cover and cook on High for 2 hours. Put the butter in a Crock Pot, heat up over medium heat add ¼ tsp. caramel extract and 2 tbsp. sugar, stir well and cook until everything melts. Pour this over caramel cream, leave everything to cool down and serve in dessert cups.

Apricot And Peaches Cream

Ingredients: Servings: 2   Cooking Time: 2 Hours

1 C. apricots, pitted and chopped
1 C. peaches, pitted and chopped
1 C. heavy cream

3 tbsp. brown sugar
1 tsp. vanilla extract

Directions:

In a blender, mix the apricots with the peaches and the other ingredients, and pulse well. Put the cream in the Crock Pot, put the lid on, cook on High for 2 hours, divide into bowls and serve.

Rhubarb Marmalade

Ingredients: Servings: 8   Cooking Time: 3 Hours

2 lb. rhubarb, chopped
2 lb. strawberries, chopped

1/3 C. water
1 C. sugar
1 tbsp. mint, chopped

Directions:

In your Crock Pot, mix water with rhubarb, strawberries, sugar and mint, stir, cover and cook on High for 3 hours. Divide into C. and serve cold.

Raisin-flax Meal Bars

Ingredients: Servings: 8   Cooking Time: 3.5 Hrs.

¼ C. raisins
1 C. oat flour
1 egg, whisked
4 oz. banana, mashed
5 oz. milk
1 tbsp. flax meal

1 tsp. ground cinnamon
½ tsp. baking soda
1 tbsp. lemon juice
1 tbsp. butter
1 tbsp. flour

Directions:

Whisk egg with mashed banana, oat flour, milk, flax meal, raising in a bowl. Stir in cinnamon, lemon juice, baking soda, and flour, then knead well. Grease the insert of the Crock Pot with butter. Make big balls out of this raisin dough and shape them into 3-4 inches bars. Place these bars in the insert of the Crock Pot. Put the cooker's lid on and set the cooking time to 3 hours on Low settings. Serve when chilled.

Greek Cream Cheese Pudding

Ingredients: Servings: 2   Cooking Time: 2 Hours

1 C. cream cheese, soft
½ C. Greek yogurt
½ tsp. baking soda
1 C. almonds, chopped

2 eggs, whisked
1 tbsp. sugar
½ tsp. almond extract

½ tsp. cinnamon
powder

Directions:
In your Crock Pot, mix the cream cheese with the yogurt, eggs and the other ingredients, whisk, put the lid on and cook on Low for 2 hours. Divide the pudding into bowls and serve.

Semolina Pie

Ingredients: Servings: 4   Cooking Time: 2 Hours

½ C. cottage cheese	1 tbsp. flour
1 tsp. vanilla extract	½ C. semolina
1 tsp. corn starch	2 tbsp. butter, melted

Directions:
Mix semolina with cottage cheese and vanilla extract. Then add corn starch, flour, and butter. Blend the mixture with the help of the blender until smooth and put in the Crock Pot. Flatten it. Close the lid and cook the semolina pie for 2 hours on High.

Apricot Marmalade

Ingredients: Servings: 2   Cooking Time: 3 Hours

1 C. apricots, chopped	2 tbsp. lemon juice
½ C. water	1 tsp. fruit pectin
1 tsp. vanilla extract	2 C. sugar

Directions:
In your Crock Pot, mix the apricots with the water, vanilla and the other ingredients, whisk, put the lid on and cook on High for 3 hours. Stir the marmalade, divide into bowls and serve cold.

Ginger Pears Mix

Ingredients: Servings: 2   Cooking Time: 2 Hours

2 pears, peeled and cored	1 C. apple juice
½ tbsp. brown sugar	1 tbsp. ginger, grated

Directions:
In your Crock Pot, mix the pears with the apple juice and the other ingredients, toss, put the lid on and cook on Low for 2 hour. Divide the mix into bowls and serve warm.

Pudding Cake

Ingredients: Servings: 8   Cooking Time: 2 Hours And 30 Minutes

1 and ½ C. sugar	2 tbsp. vegetable oil
1 C. flour	1 tsp. vanilla extract
¼ C. cocoa powder+ 2 tablespoons	1 and ½ C. hot water
½ C. chocolate almond milk	Cooking spray
2 tsp. baking powder	

Directions:
In a bowl, mix flour with 2 tbsp. cocoa, baking powder, milk, oil and vanilla extract, whisk well and spread on the bottom of the Crock Pot, greased with cooking spray. In another bowl, mix sugar with the rest of the cocoa and the water, whisk well, spread over the batter in the Crock Pot, cover, cook your cake on High for 2 hours and 30 minutes. Leave the cake to cool down, slice and serve.

Maple Roasted Pears

Ingredients: Servings: 4   Cooking Time: 6 1/4 Hours

4 ripe pears, carefully peeled and cored	1 tsp. grated ginger
1/4 C. maple syrup	1 cinnamon stick
1/4 C. white wine	2 cardamom pods, crushed
1/2 C. water	

Directions:
Combine all the ingredients in your Crock Pot. Cover with a lid and cook on low settings for 6 hours. Allow to cool before serving.

Sautéed Figs(2)

Ingredients: Servings: 6   Cooking Time: 2 Hours

6 fresh figs	2 tbsp. butter
2 tbsp. maple syrup	1 tbsp. raisins
	1 C. of water

Directions:
Put butter and figs in the Crock Pot. Add raisins and water. Close the lid and cook the meal on High for 2 hours. Then transfer the cooked figs in the plates and sprinkle with maple syrup.

Banana Almond Foster

Ingredients: Servings: 4   Cooking Time: 4 Hrs.

1 lb. banana, peeled and chopped	1 tsp. ground cinnamon
3 oz. butter	3 tbsp. coconut flakes
1 C. white sugar	½ tsp. vanilla extract
2 tsp. rum	4 tbsp. almond, crushed

Directions:
Add bananas, white sugar, rum, coconut flakes, ground cinnamon, crushed almonds, and vanilla extract to the insert of Crock Pot. Put the cooker's lid on and set the cooking time to 4 hours on Low settings. Serve with whipped cream.

Cottage Cheese Ramekins

Ingredients: Servings: 4   Cooking Time: 3 Hours

4 tsp. semolina	2 C. of cottage cheese
2 oz. raisins, chopped	2 tbsp. butter, melted
1 tsp. vanilla extract	

Directions:
Mix semolina with cottage cheese, vanilla extract, butter, and raisins. Transfer the mixture into ramekins and place the ramekins in the Crock Pot. Close the lid and cook the meal on High for 3 hours.

Pears With Grape Sauce

Ingredients: Servings: 4   Cooking Time: 1 Hr. 30 Minutes

4 pears
Juice and zest of 1 lemon
26 oz. grape juice
11 oz. currant jelly

4 garlic cloves
½ vanilla bean
4 peppercorns
2 rosemary springs

Directions:

Add grape juice, jelly, lemon juice, lemon zest, peppercorns, pears, vanilla, and rosemary in the insert of Crock Pot. Put the cooker's lid on and set the cooking time to 1.5 hours on High settings. Serve when chilled.

Apple Compote

Ingredients: Servings: 2   Cooking Time: 1 Hour

1 lb. apples, cored and cut into wedges
½ C. water
1 tbsp. sugar

1 tsp. vanilla extract
½ tsp. almond extract

Directions:

In your Crock Pot, mix the apples with the water and the other ingredients, toss, put the lid on and cook on High for 1 hour. Divide into bowls and serve cold.

Amaretti Cheesecake

Ingredients: Servings: 8   Cooking Time: 6 1/2 Hours

Crust:
6 oz. Amaretti cookies, crushed
1/4 C. butter, melted
Filling:
24 oz. cream cheese

1/2 C. sour cream
4 eggs
1/2 C. white sugar
1 tbsp. vanilla extract
1 tbsp. Amaretto liqueur

Directions:

Mix the crushed cookies with butter then transfer the mix in your crock pot and press it well on the bottom of the pot. For the filling, mix the cream cheese, sour cream, eggs, sugar, vanilla and liqueur and give it a quick mix. Pour the filling over the crust and cook for 6 hours on low settings. Allow the cheesecake to cool before slicing and serving.

Rice Vanilla Pudding

Ingredients: Servings: 6   Cooking Time: 2 Hrs.

1 tbsp. butter
7 oz. long-grain rice
4 oz. water
16 oz. milk

3 oz. sugar
1 egg
1 tbsp. cream
1 tsp. vanilla extract

Directions:

Add rice, water, egg, cream, sugar, butter, milk, and vanilla to the insert of Crock Pot. Put the cooker's lid on and set the cooking time to 2 hours on High settings. Serve when chilled.

Stewed Grapefruit

Ingredients: Servings: 6   Cooking Time: 2 Hours

1 C. water
1 C. maple syrup
64 oz. red grapefruit juice

½ C. mint, chopped
2 grapefruits, peeled and chopped

Directions:

In your Crock Pot, mix grapefruit with water, maple syrup, mint and grapefruit juice, stir, cover and cook on High for 2 hours. Divide into bowls and serve cold.

Peanut Butter Cheesecake

Ingredients: Servings: 10   Cooking Time: 8 1/2 Hours

Crust:
8 oz. graham crackers, crushed
1/2 C. butter, melted
Filling:
1 C. smooth peanut butter

20 oz. cream cheese
1/2 C. sour cream
2/3 C. light brown sugar
1 tsp. vanilla extract
4 eggs
1 pinch salt

Directions:

For the crust, mix the crackers with butter then transfer the mixture in your Crock Pot and press it well on the bottom of the pot. For the filling, mix the cream cheese, peanut butter, sour cream, sugar, vanilla, eggs and salt in a bowl. Pour the filling over the crust and cook for 8 hours on low settings. Allow the cheesecake to cool completely before serving.

Ricotta Cream

Ingredients: Servings: 10   Cooking Time: 1 Hour

½ C. hot coffee
2 and ½ tsp. gelatin
1 tsp. vanilla extract

2 C. ricotta cheese
1 tsp. espresso powder
1 tsp. sugar
1 C. whipping cream

Directions:

In a bowl, mix coffee with gelatin, stir well and leave aside until coffee is cold. In your Crock Pot, mix espresso, sugar, vanilla extract and ricotta and stir. Add coffee mix and whipping cream, cover, cook on Low for 1 hour. Divide into dessert bowls and keep in the fridge for 2 hours before serving.

Caramel Pear Pudding Cake

Ingredients: Servings: 6   Cooking Time: 4 1/2 Hours

2/3 C. all-purpose flour
1 tsp. baking powder
1/2 C. sugar
1/2 tsp. cinnamon powder

1/4 tsp. salt
1/4 C. butter, melted
1/4 C. whole milk
4 ripe pears, cored and sliced
3/4 C. caramel sauce

Directions:

Mix the flour, baking powder, sugar, salt and cinnamon in a bowl. Add the butter and milk and give it a quick mix. Place the pears in your crock pot and top with the batter. Drizzle the batter with caramel sauce and cook on low settings for 4 hours. Allow the cake to cool before serving.

Cocoa Vanilla Cake

Ingredients: Servings: 3   Cooking Time: 2 Hrs.

10 tbsp. flour
3 tbsp. butter, melted

4 eggs
¼ tsp. vanilla extract

4 tsp. sugar
1 tbsp. cocoa powder
½ tsp. baking powder

Directions:
Beat butter with eggs, cocoa powder, and all other ingredients in a mixer. Spread this cocoa batter in the insert of Crock Pot. Put the cooker's lid on and set the cooking time to 2 hours on High settings. Slice and serve.

Rich Bread Pudding

Ingredients: Servings: 6   Cooking Time: 6 1/2 Hours

6 C. bread cubes
1/4 C. golden raisins
1/2 C. dark chocolate chips
1/4 C. butter, melted
4 eggs
1 1/2 C. whole milk
1/2 C. heavy cream
1 tsp. vanilla extract
1 pinch cinnamon powder
2 tbsp. dark rum

Directions:
Mix the bread cubes, raisins and chocolate chips in your Crock Pot. Combine the butter, eggs, milk, cream, vanilla, cinnamon and dark rum and give it a good mix. Pour the mixture over the bread and bake on low settings for 6 hours. Serve the bread pudding slightly warm.

Berry Pudding

Ingredients: Servings: 2   Cooking Time: 5 Hours

¼ C. strawberries, chopped
2 tbsp. sugar
2 C. of milk
1 tbsp. corn starch
1 tsp. vanilla extract

Directions:
Mix milk with corn starch and pour liquid in the Crock Pot. Add vanilla extract, sugar, and strawberries. Close the lid and cook the pudding on low for 5 hours. Carefully mix the dessert before serving.

Red Velvet Brioche Pudding

Ingredients: Servings: 6   Cooking Time: 5 1/2 Hours

5 C. brioche cubes
2 C. whole milk
1 C. cream cheese
1 tsp. red food coloring
3 eggs
1/2 C. white sugar
1 tsp. vanilla extract
1/2 C. white chocolate chips

Directions:
Mix the brioche and white chocolate chips in your crock pot. Combine the milk, cream cheese, food coloring, eggs, sugar and vanilla in a bowl and mix well. Pour this mixture over the brioche then cook on low settings for 5 hours. The pudding is best served slightly warm.

Cherry Bowls

Ingredients: Servings: 2   Cooking Time: 1 Hour

1 C. cherries, pitted
½ C. red cherry juice
1 tbsp. sugar
2 tbsp. maple syrup

Directions:

In your Crock Pot, mix the cherries with the sugar and the other ingredients, toss gently, put the lid on, cook on High for 1 hour, divide into bowls and serve.

Cranberry Walnut Bread

Ingredients: Servings: 10   Cooking Time: 4 1/4 Hours

1 C. all-purpose flour
1 C. ground walnuts
1 1/2 tsp. baking powder
1/4 tsp. salt
2 ripe bananas, mashed
2 eggs
1/2 C. buttermilk
1 C. frozen cranberries

Directions:
Mix the flour, walnuts, baking powder and salt in a bowl. Add the bananas, eggs and buttermilk and mix well then fold in the cranberries. Pour the bread in your Crock Pot and bake for 4 hours on low settings. Allow the bread to cool in the pot before slicing and serving.

Caramel Pie

Ingredients: Servings: 6   Cooking Time: 2 Hours

1 C. vanilla cake mix
1 tsp. butter, melted
4 eggs, beaten
4 caramels, candy, crushed

Directions:
Mix vanilla cake mix with eggs and butter. Pour the liquid in the Crock Pot and sprinkle with crushed candies. Close the lid and cook the pie on high for 2 hours. Then cool it and remove from the Crock Pot. Cut the pie into 6 servings.

Lemony Figs

Ingredients: Servings: 8   Cooking Time: 6 Hrs.

3 oz. lemon
1 lb. figs
5 oz. water
2 lb. sugar
1 tsp. cinnamon
½ tsp. ground ginger

Directions:
Add figs flesh to a bowl and mash it using a fork. Transfer the flesh to the insert of Crock Pot. Stir in cinnamon, sugar, water, ginger, and lemon slices. Put the cooker's lid on and set the cooking time to 2 hours on Low settings. Blend cooked figs mixture using a hand mixer. Put the cooker's lid on and set the cooking time to 2 hours on Low settings. Serve when chilled.

Hazelnut Crumble Cheesecake

Ingredients: Servings: 8   Cooking Time: 6 1/2 Hours

Crust and topping:
3/4 C. butter, chilled and cubed
1 1/4 C. all-purpose flour
1 C. ground hazelnuts
1/4 C. buttermilk
1 pinch salt
2 tbsp. light brown sugar

Filling:
20 oz. cream cheese
1/2 C. sour cream
1/2 C. white sugar
1 tsp. vanilla extract
2 tbsp. Grand Marnier
1 tbsp. cornstarch
2 eggs

Directions:

For the crust and topping, combine all the ingredients in a food processor and pulse until a dough comes together. Cut the dough in half. Wrap one half in plastic wrap and place in the fridge. The remaining dough, roll it into a thin sheet and place it in your Crock Pot, trimming the edges if needed. For the filling, mix all the ingredients in a large bowl. Pour this mixture over the crust. For the topping, remove the dough from the fridge then grate it on a large grater over the cheesecake filling. Cover the pot and bake for 6 hours on low settings. Allow to cool completely before slicing and serving.

Pears And Grape Sauce

Ingredients: Servings: 4   Cooking Time: 1 Hour And 30 Minutes

4 pears	26 oz. grape juice
Juice and Zest of 1 lemon	4 garlic cloves
11 oz. currant jelly	½ vanilla bean
	4 peppercorns
	2 rosemary springs

Directions:
Put the jelly, grape juice, lemon zest, lemon juice, vanilla, peppercorns, rosemary and pears in your Crock Pot, cover and cook on High for 1 hour and 30 minutes. Divide everything between plates and serve.

Sweet Baked Milk

Ingredients: Servings: 5   Cooking Time: 10 Hours

4 C. of milk	½ tsp. vanilla extract
3 tbsp. sugar	

Directions:
Mix milk with sugar and vanilla extract and stir until sugar is dissolved. Then pour the liquid in the Crock Pot and close the lid. Cook the milk on Low for 10 hours.

Pomegranate And Mango Bowls

Ingredients: Servings: 2   Cooking Time: 3 Hours

2 C. pomegranate seeds	½ C. heavy cream
1 C. mango, peeled and cubed	½ tsp. vanilla extract
1 tbsp. lemon juice	2 tbsp. white sugar

Directions:
In your Crock Pot, combine the mango with the pomegranate seeds and the other ingredients, toss, put the lid on and cook on Low for 3 hours. Divide into bowls and serve cold.

Lemon Cream Dessert

Ingredients: Servings: 4   Cooking Time: 1 Hr.

1 C. heavy cream	¼ C. lemon juice
1 tsp. lemon zest, grated	8 oz. mascarpone cheese

Directions:
Whisk cream with mascarpone, lemon juice, and lemon zest in the Crock Pot. Put the cooker's lid on and set the cooking time

to 1 hour on Low settings. Divide the cream in serving glasses then refrigerate for 4 hours. Serve.

Pineapple Upside Down Cake

Ingredients: Servings: 10   Cooking Time: 5 1/4 Hours

1 C. butter, softened	1 tsp. baking powder
1/2 C. light brown sugar	1/4 tsp. salt
1/2 C. white sugar	1/2 tsp. cinnamon powder
2 eggs	2 tbsp. butter to grease the pot
1 C. all-purpose flour	1 can pineapple chunks, drained
1/2 C. ground almonds	

Directions:
Grease the pot with butter then place the pineapple chunks in the pot. For the cake, mix the softened butter, brown sugar and white sugar in a bowl. Add the eggs, one by one, mixing well after each addition. Fold in the flour, almonds, baking powder and salt, as well as cinnamon. Pour the batter over the pineapple and bake for 5 hours on low settings.

Mascarpone With Strawberry Jelly

Ingredients: Servings: 6   Cooking Time: 1 Hour

2 C. strawberries, chopped	3 tbsp. sugar
1 tbsp. gelatin	¼ C. of water
	1 C. mascarpone

Directions:
Mix strawberries with sugar and blend the mixture until smooth. Transfer it in the Crock Pot and cook on High for 1 hour. Meanwhile, mix water with gelatin. Whisk the mascarpone well. When the strawberry mixture is cooked, cool it little and add gelatin. Carefully mix it. Pour the strawberry mixture in the ramekins and refrigerate for 2 hours. Then top the jelly with whisked mascarpone.

Panna Cotta

Ingredients: Servings: 2   Cooking Time: 1.5 Hours

1 tbsp. gelatin	2 tbsp. strawberry jam
1 C. cream	
¼ C. of sugar	

Directions:
Pour cream in the Crock Pot. Add sugar and close the lid. Cook the liquid on High for 1.5 hours. Then cool it to the room temperature, add gelatin, and mix until smooth. Pour the liquid in the glasses and refrigerate until solid. Top every cream jelly with jam.

Jelly Bears

Ingredients: Servings: 4   Cooking Time: 1 Hour

1 C. of orange juice	3 tbsp. gelatin
¼ C. of water	

Directions:
Pour orange juice in the Crock Pot and cook it on High for 1 hour. Meanwhile, mix water with gelatin and leave for 10-15 minutes. When the orange juice is cooked, cool it for 10-15 minutes and

add gelatin mixture. Mix the liquid until smooth. Then pour it in the jelly molds (in the shape of bears) and refrigerate for as minimum 40 minutes.

Apple Granola Crumble

Ingredients: Servings: 4   Cooking Time: 6 1/4 Hours

4 red apples, peeled, cored and sliced
2 tbsp. honey

1 1/2 C. granola
1/2 tsp. cinnamon powder

Directions:

Mix the apples and honey in your crock pot. Top with the granola and sprinkle with cinnamon. Cover the pot and cook on low settings for 6 hours. Serve the crumble warm.

Braised Pears

Ingredients: Servings: 6   Cooking Time: 2.5 Hours

6 pears
2 C. wine

1 tbsp. sugar
1 cinnamon stick

Directions:

Cut the pears into halves and put them in the Crock Pot. Add all remaining ingredients and close the lid. Cook the pears on High for 2.5 hours. Serve the pears with hot wine mixture.

Rice Pudding

Ingredients: Servings: 6   Cooking Time: 2 Hours

1 tbsp. butter
7 oz. long grain rice
4 oz. water
16 oz. milk

3 oz. sugar
1 egg
1 tbsp. cream
1 tsp. vanilla extract

Directions:

In your Crock Pot, mix butter with rice, water, milk, sugar, egg, cream and vanilla, stir, cover and cook on High for 2 hours. Stir pudding one more time, divide into bowls and serve.

Sweet Lemon Mix

Ingredients: Servings: 4   Cooking Time: 1 Hour

2 C. heavy cream
Sugar to the taste

2 lemons, peeled and roughly chopped

Directions:

In your Crock Pot, mix cream with sugar and lemons, stir, cover and cook on Low for 1 hour. Divide into glasses and serve very cold.

Creamy Caramel Dessert

Ingredients: Servings: 2   Cooking Time: 2 Hrs.

1 and ½ tsp. caramel extract
1 C. of water
2 oz. cream cheese
2 eggs
1 and ½ tbsp. sugar

For the caramel sauce:
2 tbsp. sugar
2 tbsp. butter, melted
¼ tsp. caramel extract

Directions:

Blend cream cheese with 1 ½ tbsp. sugar, 1 ½ tsp. caramel extract, water, and eggs in a blender. Transfer this mixture to the insert of Crock Pot. Put the cooker's lid on and set the cooking time to 2 hours on High settings. Divide this cream cheese mixture into the serving cups. Now mix melted butter with caramel extract and sugar in a bowl. Pour this caramel sauce over the cream cheese mixture. Refrigerate the caramel cream for 1 hour. Serve.

Caramel

Ingredients: Servings: 10   Cooking Time: 7 Hours

1 C. of sugar
1 C. heavy cream

2 tbsp. butter

Directions:

Put sugar in the Crock Pot. Add heavy cream and butter. Close the lid and cook the caramel on Low for 7 hours. Carefully mix the cooked caramel and transfer it in the glass cans.

Almonds, Walnuts And Mango Bowls

Ingredients: Servings: 2   Cooking Time: 2 Hours

1 C. walnuts, chopped
2 tbsp. almonds, chopped
1 C. mango, peeled and roughly cubed
1 C. heavy cream

½ tsp. vanilla extract
1 tsp. almond extract
1 tbsp. brown sugar

Directions:

In your Crock Pot, mix the nuts with the mango, cream and the other ingredients, toss, put the lid on and cook on High for 2 hours. Divide the mix into bowls and serve.

Vanilla Crème Cups

Ingredients: Servings: 4   Cooking Time: 3 Hrs.

1 tbsp. vanilla extract
1 C. of sugar

½ C. heavy cream, whipped
7 egg yolks, whisked

Directions:

Mix egg yolks with sugar, vanilla extract, and cream in a mixer. Pour this creamy mixture into 4 ramekins. Pour 1 C. water into the insert of Crock Pot. Place the ramekins the cooker. Put the cooker's lid on and set the cooking time to 3 hours on Low settings. Serve.

Cocoa Cherry Compote

Ingredients: Servings: 6   Cooking Time: 2 Hours

½ C. dark cocoa powder
¾ C. red cherry juice
¼ C. maple syrup

1 lb. cherries, pitted and halved
2 tbsp. sugar
2 C. water

Directions:

In your Crock Pot, mix cocoa powder with cherry juice, maple syrup, cherries, water and sugar, stir, cover and cook on High for 2 hours. Divide into bowls and serve cold.

Coconut Poached Pears

Ingredients: Servings: 6   Cooking Time: 6 1/4 Hours

6 ripe but firm pears
2 C. coconut milk
2 C. water
1 cinnamon stick

1 star anise
3/4 C. coconut sugar
2 lemon rings

Directions:

Carefully peel and core the pears and place them in your Crock Pot.   Add the rest of the ingredients and cover with a lid. Cook on low settings for 6 hours.   Allow the pears to cool in the pot before serving.

Chocolate Whipped Cream

Ingredients: Servings: 4   Cooking Time: 2 Hours

½ C. of chocolate chips
1 C. heavy cream
1 tbsp. sugar

1 tsp. vanilla extract
½ tsp. lime zest, sliced

Directions:

Mix chocolate chips with vanilla extract and put it in the Crock Pot.   Close the lid and cook them on Low for 2 hours. Meanwhile, whip the heavy cream and mix it with sugar. Transfer the whipped cream in the serving ramekins.   Then sprinkle it with melted chocolate chips.   Top every serving with lime zest.

Cinnamon Butter

Ingredients: Servings: 6   Cooking Time: 6 Hours

2 C. apples, chopped
½ C. butter

1 tsp. ground cinnamon
2 tbsp. sugar

Directions:

Mix sugar with apples and put in the Crock Pot.   Leave the apples for 5-10 minutes or until they start to give the juice. Add ground cinnamon.   Then add butter and close the lid.   Cook the cinnamon butter on Low for 6 hours.   Then blend it with the help of the blender and transfer in the ramekins. Cool it.

Saucy Apple And Pears

Ingredients: Servings: 6   Cooking Time: 6 1/4 Hours

4 ripe pears, peeled, cored and sliced
2 Granny Smith apples, peeled, cored and sliced
1/4 C. butter

1/4 C. light brown sugar
1 C. apple juice
1 C. water
1 cinnamon stick
1 star anise

Directions:

Combine all the ingredients in your crock pot.   Cover the pot and cook on low settings for 6 hours.   Allow the dessert to cool in the pot before serving.

Cinnamon Apple Butter

Ingredients: Servings: 6   Cooking Time: 6 Hrs.

1 lb. sweet apples, peeled and chopped
6 oz. white sugar

2 oz. cinnamon stick
¼ tsp. salt
¼ tsp. ground ginger

Directions:

Add apples, white sugar, cinnamon stick, salt, and ground ginger to the insert of Crock Pot.   Put the cooker's lid on and set the cooking time to 3.5 hours on High settings.   Discard the cinnamon stick and blend the remaining apple mixture.   Put the cooker's lid on and set the cooking time to 3 hours on Low settings.   Serve when chilled.

Lentil Pudding

Ingredients: Servings: 4   Cooking Time: 6 Hours

½ C. green lentils
3 C. of milk
2 tbsp. of liquid honey

1 tsp. vanilla extract
1 tsp. cornflour

Directions:

Put all ingredients in the Crock Pot and carefully mix.   Close the lid and cook the pudding on Low for 6 hours.   Cool the pudding to the room temperature and transfer in the serving bowls.

Avocado Jelly

Ingredients: Servings: 2   Cooking Time: 1.5 Hours

1 avocado, pitted, chopped
1 C. of orange juice

1 tbsp. gelatin
3 tbsp. brown sugar

Directions:

Pour orange juice in the Crock Pot.   Add brown sugar and cook the liquid on High for 1.5 hours.   Then add gelatin and stir the mixture until smooth.   After this, blend the avocado until smooth, add orange juice liquid and mix until homogenous. Pour it in the C. and refrigerate until solid.

Dates And Rice Pudding

Ingredients: Servings: 2   Cooking Time: 3 Hours

1 C. dates, chopped
½ C. white rice
2 tbsp. brown sugar

1 C. almond milk
1 tsp. almond extract

Directions:

In your Crock Pot, mix the rice with the milk and the other ingredients, whisk, put the lid on and cook on Low for 3 hours. Divide the pudding into bowls and serve.

Jelly Cake

Ingredients: Servings: 6   Cooking Time: 2 Hours

1 C. cream
1 C. apple juice

2 tbsp. gelatin
½ C. of sugar

Directions:

Pour apple juice in the Crock Pot and cook it on High for 1 hour. Then pour the liquid in the bowl, add 1 tbsp. of gelatin and stir until homogenous.   Pour the liquid in the ice molds and freeze until solid.   Meanwhile, pour the cream in the Crock Pot.   Add sugar and cook the liquid on High for 1 hour.   After this, add gelatin, stir the liquid until smooth and cool to the room temperature. Then pour the liquid in the big bowl. Add frozen apple jelly and refrigerate the cake until smooth.

Cardamom Rice Porridge

Ingredients: Servings: 2   Cooking Time: 4 Hours

¼ C. basmati rice	1 tsp. butter
1 C. milk	1 tsp. ground
½ C. of water	cardamom

Directions:
Put all ingredients in the Crock Pot. Close the lid and cook the dessert on high for 4 hours. Cool the cooked meal and add sugar if desired.

Latte Vanilla Cake

Ingredients: Servings: 7   Cooking Time: 7 Hrs.

½ C. pumpkin puree	4 tbsp. olive oil
3 C. flour	2 tbsp. maple syrup
4 eggs	1 tbsp. vanilla extract
1 C. sugar, brown	4 tbsp. liquid honey
½ C. of coconut milk	¼ tsp. cooking spray
3 tbsp. espresso powder	

Directions:
Beat eggs with pumpkin puree, espresso powder, and brown sugar in a bowl. Stir in olive oil, coconut milk, vanilla extract, liquid honey, flour, and maple syrup. Whisk this pumpkin batter using a hand mixer until smooth. Use cooking to grease the insert of your Crock Pot and pour the batter in it. Put the cooker's lid on and set the cooking time to 7 hours on Low settings. Slice and serve when chilled.

Dark Cherry Chocolate Cake

Ingredients: Servings: 8   Cooking Time: 4 1/2 Hours

2/3 C. butter, softened	3 eggs
2/3 C. white sugar	1/4 tsp. salt
1 tsp. vanilla extract	1/4 C. cocoa powder
2/3 C. all-purpose flour	1 1/2 C. dark cherries, pitted
1 tsp. baking powder	1/2 C. water
	1/2 C. dark chocolate chips

Directions:
Mix the butter and sugar in a bowl until creamy. Stir in the eggs and vanilla and mix well then fold in the flour, baking powder, salt, baking powder and cocoa. Pour the batter in your Crock Pot and top with dark cherries. Mix the water and chocolate chips in a saucepan and cook over low heat until melted and smooth. Pour the hot sauce over the cherries and cook the cake on low settings for 4 hours. Allow the cake to cool in the pot before serving.

Chia And Orange Pudding

Ingredients: Servings: 2   Cooking Time: 1 Hour

1 tbsp. chia seeds	½ tsp. cinnamon powder
½ C. almond milk	
½ C. oranges, peeled	

and cut into segments
1 tbsp. sugar

	1 tbsp. coconut oil, melted
	2 tbsp. pecans, chopped

Directions:
In your Crock Pot, mix the chia seeds with the almond milk, orange segments and the other ingredients, toss, put the lid on and cook on High for 1 hour. Divide the pudding into bowls and serve cold.

Butternut Squash Pudding

Ingredients: Servings: 8   Cooking Time: 3 Hours

2 lbs. butternut squash, steamed, peeled and mashed	1 tsp. cinnamon powder
2 eggs	½ tsp. ginger powder
1 cupmilk	¼ tsp. cloves, ground
¾ C. maple syrup	1 tbsp. cornstarch
	Whipped cream for serving

Directions:
Toss squash with milk, eggs, maple syrup, cornstarch, cinnamon, cloves ground, and ginger in the insert of Crock Pot. Put the cooker's lid on and set the cooking time to 2 hours on Low settings. Serve with whipped cream on top.

Creamy Coconut Tapioca Pudding

Ingredients: Servings: 6   Cooking Time: 4 1/4 Hours

1 C. tapioca pearls	1 tsp. vanilla extract
1 C. coconut flakes	1/2 C. coconut sugar
2 C. coconut milk	
1 C. water	

Directions:
Combine all the ingredients in your Crock Pot. Cover the pot and cook on low settings for 4 hours. Serve the pudding warm or chilled.

Brandied Brioche Pudding

Ingredients: Servings: 8   Cooking Time: 6 1/2 Hours

10 oz. brioche bread, cubed	1/2 C. light brown sugar
4 eggs, beaten	1 tsp. vanilla extract
2 C. whole milk	
1/4 C. brandy	

Directions:
Place the brioche in a Crock Pot. Mix the eggs, milk, brandy, sugar and vanilla in a bowl then pour this mixture over the brioche. Cover the pot and cook on low settings for 6 hours. Serve the pudding slightly warm.

Egyptian Rice Pudding

Ingredients: Servings: 6   Cooking Time: 4 1/4 Hours

1 1/2 C. white rice	4 C. whole milk
1 vanilla pod, cut in half lengthwise	1/4 C. cold water
2 tbsp. cornstarch	1/2 C. sugar

1 tsp. cinnamon
powder

Directions:

Mix the rice, milk, vanilla pod and sugar in your crock pot. Cook on low settings for 3 hours. Combine the water and cornstarch in a bowl then pour this mixture over the rice pudding. Cover the pot again and cook on low settings for 1 additional hour. Serve the pudding warm or chilled, sprinkled with cinnamon powder.

Wine Dipped Pears

Ingredients: Servings: 6   Cooking Time: 1 Hr. 30 Minutes

6 green pears	A pinch of cinnamon
1 vanilla pod	7 oz. sugar
1 clove	1 glass red wine

Directions:

Add pears, cinnamon, vanilla, wine, cloves, and sugar to the insert of Crock Pot. Put the cooker's lid on and set the cooking time to 1.5 hours on High settings. Serve the pears with wine sauce.

Chocolate Fudge Cake

Ingredients: Servings: 6   Cooking Time: 2 Hours

¼ C. of sugar	1 C. flour
1 tbsp. cocoa powder	2 oz. chocolate chips
1 tsp. baking powder	1/3 C. coconut milk
	1 tbsp. coconut oil, softened

Directions:

Mix flour with sugar, cocoa powder, baking powder, and coconut milk. Stir the mixture until smooth and place in the Crock Pot. (use the baking paper to avoid burning). Then Cook the mixture on high for 2 hours. Meanwhile, mix coconut oil and coconut chips and melt them in the microwave oven. When the fudge is cooked, pour the chocolate chips mixture over it and leave to cool for 10-15 minutes as a minimum. Cut the cake into servings.

Ginger Fruit Compote

Ingredients: Servings: 6   Cooking Time: 6 1/2 Hours

2 ripe pears, peeled and cubed	1 C. fresh orange juice
2 red apples, peeled, cored and sliced	3 tbsp. light brown sugar
1/2 C. dried apricots, halved	2 C. water
4 slices fresh pineapple, cubed	1 star anise
	1 cinnamon stick
	2 whole cloves

Directions:

Combine all the ingredients in your Crock Pot. Cover the pot and cook on low settings for 6 hours. Allow the compote to cool before serving.

Quinoa Pudding

Ingredients: Servings: 2   Cooking Time: 2 Hours

1 C. quinoa	½ C. sugar
2 C. almond milk	½ tbsp. almonds, chopped
½ tbsp. walnuts, chopped	

Directions:

In your Crock Pot, mix the quinoa with the milk and the other ingredients, toss, put the lid on and cook on High for 2 hours. Divide the pudding into C. and serve.

Pavlova

Ingredients: Servings: 6   Cooking Time: 3 Hours

5 egg whites	1 tsp. vanilla extract
1 C. of sugar powder	½ C. whipped cream
1 tsp. lemon juice	

Directions:

Mix egg whites with sugar powder, lemon juice, and vanilla extract and whisk until you get firm peaks. Then line the Crock Pot with baking paper and put the egg white mixture inside. Flatten it and cook for 3 hours on low. When the egg white mixture is cooked, transfer it in the serving plate and top with whipped cream.

Cheesecake With Lime Filling

Ingredients: Servings: 10   Cooking Time: 1 Hr.

2 tbsp. butter, melted	For the filling:
2 tsp. sugar	1 lb. cream cheese
4 oz. almond meal	Zest of 1 lime
¼ C. coconut, shredded	Juice from 1 lime
Cooking spray	2 sachets lime jelly
	2 C. hot water

Directions:

Whisk coconut with butter, sugar, and almond meal in a bowl. Grease the insert of Crock Pot with cooking spray. Spread the coconut mixture in the greased cooker. Now beat cream cheese with lime zest, lime juice, and jelly in a separate bowl. Spread this cream cheese mixture over the coconut crust. Put the cooker's lid on and set the cooking time to 1 hour on High settings. Refrigerate the cooked cheesecake for 2 hours. Slice and serve.

Apricot Rice Pudding

Ingredients: Servings: 3   Cooking Time: 3 Hrs.

3 tbsp. coconut flakes	1 tbsp. butter
1 C. of rice	2 tsp. sugar
1 C. almond milk	1 tbsp. dried apricots, chopped
1 tsp. vanilla extract	

Directions:

Coconut flakes, rice, milk and all other ingredients to the insert of Crock Pot. Put the cooker's lid on and set the cooking time to 3 hours on Low settings. Allow it cool down. Serve.

Fresh Cream Mix

Ingredients: Servings: 6   Cooking Time: 1 Hour

2 C. fresh cream	Zest of 1 orange, grated
1 tsp. cinnamon powder	A pinch of nutmeg for

6 egg yolks	serving
5 tbsp. white sugar	4 tbsp. sugar
	2 C. water

Directions:

In a bowl, mix cream, cinnamon and orange zest and stir. In another bowl, mix the egg yolks with white sugar and whisk well. Add this over the cream, stir, strain and divide into ramekins. Put ramekins in your Crock Pot, add 2 C. water to the Crock Pot, cover, cook on Low for 1 hour, leave cream aside to cool down and serve.

Blondie Pie

Ingredients: Servings: 6   Cooking Time: 2.5 Hours

1 tsp. vanilla extract	1 tsp. baking powder
1 C. cream	2 oz. chocolate chips
1 C. flour	1 tbsp. coconut oil,
1 egg, beaten	softened
¼ C. of sugar	

Directions:

Mix vanilla extract, cream, flour, and egg. Then add sugar, baking powder, and coconut oil. When the mixture is smooth, add chocolate chips and mix them with the help of the spatula. Then pour the mixture in the Crock Pot and close the lid. Cook the pie on High for 2.5 hours.

Summer Fruits Compote

Ingredients: Servings: 6   Cooking Time: 3 Hours

1 C. apricots, pitted, chopped	1 C. strawberries
½ C. cherries, pitted	¼ C. blackberries
	½ C. of sugar
	8 C. of water

Directions:

Put all ingredients in the Crock Pot. Cook compote on High for 3 hours. Cool it and serve with ice cubes.

POULTRY RECIPES

Creamy Duck Breast

Ingredients: Servings: 1   Cooking Time: 4 Hours

1 medium duck breast, skin scored	½ tsp. orange extract
1 tbsp. sugar	Salt and black pepper to the taste
1 tbsp. heavy cream	1 C. baby spinach
2 tbsp. butter, melted	¼ tsp. sage, dried

Directions:

In your Crock Pot, mix butter with duck breast, cream, sugar, orange extract, salt, pepper and sage, stir, cover and cook on High for 4 hours. Add spinach, toss, leave aside for a few minutes, transfer to a plate and serve.

Chicken Pate

Ingredients: Servings: 6   Cooking Time: 8 Hours

1 carrot, peeled	2 C. of water
1 tsp. salt	2 tbsp. coconut oil
1-lb. chicken liver	

Directions:

Chop the carrot roughly and put it in the Crock Pot. Add chicken liver and water. Cook the mixture for 8 hours on Low. Then drain water and transfer the mixture in the blender. Add coconut oil and salt. Blend the mixture until smooth. Store the pate in the fridge for up to 7 days.

Crock Pot Chicken Thighs

Ingredients: Servings: 6   Cooking Time: 4 Hours

5 lb. chicken thighs	½ C. white vinegar
Salt and black pepper to the taste	4 garlic cloves, minced
1 tsp. black peppercorns	3 bay leaves
	½ C. soy sauce

Directions:

In your Crock Pot mix chicken, vinegar, soy sauce, salt, pepper, garlic, peppercorns and bay leaves, stir, cover and cook on High for 4 hours. Discard bay leaves, stir, divide chicken mix between plates and serve.

Chili Sausages

Ingredients: Servings: 4   Cooking Time: 3 Hours

1-lb. chicken sausages, roughly chopped	1 tbsp. chili powder
	1 tsp. tomato paste
½ C. of water	

Directions:

Sprinkle the chicken sausages with chili powder and transfer in the Crock Pot. Then mix water and tomato paste and pour the liquid over the chicken sausages. Close the lid and cook the meal on High for 3 hours.

Asian Sesame Chicken

Ingredients: Servings: 12   Cooking Time: 8 Hours

12 chicken thighs, bones and skin removed	3 tbsp. water
	3 tbsp. soy sauce
2 tbsp. sesame oil	1 thumb-size ginger, sliced thinly

Directions:

Place all ingredients in the crockpot. Stir all ingredients to combine. Close the lid and cook on low for 8 hours or on high for 6 hours. Once cooked, garnish with toasted sesame seeds.

Ginger Turkey Mix

Ingredients: Servings: 2   Cooking Time: 6 Hours

1 lb. turkey breast, skinless, boneless and roughly cubed	A pinch of salt and black pepper
1 tbsp. ginger, grated	1 tsp. chili powder
2 tsp. olive oil	2 garlic cloves, minced
1 C. tomato passata	1 tbsp. cilantro, chopped
½ C. chicken stock	

Directions:

Grease the Crock Pot with the oil and mix the turkey with the ginger and the other ingredients inside. Put the lid on, cook on High for 6 hours, divide between plates and serve.

Chicken Drumsticks With Zucchini

Ingredients: Servings: 4   Cooking Time: 7 Hours

4 chicken drumsticks	½ tsp. salt
1 tsp. ground black pepper	1 C. of water
½ tsp. ground turmeric	1 large zucchini, chopped

Directions:

Put all ingredients in the Crock Pot. Close the lid and cook the meal on Low for 7 hours.

Shredded Soy Lemon Chicken

Ingredients: Servings: 8   Cooking Time: 8 Hours

2 lb. chicken breasts, bones and skin removed	½ C. soy sauce
1 C. water	1 onion, chopped finely
¼ C. lemon juice	2 tbsp. sesame oil
4 cloves of garlic, minced	Salt and pepper to taste

Directions:

Place all ingredients in the CrockPot. Close the lid and cook on high for 6 hours or on low for 8 hours. Once the chicken is very tender, shred the meat using two forks. Serve with the sauce.

Garlic Duck

Ingredients: Servings: 4   Cooking Time: 5 Hours

1 tbsp. minced garlic	1-lb. duck fillet
1 tbsp. butter, softened	1 tsp. dried thyme
	1/3 C. coconut cream

Directions:

Mix minced garlic with butter, and dried thyme. Then rub the suck fillet with garlic mixture and place it in the Crock Pot. Add coconut cream and cook the duck on High for 5 hours. Then slice the cooked duck fillet and sprinkle it with hot garlic coconut milk.

Chicken Vegetable Curry

Ingredients: Servings: 6   Cooking Time: 8 Hours

1-lb. chicken breasts, bones removed	1 tbsp. butter
1 package frozen vegetable mix	1 C. water
	2 tbsp. curry powder

Directions:

Place all ingredients in the crockpot. Stir to combine everything. Close the lid and cook on low for 8 hours or on high for 6 hours.

Chicken Sausage Stew

Ingredients: Servings: 4   Cooking Time: 5 Hours

4 chicken breasts, skinless and boneless	A drizzle of olive oil
6 Italian sausages, sliced	1 tsp. garlic powder
5 garlic cloves, minced	29 oz. canned tomatoes, chopped
1 white onion, chopped	15 oz. tomato sauce
1 tsp. Italian seasoning	1 C. of water
	½ C. balsamic vinegar

Directions:

Place sausage and chicken slices in the Crock Pot. Add onion, garlic, oil and all other ingredients to the chicken. Put the cooker's lid on and set the cooking time to 5 hours High settings. Serve warm.

Parsley Chicken Mix

Ingredients: Servings: 2   Cooking Time: 5 Hours

1 lb. chicken breast, skinless, boneless and sliced	1 tbsp. lemon juice
½ C. parsley, chopped	½ C. chicken stock
2 tbsp. olive oil	¼ C. black olives, pitted and halved
1 tbsp. pine nuts	1 tsp. hot paprika
	A pinch of salt and black pepper

Directions:

In a blender, mix the parsley with the oil, pine nuts and lemon juice and pulse well. In your Crock Pot, mix the chicken with the parsley mix and the remaining ingredients, toss, put the lid on and cook on High for 5 hours. Divide everything between plates and serve.

Crockpot Kalua Chicken

Ingredients: Servings: 4   Cooking Time: 8 Hours

2 lb. chicken thighs, bones and skin removed	1 tbsp. liquid smoke
1 tbsp. salt	¼ C. water

Directions:

Place all ingredients in the CrockPot. Close the lid and cook on high for 6 hours or on low for 8 hours. Once cooked, serve with organic sour cream, avocado slices, and cilantro if desired.

Chicken And Peppers

Ingredients: Servings: 2   Cooking Time: 6 Hours

1 lb. chicken breasts, skinless, boneless and cubed	1 tsp. olive oil
¼ C. tomato sauce	½ tsp. coriander, ground
2 red bell peppers, cut into strips	1 tsp. Italian seasoning
½ tsp. rosemary, dried	A pinch of cayenne pepper
	1 C. chicken stock

Directions:

In your Crock Pot, mix the chicken with the peppers, tomato sauce and the other ingredients, toss, put the lid on and cook on Low for 6 hours.   divide everything between plates and serve.

Garlic Turkey

Ingredients: Servings: 2   Cooking Time: 6 Hours

1 lb. turkey breast, skinless, boneless and cubed
1 tbsp. avocado oil
2 tbsp. tomato paste
2 tbsp. garlic, minced

½ C. chicken stock
½ tsp. chili powder
½ tsp. oregano, dried
A pinch of salt and black pepper
1 tbsp. parsley, chopped

Directions:
In your Crock Pot, mix the turkey with the oil, stock, tomato paste and the other ingredients, toss, put the lid on and cook on Low for 6 hours.   Divide the mix between plates and serve with a side salad.

Lettuce And Chicken Salad

Ingredients: Servings: 6   Cooking Time: 7 Hours

2 oz. scallions, chopped
2 C. lettuce, chopped
2 oz. Mozzarella, chopped

½ C. of soy sauce
1 tbsp. olive oil
8 oz. chicken fillet, chopped

Directions:
Pour soy sauce in the Crock Pot.   Add chicken and close the lid. Cook the chicken on low for 7 hours.   Drain soy sauce and transfer the chicken in the salad bowl.   Add all remaining ingredients and stir the salad well.

Duck With Potatoes

Ingredients: Servings: 4   Cooking Time: 6 Hours

1 duck, cut into small chunks
Salt and black pepper to the taste
1 potato, cut into cubes
1-inch ginger root, sliced

4 garlic cloves, minced
4 tbsp. sugar
4 tbsp. soy sauce
2 green onions, chopped
4 tbsp. sherry wine
¼ C. of water

Directions:
Add duck pieces, garlic and all other ingredients to the Crock Pot. Put the cooker's lid on and set the cooking time to 6 hours on Low settings.   Serve warm.

Scallions And Chicken Salad

Ingredients: Servings: 4   Cooking Time: 3 Hours

4 oz. scallions, chopped
2 eggs, hard-boiled, cooked, chopped
2 tbsp. mayonnaise

1 tbsp. plain yogurt
5 oz. chicken fillet
1 C. of water
1 tsp. ground black pepper

Directions:
Put the chicken in the Crock Pot. Add water.   Close the lid and cook the chicken on high for 3 hours.   Then shred the chicken and add all remaining ingredients from the list above.   Carefully mix the salad.

Jamaican Chicken

Ingredients: Servings: 3   Cooking Time: 4 Hours

12 oz. chicken fillet
½ tsp. ground coriander
½ tsp. dried cilantro

½ tsp. lemon zest
1 jalapeno, sliced
1 tsp. olive oil
1 C. tomato juice

Directions:
Rub the chicken fillet with ground coriander, cilantro, lemon zest, and olive oil.   Put the chicken in the Crock Pot.   Add tomato juice and jalapeno.   Cook the meal on High for 4 hours.

Turkey Soup

Ingredients: Servings: 4   Cooking Time: 3 Hours

3 celery stalks, chopped
1 yellow onion, chopped
1 tbsp. olive oil
Salt and black pepper to the taste

6 C. turkey stock
¼ C. parsley, chopped
3 C. baked spaghetti squash, chopped
3 C. turkey, cooked and shredded

Directions:
In your Crock Pot, mix oil with celery, onion, stock, salt, pepper, squash, turkey and parsley, stir, cover, cook on High for 3 hours, ladle into bowls and serve.

Bacon Chicken

Ingredients: Servings: 4   Cooking Time: 7 Hours

4 bacon slices, cooked
4 chicken drumsticks
½ C. of water

¼ tomato juice
1 tsp. salt
½ tsp. ground black pepper

Directions:
Sprinkle the chicken drumsticks with the salt and ground black pepper.   Then wrap every chicken drumstick in the bacon and arrange it in the Crock Pot.   Add water and tomato juice.   Cook the meal on Low for 7 hours.

Chicken Mix

Ingredients: Servings: 4   Cooking Time: 8 Hours

1 C. carrot, chopped
1-lb. chicken wings
1 C. of water
½ C. tomato juice

1 tsp. salt
1 tsp. dried rosemary

Directions:
Put chicken wings in the Crock Pot.   Add carrot, tomato juice, water, salt, and dried rosemary.   Close the lid and cook the meal on low for 8 hours.

Turkey Gumbo

Ingredients: Servings: 4   Cooking Time: 7 Hours

1 lb. turkey wings
Salt and black pepper to the taste
1 yellow onion, chopped
1 yellow bell pepper, chopped
3 garlic cloves, chopped

5 oz. water
2 tbsp. chili powder
1 and ½ tsp. cumin, ground
A pinch of cayenne pepper
2 C. veggies stock

Directions:

In your Crock Pot, mix turkey with salt, pepper, onion, bell pepper, garlic, chili powder, cumin, cayenne and stock, stir, cover and cook on Low for 7 hours.   Divide everything between plates and serve.

Chicken And Sauce(2)

Ingredients: Servings: 4   Cooking Time: 5 Hours

1 chicken, cut into medium pieces
Salt and black pepper to the taste
1 tbsp. olive oil
½ tsp. sweet paprika
½ tsp. marjoram, dried

¼ C. white wine
¼ C. chicken stock
2 tbsp. white vinegar
¼ C. apricot preserves
1 and ½ tsp. ginger, grated
2 tbsp. honey

Directions:

In your Crock Pot, mix chicken with salt, pepper, oil, paprika, wine, marjoram, stock, vinegar, apricots preserves, ginger and honey, stir, cover and cook on Low for 5 hours.   Divide between plates and serve.

Puerto Rican Chicken

Ingredients: Servings: 6   Cooking Time: 8 Hours

8 oz. chicken breast
7 oz. chicken filler
6 oz. chicken wings
½ tsp. ground cumin
1 tsp. cilantro
1 tbsp. fresh thyme leaves
1 tsp. ground coriander

1 tbsp. ground celery root
2 jalapeno
6 tbsp. dry wine
3 oz. lemon wedges
3 red potatoes
1 yellow onion
1 tbsp. olive oil

Directions:

Add chicken wings, fillet, and breast to the Crock Pot.   Blend all the veggies in a blender and add it to the cooker.   Stir in all tomatoes and all other ingredients to the chicken.   Put the cooker's lid on and set the cooking time to 8 hours on Low settings.   Mix well and serve warm.

Thyme Whole Chicken

Ingredients: Servings: 6   Cooking Time: 9 Hours

1.5-lb. whole chicken
1 tbsp. dried thyme

1 tbsp. olive oil
1 tsp. salt
1 C. of water

Directions:

Chop the whole chicken roughly and sprinkle with dried thyme, olive oil, and salt.   Then transfer it in the Crock Pot, add water. Cook the chicken on low for 9 hours.

Creamy Turkey Mix

Ingredients: Servings: 2   Cooking Time: 7 Hours

1 lb. turkey breast, skinless, boneless and cubed
1 tsp. turmeric powder
½ tsp. garam masala
½ C. heavy cream
1 red onion, chopped

½ C. chicken stock
4 garlic cloves, minced
¼ C. chives, chopped
A pinch of salt and black pepper
1 tbsp. chives, chopped

Directions:

In your Crock Pot, mix the turkey with turmeric, garam masala and the other ingredients except the cream, toss, put the lid on and cook on Low for 6 hours.   Add the cream, toss, put the lid on again, cook on Low for 1 more hour, divide everything between plates and serve.

Turkey And Avocado

Ingredients: Servings: 2   Cooking Time: 6 Hours

1 lb. turkey breasts, skinless, boneless and cubed
1 C. avocado, peeled, pitted and cubed
1 C. tomatoes, cubed

1 tbsp. chives, chopped
½ tsp. chili powder
4 garlic cloves, minced
¼ C. chicken stock

Directions:

In Crock Pot, mix the turkey with the tomatoes, chives and the other ingredients except the avocado, toss, put the lid on and cook on Low for 5 hours and 30 minutes.   Add the avocado, toss, cook on Low for 30 minutes more, divide everything between plates and serve.

Poultry Stew

Ingredients: Servings: 6   Cooking Time: 8 Hours

3 garlic cloves, peeled and minced
3 carrots, cut into 3 parts
1 lb. chicken fillet, diced
1 lb. duck fillet, diced

1 tbsp. smoked paprika
¼ C. of soy sauce
1 tbsp. honey
1 tsp. nutmeg
1 tsp. fresh rosemary
1 tsp. black peas
2 C. of water

Directions:

Add chicken, duck, and all other ingredients to the Crock Pot. Put the cooker's lid on and set the cooking time to 8 hours on Low settings.   Serve warm.

Lemon Turkey And Spinach

Ingredients: Servings: 4   Cooking Time: 7 Hours

1 lb. turkey breasts, skinless, boneless and roughly cubed
1 C. baby spinach
2 spring onions, chopped
½ tsp. chili powder

Juice of ½ lemon
1 C. chicken stock
1 tbsp. oregano, chopped
A pinch of salt and black pepper
1 tsp. garam masala

Directions:
In your Crock Pot, mix the turkey with the lemon juice, spring onions and the other ingredients except the baby spinach, toss, put the lid on and cook on Low for 6 hours and 30 minutes. Add the spinach, cook everything on Low for 30 minutes more, divide between plates and serve.

Chicken Piccata

Ingredients: Servings: 4   Cooking Time: 8 Hours

4 chicken breasts, skin and bones removed
Salt and pepper to taste

¼ C. butter, cubed
¼ C. chicken broth
1 tbsp. lemon juice

Directions:
Place all ingredients in the crockpot. Give a good stir to combine everything. Close the lid and cook on low for 8 hours or on high for 6 hours.

Chicken And Mango Mix

Ingredients: Servings: 2   Cooking Time: 5 Hours

1 lb. chicken breast, skinless, boneless and sliced
1 C. mango, peeled and cubed
4 scallions, chopped
1 tbsp. avocado oil
½ tsp. chili powder

½ tsp. rosemary, dried
1 C. chicken stock
1 tbsp. sweet paprika
A pinch of salt and black pepper
1 tbsp. chives, chopped

Directions:
In your Crock Pot, mix the chicken with the mango, scallions, chili powder and the other ingredients, toss, put the lid on and cook on Low for 5 hours. Divide the mix between plates and serve.

Citrus Glazed Chicken

Ingredients: Servings: 4   Cooking Time: 4 Hours

2 lbs. chicken thighs, skinless, boneless and cut into pieces
Salt and black pepper to the taste
3 tbsp. olive oil
¼ C. flour
For the sauce:
2 tbsp. fish sauce

¼ C. of orange juice
2 tsp. sugar
1 tbsp. orange zest
¼ tsp. sesame seeds
2 tbsp. scallions, chopped
½ tsp. coriander, ground

1 and ½ tsp. orange extract
1 tbsp. ginger, grated

1 C. of water
¼ tsp. red pepper flakes
2 tbsp. soy sauce

Directions:
Whisk flour with black pepper, salt, and chicken pieces in a bowl to coat well. Add chicken to a pan greased with oil and sear it over medium heat until golden brown. Transfer the chicken to the Crock Pot. Blend orange juice, fish sauce, soy sauce, ginger, water, coriander, orange extract, and stevia in a blender jug. Pour this fish sauce mixture over the chicken and top it with orange zest, scallions, sesame seeds, and pepper flakes. Put the cooker's lid on and set the cooking time to 4 hours on High settings. Serve warm.

Orange Chicken(1)

Ingredients: Servings: 4   Cooking Time: 8 Hours

1 orange, chopped
1 tsp. ground turmeric
1 tsp. peppercorn
1 tsp. olive oil

1 tsp. salt
1 C. of water
1-lb. chicken breast, skinless, boneless, sliced

Directions:
Put all ingredients in the Crock Pot and gently mix them. Close the lid and cook the meal on Low for 8 hours. When the time is finished, transfer the chicken in the serving bowls and top with orange liquid from the Crock Pot.

Spicy Almond-crusted Chicken Nuggets In The Crockpot

Ingredients: Servings: 6   Cooking Time: 8 Hours

¼ C. butter, melted
1 ½ C. almond meal
1 ½ C. grated parmesan cheese

1 ½ lb. boneless chicken breasts, cut into strips
2 eggs, beaten

Directions:
Place foil at the bottom of the crockpot. Combine the almond meal and parmesan cheese. Dip the chicken strips into the eggs and dredge into the parmesan and cheese mixture. Place carefully in the crockpot. Close the lid and cook on low for 8 hours or on high for 6 hours.

Chicken With Peach And Orange Sauce

Ingredients: Servings: 8   Cooking Time: 6 Hours

6 chicken breasts, skinless and boneless
15 oz. canned peaches and their juice

12 oz. orange juice
2 tbsp. lemon juice
1 tsp. soy sauce

Directions:
In your Crock Pot, mix chicken with orange juice, lemon juice, peaches and soy sauce, toss, cover and cook on Low for 6 hours. Divide chicken breasts on plates, drizzle peach and orange sauce all over and serve.

Chicken Potato Casserole

Ingredients: Servings: 6   Cooking Time: 10 Hours

10 oz. ground chicken	8 oz. Parmesan, shredded
4 large potatoes, peeled and sliced	1 tsp. paprika
2 egg, beaten	1 tsp. cilantro
1 large onion, diced	½ tsp. nutmeg
1 tsp. ground black pepper	1 tsp. butter
1 C. heavy cream	1 carrot, grated

Directions:

Grease the base of the Crock Pot with butter. Spread the ground chicken in the cooker and top it with potatoes and onion. Whisk egg with cream, cilantro, nutmeg, paprika, and black pepper in a bowl. Pour this cream-egg mixture over the veggies and top it with grated carrot and ½ of the shredded cheese. Put the cooker's lid on and set the cooking time to 10 hours on Low settings. Garnish with remaining cheese. Serve.

Parmesan Chicken Fillet

Ingredients: Servings: 4   Cooking Time: 7 Hours

10 oz. chicken fillet	1 white onion, sliced
6 oz. Parmesan, shredded	½ C. bread crumbs
1 tbsp. lemon juice	3 tbsp. chicken stock
2 tomatoes, chopped	1 tsp. ground black pepper
1 tbsp. butter, melted	

Directions:

Add chicken, onion, and all other ingredients to the Crock Pot. Put the cooker's lid on and set the cooking time to 7 hours on Low settings. Serve warm.

Sweet And Hot Chicken Wings

Ingredients: Servings: 6   Cooking Time: 4 Hours

12 chicken wings, cut into 24 pieces	¼ C. honey
1 lb. celery, cut into thin matchsticks	Salt to the taste
4 tbsp. hot sauce	¼ C. tomato puree
	1 C. yogurt
	1 tbsp. parsley, chopped

Directions:

In your Crock Pot, mix chicken with celery, honey, hot sauce, salt, tomato puree and parsley, stir, cover and cook on High for 3 hours and 30 minutes. Add yogurt, toss, cover, cook on High for 30 minutes more, divide between plates and serve

Coriander And Turmeric Chicken

Ingredients: Servings: 2   Cooking Time: 6 Hours

1 lb. chicken breasts, skinless, boneless and cubed	1 tbsp. olive oil
	1 tbsp. lime zest, grated
1 tbsp. coriander, chopped	1 C. lime juice
½ tsp. turmeric	1 tbsp. chives, chopped
	¼ C. tomato sauce

powder
2 scallions, minced

Directions:

In your Crock Pot, mix the chicken with the coriander, turmeric, scallions and the other ingredients, toss, put the lid on and cook on Low for 6 hours. Divide the mix between plates and serve right away.

African Chicken Meal

Ingredients: Servings: 6   Cooking Time: 8 Hours

13 oz. chicken breast	1 tbsp. tomato sauce
1 tsp. peanut oil	1 C. tomatoes, canned
1 tsp. ground black pepper	1 tbsp. kosher salt
1 tsp. oregano	¼ tsp. ground cardamom
1 chili pepper	½ tsp. ground anise
1 carrot	

Directions:

Rub the chicken breast with peanut oil then and sear for 1 minute per side in the skillet. Transfer the chicken to the Crock Pot. Add tomato sauce, salt, and all other ingredients to the cooker. Put the cooker's lid on and set the cooking time to 8 hours on Low settings. Serve.

Chicken And Asparagus

Ingredients: Servings: 2   Cooking Time: 5 Hours

1 lb. chicken breast, skinless, boneless and cubed	A pinch of salt and black pepper
1 C. asparagus, sliced	1 tsp. garam masala
1 tbsp. olive oil	1 C. chicken stock
2 scallions, chopped	1 C. tomatoes, cubed
	1 tbsp. parsley, chopped

Directions:

In your Crock Pot, mix the chicken with the asparagus, oil and the other ingredients except the asparagus, toss, put the lid on and cook on High for 4 hours. Add the asparagus, toss, cook on High for 1 more hour, divide everything between plates and serve.

Crockpot Tomato And Coconut Chicken

Ingredients: Servings: 6   Cooking Time: 8 Hours

2 lb. organic chicken thighs, bones and skin removed	1 onion, chopped
	1 tsp. ginger, minced
1 can full fat coconut milk, unsweetened	1 tsp. cumin
1 C. tomato, chopped and pureed	½ tsp. garam masala
2 cloves of garlic, chopped	½ tsp. cinnamon
1 tbsp. red curry paste	¼ tsp. cayenne pepper
2 ½ tsp. yellow curry powder	Salt and pepper to taste
	1 bunch kale leaves, stems removed

Directions:

Place all ingredients except for the kale in the CrockPot. Close the lid and cook on high for 5 hours or on low for 8 hours. An hour before the cooking time ends, add in the kale leaves. Continue cooking until the chicken is cooked through.

Horseradish Chicken Wings

Ingredients: Servings: 4   Cooking Time: 6 Hours

3 tbsp. horseradish, grated	1 tsp. ketchup
1 tbsp. mayonnaise	½ C. of water
	1-lb. chicken wings

Directions:
Mix chicken wings with ketchup, horseradish, and mayonnaise, Put them in the Crock Pot and add water.   Cook the meal on Low for 6 hours.

Buffalo Chicken Tenders

Ingredients: Servings: 4   Cooking Time: 3.5 Hours

12 oz. chicken fillet	½ C. of coconut milk
3 tbsp. buffalo sauce	1 jalapeno pepper, chopped

Directions:
Cut the chicken fillet into tenders and sprinkle the buffalo sauce. Put the chicken tenders in the Crock Pot.   Add coconut milk and jalapeno pepper.   Close the lid and cook the meal on high for 3.5 hours.

Paella

Ingredients: Servings: 6   Cooking Time: 4 Hours

12 oz. chicken fillet, chopped	2 C. chicken stock
4 oz. chorizo, chopped	1 tsp. dried cilantro
½ C. white rice	1 tsp. chili flakes
1 tsp. garlic, diced	Cooking spray

Directions:
Spray the skillet with cooking spray and put the chorizo inside. Roast the chorizo for 2 minutes per side and transfer in the Crock Pot.   Then put rice in the Crock Pot.   Then add all remaining ingredients and carefully stir the paella mixture.   Cook it on High for 4 hours.

Chicken, Peppers And Onions

Ingredients: Servings: 4   Cooking Time: 8 Hours

1 tbsp. olive oil	1-lb. boneless chicken breasts, sliced
½ C. shallots, peeled	
½ C. green and red peppers, diced	Salt and pepper to taste

Directions:
Heat oil in a skillet over medium flame.   Sauté the shallots until fragrant and translucent. Allow to cook so that the outer edges of the shallots turn slightly brown.   Transfer into the crockpot. Add the chicken breasts and the peppers.   Season with salt and pepper to taste.   Add a few tbsp. of water.   Close the lid and cook on low for 8 hours or on high for 6 hours.

Peppercorn Chicken Thighs

Ingredients: Servings: 6   Cooking Time: 4 Hours

5 lbs. chicken thighs	½ C. white vinegar
Salt and black pepper to the taste	4 garlic cloves, minced
1 tsp. black peppercorns	3 bay leaves
	½ C. of soy sauce

Directions:
Add chicken, peppercorns, and all other ingredients to the Crock Pot.   Put the cooker's lid on and set the cooking time to 4 hours on High settings.   Discard the bay leaves.   Serve warm.

Chicken Stuffed With Plums

Ingredients: Servings: 6   Cooking Time: 4 Hours

6 chicken fillets	1 tsp. salt
1 C. plums, pitted, sliced	1 tsp. white pepper
1 C. of water	

Directions:
Beat the chicken fillets gently and rub with salt and white pepper. Then put the sliced plums on the chicken fillets and roll them. Secure the chicken rolls with toothpicks and put in the Crock Pot. Add water and close the lid.   Cook the meal on High for 4 hours. Then remove the chicken from the Crock Pot, remove the toothpicks and transfer in the serving plates.

Chicken Wings In Vodka Sauce

Ingredients: Servings: 4   Cooking Time: 6 Hours

1-lb. chicken wings	1 tbsp. olive oil
½ C. vodka sauce	

Directions:
Put all ingredients in the Crock Pot and mix well.   Close the lid and cook the meal on Low for 6 hours.

Chicken Parm

Ingredients: Servings: 3   Cooking Time: 4 Hours

9 oz. chicken fillet	3 oz. Parmesan, grated
1/3 C. cream	1 tsp. olive oil

Directions:
Brush the Crock Pot bowl with olive oil from inside.   Then slice the chicken fillet and place it in the Crock Pot.   Top it with Parmesan and cream.   Close the lid and cook the meal on High for 4 hours.

Lime And Pepper Chicken

Ingredients: Servings: 4   Cooking Time: 8 Hours

Salt and pepper to taste	½ C. lime juice
3 tbsp. sucralose or stevia sweetener	4 chicken breasts, bones removed
	1 tbsp. olive oil

Directions:

In a mixing bowl, combine the lime juice, salt, pepper, and sucralose. Marinate the chicken breasts for a few hours in the fridge. Add the oil and give a good mix. Close the lid and cook on low for 8 hours or on high for 6 hours.

Tomato Chicken And Chickpeas

Ingredients: Servings: 2   Cooking Time: 7 Hours

1 tbsp. olive oil
1 red onion, chopped
1 C. canned chickpeas, drained
1 lb. chicken breast, skinless, boneless and cubed
½ C. cherry tomatoes, halved

½ C. tomato sauce
½ tsp. rosemary, dried
½ tsp. turmeric powder
1 C. chicken stock
A pinch of salt and black pepper
1 tbsp. chives, chopped

Directions:

Grease the Crock Pot with the oil and mix the chicken with the onion, chickpeas and the other ingredients inside the pot. Put the lid on, cook on Low for 7 hours, divide between plates and serve.

Salsa Chicken Wings

Ingredients: Servings: 5   Cooking Time: 6 Hours

2-pounds chicken wings

2 C. salsa
½ C. of water

Directions:

Put all ingredients in the Crock Pot. Carefully mix the mixture and close the lid. Cook the chicken wings on low for 6 hours.

Cauliflower Chicken

Ingredients: Servings: 6   Cooking Time: 7 Hours

2 C. cauliflower, chopped
1-lb. ground chicken
1 tsp. chili powder

1 tsp. ground turmeric
1 tsp. salt
1 C. of water
3 tbsp. plain yogurt

Directions:

Mix ground chicken with chili powder, ground turmeric, and salt. Then mix the chicken mixture with cauliflower and transfer in the Crock Pot. Add plain yogurt and water. Close the lid and cook the meal on Low for 7 hours.

Lemongrass Chicken Thighs

Ingredients: Servings: 6   Cooking Time: 4 Hours

6 chicken thighs
1 tbsp. dried sage
1 tsp. ground paprika

1 tsp. salt
2 tbsp. sesame oil
1 C. of water

Directions:

Mix dried sage with salt, and ground paprika. Then rub the chicken thighs with the sage mixture and transfer in the Crock Pot. Sprinkle the chicken with sesame oil and water. Close the chicken on High for 4 hours.

Stuffed Pasta

Ingredients: Servings: 6   Cooking Time: 4 Hours

12 oz. cannelloni
9 oz. ground chicken
1 tsp. Italian seasonings

2 oz. Parmesan, grated
½ C. tomato juice
½ C. of water

Directions:

Mix the ground chicken with Italian seasonings and fill the cannelloni. Put the stuffed cannelloni in the Crock Pot. Add all remaining ingredients and close the lid. Cook the meal on High for 4 hours.

Chicken And Chickpeas

Ingredients: Servings: 4   Cooking Time: 4 Hours

1 yellow onion, chopped
4 garlic cloves, minced
1 tbsp. ginger, grated
1 and ½ tsp. paprika
1 tbsp. cumin, ground
1 and ½ tsp. coriander, ground
1 tsp. turmeric, ground
Salt and black pepper to the taste

2 tbsp. butter
A pinch of cayenne pepper
15 oz. canned tomatoes, crushed
¼ C. lemon juice
1 lb. spinach, chopped
3 lb. chicken drumsticks and thighs
½ C. cilantro, chopped
½ C. chicken stock
15 oz. canned chickpeas, drained
½ C. heavy cream

Directions:

Grease your Crock Pot with the butter, add onion, garlic, ginger, paprika, cumin, coriander, turmeric, salt, pepper, cayenne, tomatoes, lemon juice, spinach, chicken, stock, chickpeas and heavy cream, cover and cook on High for 4 hours. Add cilantro, stir everything, divide between plates and serve.

Turmeric Meatballs

Ingredients: Servings: 4   Cooking Time: 2.5 Hours

1-lb. ground chicken
1 tbsp. ground turmeric
1 tsp. salt

½ tsp. ground ginger
1 tbsp. corn starch
½ C. cream

Directions:

Mix ground chicken with ground turmeric, ginger, salt, and corn starch. Then make the medium-size meatballs. Preheat the skillet well. Put the meatballs in the hot skillet and cook them for 30 seconds per side. Then transfer the meatballs in the Crock Pot, add cream, and close the lid. Cook the meatballs on High for 2.5 hours.

Chicken Cordon Bleu

Ingredients: Servings: 4   Cooking Time: 3.5 Hours

4 ham slices
1-lb. chicken fillet
4 Cheddar cheese
slices
1 egg, beaten

1 tsp. salt
1 tsp. ground black
pepper
½ C. of water
1 tbsp. olive oil

Directions:

Cut the chicken fillet into 4 servings.   Then beat every chicken fillet and sprinkle with salt and ground black pepper.   Put the ham and cheese on the fillets and roll them.   Secure the chicken fillets with toothpicks and sprinkle with olive oil.   Place the chicken fillets in the Crock Pot.   Add water and close the lid. Cook the meal on High for 3.5 hours.

Carrot Meatballs

Ingredients: Servings: 6   Cooking Time: 6 Hours

1 C. carrot, shredded
14 oz. ground chicken
1 tsp. cayenne pepper

½ C. of water
1 tbsp. butter
1 tsp. salt
1 tsp. ground cumin

Directions:

Mix carrot with ground chicken   Then add cayenne pepper, salt, and ground cumin.   After this, make the small meatballs and put them in the Crock Pot.   Add water and butter.   Close the lid and cook the meatballs on low for 6 hours.

Paprika Chicken And Artichokes

Ingredients: Servings: 2   Cooking Time: 7 Hours And 10 Minutes

1 lb. chicken breast,
skinless, boneless
and cut into strips
1 C. canned artichoke
hearts, drained and
halved
2 garlic cloves,
minced

3 scallions, chopped
1 tbsp. olive oil
1 tbsp. sweet paprika
1 C. chicken stock
½ C. parsley,
chopped

Directions:

Heat up a pan with the oil over medium-high heat, add the scallions, garlic and the chicken, brown for 10 minutes and transfer to the Crock Pot.   Add the rest of the ingredients, toss, put the lid on and cook on Low for 7 hours.   Divide everything between plates and serve.

Sesame Chicken Wings

Ingredients: Servings: 4   Cooking Time: 4 Hours

1 lb. chicken wings
½ C. fresh parsley,
chopped
1 tsp. salt
1 tsp. ground black
pepper

¼ C. milk
1 tbsp. sugar
5 tbsp. honey
2 tbsp. sesame seeds
¼ C. chicken stock
1 tsp. soy sauce

Directions:

Rub the chicken wings with salt and black pepper.   Add this chicken to the Crock Pot along with chicken stock and parsley. Put the cooker's lid on and set the cooking time to 4 hours on High settings.   Mix milk with honey, sugar, and sesame seeds in a bowl.   Transfer the chicken to a baking tray.   Pour the sesame mixture over the chicken wings.   Bake them for 10 minutes at 350 degrees F in a preheated oven.   Enjoy.

Chopped Chicken Liver Balls

Ingredients: Servings: 6   Cooking Time: 4 Hours

1 egg, beaten
3 tbsp. semolina
1 tsp. Italian
seasonings

1 tbsp. flour
½ tsp. salt
1-lb. liver, minced
1/3 C. water

Directions:

Mix egg with semolina, Italian seasonings, flour, salt, and minced liver.   When the mixture is homogenous, make the medium size balls and put them in the Crock Pot.   Add water and close the lid.   Cook the liver balls on High for 4 hours.

Rosemary Chicken Thighs

Ingredients: Servings: 2   Cooking Time: 7 Hours

1 lb. chicken thighs,
boneless
1 tsp. rosemary, dried
½ tsp. sweet paprika
½ tsp. garam masala

1 tbsp. olive oil
½ C. chicken stock
A pinch of salt and
black pepper
1 tbsp. cilantro,
chopped

Directions:

In your Crock Pot, mix the chicken with the rosemary, paprika and the other ingredients, toss, put the lid on and cook on Low for 7 hours/   Divide the chicken between plates and serve with a side salad.

Lemon Chicken Thighs

Ingredients: Servings: 4   Cooking Time: 7 Hours

4 chicken thighs,
skinless, boneless
1 lemon, sliced
1 tsp. ground black
pepper

½ tsp. ground
nutmeg
1 tsp. olive oil
1 C. of water

Directions:

Rub the chicken thighs with ground black pepper, nutmeg, and olive oil.   Then transfer the chicken in the Crock Pot.   Add lemon and water.   Close the lid and cook the meal on LOW for 7 hours.

Chicken And Sauce(1)

Ingredients: Servings: 8   Cooking Time: 4 Hours

1 whole chicken, cut
into medium pieces
1 tbsp. olive oil
1 and ½ tbsp. lemon
juice
1 C. chicken stock

1 tsp. cinnamon
powder
Salt and black pepper
to the taste
1 tbsp. sweet paprika
1 tsp. onion powder

1 tbsp. cilantro,
chopped

Directions:

In your Crock Pot, mix chicken with oil, lemon juice, stock, cilantro, cinnamon, salt, pepper, paprika and onion powder, stir, cover and cook on High for 4 hours. Divide chicken between plates and serve with cooking sauce drizzled on top.

Chicken And Green Onion Sauce

Ingredients: Servings: 4   Cooking Time: 4 Hours

2 tbsp. butter, melted
4 chicken breast
halves, skinless and
boneless

4 green onions,
chopped
Salt and black pepper
to the taste
8 oz. sour cream

Directions:

In your Crock Pot, mix chicken with melted butter, green onion, salt, pepper and sour cream, cover and cook on High for 4 hours. Divide chicken between plates, drizzle green onions sauce all over and serve.

Alfredo Chicken

Ingredients: Servings: 4   Cooking Time: 2 Hours And 30 Minutes

1 lb. chicken breasts,
skinless and boneless
4 tbsp. soft butter
1 C. chicken stock
Salt and black pepper
to the taste

2 C. heavy cream
½ tsp. Italian
seasoning
½ tsp. garlic powder
1/3 C. parmesan,
grated
½ lb. rigatoni

Directions:

In your Crock Pot, mix chicken with butter, stock, cream, salt, pepper, garlic powder and Italian seasoning, stir, cover and cook on High for 2 hours. Shred meat, return to Crock Pot, also add rigatoni and parmesan, cover and cook on High for 30 minutes more. Divide between plates and serve.

Rosemary Chicken In Yogurt

Ingredients: Servings: 4   Cooking Time: 6 Hours

1 C. plain yogurt
1 tbsp. dried
rosemary
2 tbsp. olive oil

1 tsp. onion powder
1-lb. chicken breast,
skinless, boneless,
chopped

Directions:

Rub the chicken breast with onion powder, dried rosemary, and olive oil. Transfer the chicken in the Crock Pot. Add plain yogurt and close the lid. Cook the chicken on low for 6 hours. When the meal is cooked, transfer it in the plates and top with hot yogurt mixture from the Crock Pot.

Chicken And Mustard Sauce

Ingredients: Servings: 3   Cooking Time: 4 Hours

8 bacon strips,
cooked and chopped
Salt and black pepper
to the taste
1 C. yellow onion,
chopped
1 tbsp. olive oil

1/3 C. Dijon mustard
1 and ½ C. chicken
stock
3 chicken breasts,
skinless and boneless
¼ tsp. sweet paprika

Directions:

In a bowl, mix paprika with mustard, salt and pepper and stir well. Spread this on chicken breasts and massage. Heat up a pan with the oil over medium-high heat, add chicken breasts, cook for 2 minutes on each side and transfer to your Crock Pot. Add stock, bacon and onion, stir, cover and cook on High for 4 hours. Divide chicken between plates, drizzle mustard sauce all over and serve.

Chicken And Tomatillos

Ingredients: Servings: 6   Cooking Time: 4 Hours

1 lb. chicken thighs,
skinless and boneless
2 tbsp. olive oil
1 yellow onion,
chopped
1 garlic clove, minced
4 oz. canned green
chilies, chopped
A handful cilantro,
chopped
Salt and black pepper
to the taste

15 oz. canned
tomatillos, chopped
5 oz. canned
garbanzo beans,
drained
15 oz. rice, cooked
5 oz. tomatoes,
chopped
15 oz. cheddar cheese,
grated
4 oz. black olives,
pitted and chopped

Directions:

In your Crock Pot, mix oil with onions, garlic, chicken, chilies, salt, pepper, cilantro and tomatillos, stir, cover the Crock Pot and cook on High for 3 hours Take chicken out of the Crock Pot, shred, return to Crock Pot, add rice, beans, cheese, tomatoes and olives, cover and cook on High for 1 more hour. Divide between plates and serve.

Mexican Chicken In Crockpot

Ingredients: Servings: 4   Cooking Time: 8 Hours

2 tbsp. butter
1 can diced tomatoes,
undrained
2 C. chicken, cubed

Salt and pepper to
taste
1 tsp. cumin

Directions:

Place all ingredients in the crockpot. Mix everything to combine. Close the lid and cook on low for 8 hours or on high for 5 hours.

Coca Cola Dipped Chicken

Ingredients: Servings: 4   Cooking Time: 4 Hours

1 yellow onion,
minced
1 tbsp. balsamic
vinegar
1 chili pepper,
chopped

4 chicken drumsticks
15 oz. coca cola
Salt and black pepper
to the taste
2 tbsp. olive oil

Directions:

Add chicken to a pan greased with oil and sear it until golden brown from both the sides. Transfer the chicken to the Crock Pot. Stir in coca-cola, chili, onion, vinegar, black pepper, and salt to the cooker. Put the cooker's lid on and set the cooking time to 4 hours on High settings. Serve warm.

Chickpea And Chicken Bowl

Ingredients: Servings: 7   Cooking Time: 3 Hours

2 C. chickpeas, cooked	1 tsp. taco seasonings
1-lb. chicken fillet, sliced	1 C. fresh cilantro, chopped
½ C. plain yogurt	½ C. of water

Directions:

Mix chicken slices with taco seasonings and transfer in the Crock Pot. Add water and close the lid. Cook the chicken on High for 3 hours. Then drain water and transfer the chicken in the bowls. Add chickpeas and top with fresh cilantro and plain yogurt.

Chocolaty Chicken Mash

Ingredients: Servings: 7   Cooking Time: 3 Hours 10 Minutes

4 oz. milk chocolate	1 C. of water
½ C. heavy cream	1 tbsp. sesame oil
14 oz. ground chicken	1 tsp. cumin seeds
1 tsp. salt	¼ C. baby carrot, chopped
1 tbsp. tomato sauce	
1 tsp. hot chili sauce	

Directions:

Mix the ground chicken with tomato sauce, salt, water, cumin seeds, sesame oil, and hot chili sauce in a bowl. Spread the chicken in the Crock Pot and top with baby carrots. Put the cooker's lid on and set the cooking time to 3 hours on High settings. Stir the chicken after 1 hour of cooking. Melt the milk chocolate in a bowl by heating in the microwave. Stir in cream and mix well, then add this mixture to the Crock Pot. Mix it with ground chicken. Put the cooker's lid on and set the cooking time to 10 minutes on High settings. Serve.

Oregano Chicken Breast

Ingredients: Servings: 4   Cooking Time: 4 Hours

1-lb. chicken breast, skinless, boneless, roughly chopped	1 bay leaf
	1 tsp. peppercorns
	1 tsp. salt
1 tbsp. dried oregano	2 C. of water

Directions:

Pour water in the Crock Pot and add peppercorns and bay leaf. Then sprinkle the chicken with the dried oregano and transfer in the Crock Pot. Close the lid and cook the meal on High for 4 hours.

Chicken Mushrooms Stroganoff

Ingredients: Servings: 4   Cooking Time: 4 Hours

2 garlic cloves, minced	1 C. chicken stock
	1 C. of coconut milk

8 oz. mushrooms, roughly chopped
¼ tsp. celery seeds
1 yellow onion, chopped
1 lb. chicken breasts, cut into pieces
1 and ½ tsp. thyme, dried
2 tbsp. parsley, chopped
Salt and black pepper to the tasted
Already cooked pasta for serving

Directions:

Add chicken, salt, onion, black pepper, garlic, coconut milk, stock, thyme, half of the parsley, celery seeds, and mushrooms to the Crock Pot. Put the cooker's lid on and set the cooking time to 4 hours on High settings. Stir in pasta and parsley. Serve.

Chicken And Lentils Meatballs

Ingredients: Servings: 4   Cooking Time: 2.5 Hours

½ C. red lentils, cooked	½ tsp. salt
10 oz. ground chicken	2 tbsp. flour
1 tsp. ground black pepper	1 tsp. sesame oil
	½ C. chicken stock

Directions:

Mix lentils with ground chicken. Add ground black pepper, salt, and flour. Make the meatballs and put them in the hot skillet. Add sesame oil and roast the meatballs for 1 minute per side on high heat. Pour chicken stock in the Crock Pot. Add meatballs and cook them on High for 2.5 hours.

Rosemary Rotisserie Chicken

Ingredients: Servings: 12   Cooking Time: 12 Hours

1-gallon water	¾ C. salt
2 tbsp. rosemary and other herbs of your choice	½ C. butter
	1 whole chicken, excess fat removed

Directions:

In a pot, combine the water, salt, sugar, and herbs. Stir to dissolve the salt and sugar. Submerge the chicken completely and allow to sit in the brine for 12 hours inside the fridge. Line the crockpot with tin foil. Place the chicken and cook on low for 12 hours or on high for 7 hours.

Algerian Chicken

Ingredients: Servings: 2   Cooking Time: 4 Hours

6 oz. chicken breast, skinless, boneless, sliced	1 tsp. harissa
	1 tbsp. sesame oil
1 tsp. peanut oil	1 C. tomatoes, canned
1 tsp. tomato paste	¼ C. of water

Directions:

Mix tomato paste with harissa, peanut oil, and sesame oil. Whisk the mixture and mix it with sliced chicken breast. After this, transfer the chicken in the Crock Pot in one layer. Add water and close the lid. Cook the chicken on High for 4 hours.

Sweet Potato Jalapeno Stew

Ingredients: Servings: 8   Cooking Time: 8 Hours

1 yellow onion, chopped	3 C. chicken stock
½ C. red beans, dried	2 jalapeno peppers, chopped
2 red bell peppers, chopped	Salt and black pepper to the taste
2 tbsp. ginger, grated	½ tsp. cumin, ground
4 garlic cloves, minced	½ tsp. coriander, ground
2 lbs. sweet, peeled and cubed	¼ tsp. cinnamon powder
14 oz. canned tomatoes, chopped	To Garnish:
	¼ C. peanuts, roasted and chopped
	Juice of ½ lime

Directions:
Add red beans along with all other ingredients to the Crock Pot. Put the cooker's lid on and set the cooking time to 8 hours on Low settings. Garnish with peanuts and lime juice. Serve warm.

Chicken Stuffed With Beans

Ingredients: Servings: 12   Cooking Time: 10 Hours

21 oz. whole chicken	1 tsp. oregano
1 chili pepper, chopped	1 tsp. apple cider vinegar
1 C. soybeans, canned	1 tsp. olive oil
2 red onion, peeled and diced	1 tbsp. dried basil
1 carrot, peeled and diced	1 tsp. paprika
1 tsp. onion powder	¼ tsp. ground red pepper
1 tsp. cilantro, chopped	½ C. fresh dill
	2 potatoes, peeled and diced
	4 tbsp. tomato sauce

Directions:
Blend chili pepper, onion powder, cilantro, oregano, olive oil, red pepper, tomato sauce, dill, paprika, basil, and vinegar in a blender. Stuff the whole chicken with soybeans, and vegetables. Brush it with the blender spice-chili mixture liberally. Place the spiced chicken in the Crock Pot and pour the remaining spice mixture over it. Put the cooker's lid on and set the cooking time to 10 hours on Low settings. Slice and serve.

Crockpot Chicken Curry

Ingredients: Servings: 6   Cooking Time: 8 Hours

2 lb. chicken breasts, bones removed	4 tbsp. curry powder
1 can coconut milk	Salt and pepper to taste
1 onion, chopped	

Directions:

Place all ingredients in the crockpot. Give a good stir to incorporate everything. Close the lid and cook on low for 8 hours or 6 hours on high.

Turkey With Zucchini

Ingredients: Servings: 4   Cooking Time: 8 Hours

1-lb. ground turkey	2 green onions, sliced
2 red peppers cut into strips	1 large zucchini, sliced
Salt and pepper to taste	

Directions:
Place the ground turkey and red peppers in the crockpot. Season with salt and pepper to taste. Close the lid and cook on low for 8 hours or on high for 6 hours. An hour before the cooking time is done, stir in the green onions and zucchini. Cook further until the vegetables are soft.

Basic Shredded Chicken

Ingredients: Servings: 12   Cooking Time: 8 Hours

6 lb. chicken breasts, bones and skin removed	1 tsp. salt
½ tsp. black pepper	5 C. homemade chicken broth
	4 tbsp. butter

Directions:
Place all ingredients in the CrockPot. Close the lid and cook on high for 6 hours or on low for 8 hours. Shred the chicken meat using two forks. Return to the CrockPot and cook on high for another 30 minutes.

Saucy Chicken

Ingredients: Servings: 4   Cooking Time: 5 Hours

1 chicken, cut into medium pieces	¼ C. chicken stock
Salt and black pepper to the taste	2 tbsp. white vinegar
1 tbsp. olive oil	¼ C. apricot preserves
½ tsp. sweet paprika	
¼ C. white wine	1 and ½ tsp. ginger, grated
½ tsp. marjoram, dried	2 tbsp. honey

Directions:
Add chicken, marjoram, and all other ingredients to the Crock Pot. Put the cooker's lid on and set the cooking time to 5 hours on Low settings. Serve warm.

Party Chicken Wings

Ingredients: Servings: 4   Cooking Time: 4 Hours

1-lb. chicken wings	2 tbsp. butter
3 tbsp. hot sauce	¼ C. of soy sauce

Directions:
Put all ingredients in the Crock Pot and close the lid. Cook the chicken wings on High for 4 hours. Then transfer the chicken wings in the big bowl and sprinkle with hot sauce gravy from the Crock Pot.

Pulled Maple Chicken

Ingredients: Servings: 2   Cooking Time: 6 Hours

2 tomatoes, chopped	1 tbsp. maple syrup
2 red onions, chopped	1 tsp. chili powder
2 chicken breasts, skinless and boneless	1 tsp. basil, dried
	3 tbsp. water
2 garlic cloves, minced	1 tsp. cloves, ground

Directions:

Place chicken along with all other ingredients in the Crock Pot. Put the cooker's lid on and set the cooking time to 6 hours on Low settings. Shred the cooked chicken and serve with the veggies. Enjoy.

Basil Chicken

Ingredients: Servings: 4   Cooking Time: 7 Hours

2 tbsp. balsamic vinegar	1 tsp. dried oregano
1 C. of water	1-lb. chicken fillet, sliced
1 tsp. dried basil	1 tsp. mustard

Directions:

Mix chicken fillet with mustard and balsamic vinegar. Add dried basil, oregano, and transfer in the Crock Pot. Add water and close the lid. Cook the chicken on low for 7 hours.

BEEF, PORK & LAMB RECIPES

Pineapple Pork

Ingredients: Servings: 4   Cooking Time: 4.5 Hours

½ C. pineapple, canned, chopped	1 tsp. smoked paprika
10 oz. pork sirloin, sliced	½ tsp. chili flakes
½ C. of water	1 tsp. butter

Directions:

Melt the butter in the skillet and add sliced pork sirloin. Sprinkle it with smoked paprika and chili flakes and roast for 5 minutes on high heat. Then transfer the meat in the Crock Pot, add water and pineapple. Close the lid and cook the meal on High for 5 hours.

Pesto Lamb Chops

Ingredients: Servings: 2   Cooking Time: 6 Hours

1 lb. lamb chops	2 tbsp. olive oil
2 tbsp. basil pesto	A pinch of salt and black pepper
1 tbsp. sweet paprika	½ C. beef stock

Directions:

In your Crock Pot, mix the lamb chops with the pesto, paprika and the other ingredients, toss, put the lid on and cook on Low for 6 hours. Divide the mix between plates and serve.

Radish And Pork Ragu

Ingredients: Servings: 4   Cooking Time: 7 Hours

2 C. radish, halved	2 tbsp. sesame oil
1 C. of water	1 tsp. sesame seeds
1 tbsp. dried dill	8 oz. pork tenderloin, sliced
½ tsp. dried basil	
1 tsp. salt	

Directions:

Put all ingredients in the Crock Pot. Carefully mix them and close the lid. Cook the pork ragu on Low for 7 hours.

Beef Dip

Ingredients: Servings: 6   Cooking Time: 10 Hours

½ C. heavy cream	1 tsp. garlic powder
1 onion, diced	4 oz. dried beef, chopped
1 tsp. cream cheese	
½ C. Cheddar cheese, shredded	½ C. of water

Directions:

Put all ingredients in the Crock Pot. Gently stir the ingredients and close the lid. Cook the dip on Low for 10 hours.

Creamy Beef

Ingredients: Servings: 2   Cooking Time: 6 Hours

1 lb. beef stew meat, cubed	1 red onion, sliced
1 C. heavy cream	3 scallions, chopped
½ tsp. turmeric powder	1 tbsp. chives, chopped
2 tbsp. olive oil	A pinch of salt and black pepper

Directions:

In your Crock Pot, mix the beef with the cream, onion and the other ingredients, toss, put the lid on and cook on Low for 6 hours. Divide everything between plates and serve.

Sausages In Sweet Currant Sauce

Ingredients: Servings: 4   Cooking Time: 4.5 Hours

1 tbsp. butter	1 C. of water
1 C. fresh currant	1-lb. beef sausages
1 tbsp. brown sugar	1 tbsp. sunflower oil

Directions:

Mix currants with brown sugar and blend with the help of the immersion blender until smooth. Pour the liquid in the Crock Pot. Add all remaining ingredients and close the lid. Cook the sausages on High for 5 hours.

Ginger Beef

Ingredients: Servings: 2   Cooking Time: 4.5 Hours

10 oz. beef brisket, sliced	1 tbsp. olive oil
1 tsp. minced ginger	1 tbsp. lemon juice
1 tsp. ground coriander	1 C. of water

Directions:

In the bowl mix lemon juice and olive oil. Then mix beef brisket with ground coriander and minced ginger. Sprinkle the meat with oil mixture and transfer in the Crock Pot. Add water and cook the meal on High for 5 hours.

Lamb Leg Mushrooms Satay

Ingredients: Servings: 8   Cooking Time: 8 Hrs.

1 and ½ lbs. lamb leg, bone-in	6 garlic cloves, minced
2 carrots, sliced	2 tbsp. tomato paste
½ lbs. mushrooms, sliced	1 tsp. olive oil
4 tomatoes, chopped	Salt and black pepper to the taste
1 small yellow onion, chopped	Handful parsley, chopped

Directions:

Add lamb, carrots, and all other ingredients to the Crock Pot. Put the cooker's lid on and set the cooking time to 8 hours on Low settings. Serve warm.

Tender Glazed Pork Ribs

Ingredients: Servings: 4   Cooking Time: 7 Hours

1-lb. baby back pork ribs	1 tbsp. tamarind
1 orange, sliced	½ C. apple juice
1 tsp. liquid honey	1 anise pod
	1 tbsp. tomato sauce

Directions:

Put the baby back ribs in the Crock Pot. Add tamarind, apple juice, tomato sauce, and anise pod. Then add sliced orange and close the lid. Cook the pork ribs on low for 6 hours. Then sprinkle the meat with liquid honey and cook on high for 1 hour.

Taco Pork

Ingredients: Servings: 5   Cooking Time: 5 Hours

1-lb. pork shoulder, chopped	1 tbsp. lemon juice
1 tbsp. taco seasonings	1 C. of water

Directions:

Mix pork shoulder with taco seasonings and place in the Crock Pot. Add water and cook it on High for 5 hours. After this, transfer the cooked meat in the bowl and shred gently with the help of the fork. Add lemon juice and shake gently.

Garlic-parmesan Beef

Ingredients: Servings: 2   Cooking Time: 4 Hours

1 oz. Parmesan, grated	1 tsp. olive oil
1 carrot, grated	1 tsp. chili powder
8 oz. ground beef	
½ C. of water	

Directions:

Mix the ground beef with carrot and transfer it in the Crock Pot. Add olive oil, chili powder, and water. Close the lid and cook

the beef on high for 4 hours. After this, add parmesan and carefully mix the meal.

Beef Chuck Roast

Ingredients: Servings: 6   Cooking Time: 8 Hours And 30 Minutes

4 lb. beef chuck roast	10 thyme springs
1 C. veggie stock	1 yellow onion, roughly chopped
1 tbsp. coconut oil	
1 bay leaf	2 celery ribs, roughly chopped
4 garlic cloves, minced	1 cauliflower head, florets separated
1 carrot, roughly chopped	Salt and black pepper to the taste

Directions:

Season beef with salt and some black pepper. Heat up a pan with the oil over medium-high heat, add beef roast, brown for 5 minutes on each side, transfer to your Crock Pot, add thyme springs, stock, bay leaf, garlic, celery, onion and carrot, cover and cook on Low for 8 hours. Add cauliflower, cover Crock Pot again, cook on High for 20 minutes more, divide everything between plates and serve.

Garlic Beef Sausages

Ingredients: Servings: 2   Cooking Time: 3 Hours

8 oz. beef sausages	1 tsp. dried thyme
1 tsp. garlic powder	2 tbsp. avocado oil
1 garlic clove, crushed	½ C. of water

Directions:

Chop the sausages roughly and sprinkle with garlic powder and dried thyme. Then heat the avocado oil in the skillet. Add the chopped sausages and roast for 1 minute per side. Transfer the sausages in the Crock Pot. Add all remaining ingredients and close the lid. Cook the sausages on High for 3 hours.

Rich Lamb Shanks

Ingredients: Servings: 4   Cooking Time: 7 Hours

2 tbsp. olive oil	4 lamb shanks
1 yellow onion, finely chopped	1 tsp. oregano, dried
3 carrots, roughly chopped	1 tomato, roughly chopped
2 garlic cloves, minced	4 oz. chicken stock
2 tbsp. tomato paste	Salt and black pepper to the taste

Directions:

In your Crock Pot, mix lamb with oil, onion, garlic, carrots, tomato paste, tomato, oregano, stock, salt and pepper, stir, cover and cook on Low for 7 hours. Divide into bowls and serve hot.

Short Ribs

Ingredients: Servings: 6   Cooking Time: 10 Hours

3 lb. beef short ribs	2 tbsp. tapioca, crushed
1 fennel bulb, cut into wedges	2 tbsp. tomato paste

2 yellow onions, cut into wedges
1 C. carrot, sliced
14 oz. canned tomatoes, chopped
1 C. dry red wine
1 tsp. rosemary, dried
Salt and black pepper to the taste
4 garlic cloves, minced

Directions:
In your Crock Pot, mix short ribs with fennel, onions, carrots, tomatoes, wine, tapioca, tomato paste, salt, pepper, rosemary and garlic, cover and cook on Low for 10 hours. Divide everything between plates and serve.

Lamb Casserole

Ingredients: Servings: 2   Cooking Time: 7 Hours

2 garlic cloves, minced
1 red onion, chopped
1 tbsp. olive oil
1 celery stick, chopped
10 oz. lamb fillet, cut into medium pieces
Salt and black pepper to the taste
1 and ¼ C. lamb stock
2 carrots, chopped
½ tbsp. rosemary, chopped
1 leek, chopped
1 tbsp. mint sauce
1 tsp. sugar
1 tbsp. tomato puree
½ cauliflower, florets separated
½ celeriac, chopped
2 tbsp. butter

Directions:
Heat up a Crock Pot with the oil over medium heat, add garlic, onion and celery, stir and cook for 5 minutes. Add lamb pieces, stir, brown for 3 minutes and transfer everything to your Crock Pot. Add carrot, leek, rosemary, stock, tomato puree, mint sauce, sugar, cauliflower, celeriac, butter, salt and black pepper, cover and cook on Low for 7 hours. Divide lamb and all the veggies between plates and serve.

Braised Lamb Shank

Ingredients: Servings: 4   Cooking Time: 10 Hours

4 lamb shanks
1 C. of water
½ C. tomato juice
1 tbsp. cornflour
1 tsp. salt
1 tsp. cayenne pepper
1 onion, chopped
½ carrot, chopped

Directions:
Mix tomato juice with cornflour and pour the liquid in the Crock Pot. Add lamb shanks, water, salt, cayenne pepper, onion, and carrot. Close the lid and cook the meat on low for 10 hours.

Jalapeno Basil Pork Chops

Ingredients: Servings: 4   Cooking Time: 12 Hours

½ C. jalapeno peppers, chopped
4 pork loin, chopped
½ C. dry white wine
¼ C. fresh basil
Salt and pepper to taste

Directions:
Place all ingredients in the crockpot. Give a good stir to combine all ingredients. Cook on low for 12 hours or on high for 8 hours.

Rosemary Lamb Shoulder

Ingredients: Servings: 3   Cooking Time: 9 Hours

1 tbsp. fresh rosemary
½ C. apple cider vinegar
1 tbsp. olive oil
9 oz. lamb shoulder
1 C. of water
1 tsp. ground black pepper
2 garlic cloves, peeled

Directions:
Rub the lamb shoulder with olive oil and fresh rosemary. Then put the lamb shoulder in the apple cider vinegar and leave for 30 minutes to marinate. After this, transfer the lamb shoulder in the Crock Pot. Add water, ground black pepper, and garlic cloves. Close the lid and cook the meat on low for 9 hours.

Pork In Onion Gravy

Ingredients: Servings: 4   Cooking Time: 9 Hours

2 C. onion, sliced
1 tsp. smoked paprika
½ tsp. dried parsley
2 tbsp. butter
1 C. cream
12 oz. pork loin, sliced

Directions:
Grease the Crock Pot bottom with butter. Put the onion inside in one layer. After this, add sliced pork loin and sprinkle it with smoked paprika and dried parsley. Add cream and close the lid. Cook the meal on Low for 9 hours.

Baked Sirloin In Crockpot

Ingredients: Servings: 8   Cooking Time: 12 Hours

2 lb. sirloin steak, cut into 1-inch pieces
Salt and pepper to taste
1 ½ tbsp. cumin
2 small red onions, cut into wedges
2 red bell peppers, cut into strips

Directions:
Season the steak with cumin, salt, and pepper. Grease a skillet and heat over medium flame. Sear the steak for 2 minutes on each side. Add the onions and sear until the edges turn brown. Place into the crockpot. Add a few tbsp. of water. Close the lid and cook on low for 10 hours or on high for 7 hours. An hour before the cooking time ends, stir in the red bell peppers. Cook until the bell peppers become soft.

Crockpot Pork Roast

Ingredients: Servings: 4   Cooking Time: 12 Hours

1-lb. pork loin roast, bones removed
3 tbsp. olive oil
1 tsp. thyme leaves
1 tsp. marjoram leaves
½ tbsp. dry mustard

Directions:
Line the bottom of the crockpot with foil. Combine all ingredients in a bowl. Massage the pork to coat all surface with the spices. Place in the crockpot and cook on low for 12 hours or on high for 8 hours.

Crockpot Creamy Beef Bourguignon

Ingredients: Servings: 8   Cooking Time: 10 Hours

3 beef steaks, cut into large chunks
3 tbsp. lard
3 cloves of garlic, minced
1 onion, diced
1 tbsp. organic tomato puree

4 C. white mushrooms, sliced
1 C. homemade chicken stock
Salt and pepper to taste
½ C. heavy cream

Directions:

Place all ingredients except the cream in the CrockPot. Give a good stir. Close the lid and cook on high for 8 hours or on low for 10 hours.

Pork Liver Kebabs

Ingredients: Servings: 6   Cooking Time: 3.5 Hours

15 oz. pork liver, roughly chopped
1 tsp. onion powder
1 tsp. garlic powder
½ tsp. salt

2 bell peppers, roughly chopped
1 tbsp. cornflour
1 C. of water
1 tbsp. coconut oil

Directions:

Sprinkle the pork liver with onion powder, garlic powder, cornflour, and salt. Then string the liver int skewers (wooden sticks) and sprinkle with coconut oil. Arrange the skewers in the Crock Pot. Add water and close the lid. Cook them on High for 3.5 hours.

Crockpot Pork Chili Verde

Ingredients: Servings: 9   Cooking Time: 10 Hours

1 C. tomatoes, chopped
1 C. onions, quartered
4 cloves of garlic, chopped
2 green chili peppers
½ tsp. oregano

½ tsp. cumin
2 lb. pork stew meat, bones removed
3 tbsp. butter, melted
3 tbsp. cilantro, chopped

Directions:

In a blender, place the tomatoes, onions, garlic, chili peppers, oregano, and cumin. Blend until smooth. Pour into the CrockPot and add the meat and butter. Close the lid and cook on high for 8 hours or on low for 10 hours. Garnish with cilantro once cooked.

Beef With Peas And Corn

Ingredients: Servings: 2   Cooking Time: 7 Hours

1 lb. beef stew meat, cubed
½ C. corn
½ C. fresh peas
1 tbsp. lime juice

2 scallions, chopped
1 C. beef stock
2 tbsp. tomato paste
½ C. chives, chopped

Directions:

In your Crock Pot, mix the beef with the corn, peas and the other ingredients, toss, put the lid on and cook on Low for 7 hours. Divide the mix between plates and serve right away.

Easy Crockpot Meatballs

Ingredients: Servings: 6   Cooking Time: 10 Hours

2 tbsp. olive oil
2 lb. ground beef
1 tbsp. cumin
1 tsp. paprika
2 eggs, beaten

3 cloves of garlic, minced
1 tbsp. dried parsley
Salt and pepper to taste

Directions:

Grease the bottom of the CrockPot with olive oil. Place all ingredients in the mixing bowl. Form small balls using your hands and place inside the CrockPot. Close the lid and cook on high for 6 hours or on low for 10 hours. Halfway through the cooking time, turn or flip the meatballs. Close the lid and continue cooking until meat is cooked through.

Stuffed Mushrooms With Ground Pork

Ingredients: Servings: 4   Cooking Time: 4 Hours

2 C. cremini mushrooms caps
1 C. ground pork
1 onion, minced

¼ C. butter
1 tsp. salt
¼ C. of water

Directions:

Mix ground pork with minced onion and salt. Then fill the cremini mushroom caps with ground pork mixture and put in the Crock Pot. Add butter and water. Cook the mushroom caps on High for 4 hours.

Herbed Cinnamon Beef

Ingredients: Servings: 6   Cooking Time: 5 Hrs.

4 lbs. beef brisket
2 oranges, sliced
2 garlic cloves, minced
2 yellow onions, thinly sliced
11 oz. celery, thinly sliced

1 tbsp. dill, dried
3 bay leaves
4 cinnamon sticks, cut into halves
Salt and black pepper to the taste
17 oz. veggie stock

Directions:

Add beef, orange slices, and all other ingredients to the insert of Crock Pot. Put the cooker's lid on and set the cooking time to 5 hours on High settings. Serve warm.

Beef Pot Roast

Ingredients: Servings: 6   Cooking Time: 12 Hours

2 lb. shoulder pot roast, bones removed
Salt and pepper to taste
¼ C. water

1 package mushrooms, sliced
1 tbsp. Worcestershire sauce

Directions:

Place all ingredients in the crockpot. Give a good stir. Close the lid and cook on low for 12 hours or on high for 10 hours.

Beef With Green Beans And Cilantro

Ingredients: Servings: 2   Cooking Time: 7 Hours

1 lb. beef stew meat, cubed
1 C. green beans, trimmed and halved
1 red onion, sliced
½ tsp. chili powder
½ tsp. rosemary, chopped
2 tsp. olive oil
1 C. beef stock
1 tbsp. cilantro, chopped

Directions:
In your Crock Pot, mix the beef with the green beans, onion and the other ingredients, toss, put the lid on and cook on Low for 7 hours. Divide the mix between plates and serve right away.

One Pot Pork Chops

Ingredients: Servings: 6   Cooking Time: 10 Hours

2 C. broccoli florets
½ C. green and red bell peppers
6 pork chops
1 onion, sliced
Salt and pepper to taste

Directions:
Place all ingredients in the crockpot. Give a stir to mix everything. Close the lid and cook on low for 10 hours or on high for 8 hours.

Barbecue Crockpot Meatloaf

Ingredients: Servings: 6   Cooking Time: 10 Hours

1-lb. ground beef
1 C. cheddar cheese
Salt and pepper to taste
2 eggs, beaten
2 tbsp. liquid smoke

Directions:
Place all ingredients in a mixing bowl. Scoop the mixture into greased ramekins. Place the ramekins inside the crockpot. Pour water into the crockpot such that 1/8 of the ramekins are soaked. Close the lid and cook on low for 10 hours or on high for 7 hours.

Crockpot Beef Picadillo

Ingredients: Servings: 8   Cooking Time: 10 Hours

2 lb. ground beef
1 ½ tbsp. chili powder
2 tbsp. dried oregano
1 tsp. cinnamon powder
1 C. tomatoes, chopped
1 red onions, chopped
2 Anaheim peppers, seeded and chopped
20 green olives, pitted and chopped
8 cloves of garlic, minced
Salt and pepper to taste

Directions:
Place all ingredients in the CrockPot. Give a good stir. Close the lid and cook on high for 8 hours or on low for 10 hours.

Bbq Ribs

Ingredients: Servings: 4   Cooking Time: 4 Hours

1-lb. pork ribs, roughly chopped
1 tsp. minced garlic
½ C. BBQ sauce
1 tbsp. olive oil
¼ C. plain yogurt

Directions:
Mix BBQ sauce with plain yogurt and minced garlic and pour it in the Crock Pot. Then pour olive oil in the skillet and heat well. Add pork ribs and roast them for 3 minutes per side on high heat. Transfer the pork ribs in the Crock Pot and carefully mix. Close the lid and cook them on High for 4 hours.

Cayenne Lamb Mix

Ingredients: Servings: 2   Cooking Time: 4 Hours

1 lb. lamb stew meat, cubed
½ C. tomato sauce
½ tsp. cayenne pepper
1 red onion, sliced
2 tsp. olive oil
½ tsp. sweet paprika
A pinch of salt and black pepper
1 tbsp. cilantro, chopped

Directions:
In your Crock Pot, mix the lamb with the tomato sauce, cayenne and the other ingredients, toss, put the lid on and cook on High for 4 hours.. Divide the mix between plates and serve.

Spiced Pork Belly

Ingredients: Servings: 8   Cooking Time: 12 Hours

1 tbsp. olive oil
2-lb. pork belly
3 cloves of garlic, crushed
½ tsp. ground black pepper
½ tsp. turmeric
½ tsp. ground cumin
½ tbsp. lemon juice
½ tbsp. salt

Directions:
Line the bottom of the CrockPot with aluminum foil. Grease the foil with olive oil. Place all ingredients in a mixing bowl. Massage and allow to marinate in the fridge for 2 hours. Place inside the CrockPot. Close the lid and cook on high for 10 hours or on low for 12 hours.

Pork With Apples

Ingredients: Servings: 4   Cooking Time: 8 Hrs.

A pinch of nutmeg, ground
2 lbs. pork tenderloin
4 apples, cored and sliced
2 tbsp. maple syrup

Directions:
Add apples to the insert of the Crock Pot. Drizzle nutmeg over the apples then add pork along with remaining ingredients. Put the cooker's lid on and set the cooking time to 8 hours on Low settings. Slice the pork and return to the apple mixture. Mix well and serve warm.

Bulgogi

Ingredients: Servings: 6   Cooking Time: 8 Hours

1-lb. beef chuck roast
5 tbsp. soy sauce
2 tbsp. sesame oil
1 tsp. ground black

2 tbsp. rice vinegar
2 tbsp. cornflour
2 C. beef stock

pepper
1 tsp. chili powder
1 onion, sliced
1 tsp. sriracha

Directions:

Chop the beef and put it in the Crock Pot. Then add soy sauce, rice vinegar, cornflour, sesame oil, ground black pepper, chili powder, onion, and sriracha. Mix the mixture well and add beef stock. Close the lid and cook the meal on low for 8 hours.

Pork Casserole

Ingredients: Servings: 4   Cooking Time: 8 Hours

1 C. cauliflower, chopped
1 tsp. ground black pepper
1 tsp. cayenne pepper

7 oz. pork mince
1 C. Cheddar cheese, shredded
½ C. cream
1 tsp. sesame oil

Directions:

Brush the Crock Pot bowl with sesame oil from inside. Then mix minced pork with ground black pepper and cayenne pepper. Place the meat in the Crock Pot and flatten gently. After this, top it with cauliflower and Cheddar cheese. Add cream and close the lid. Cook the casserole on Low for 8 hours.

Chinese Pork Ribs

Ingredients: Servings: 6   Cooking Time: 12 Hours

¼ C. soy sauce
2 cloves of garlic
2 tbsp. Chinese five-spice powder

4 lb. pork ribs, bone in
3 tbsp. sugar-free ketchup

Directions:

Combine everything in the crockpot. Close the lid and cook on low for 12 hours or on high for 8 hours.

Crockpot Asian Pot Roast

Ingredients: Servings: 6   Cooking Time: 10 Hours

2 lb. beef chuck roast, excess fat trimmed
1 ½ tsp. salt
3.4 tsp. ground black pepper
2 tbsp. basil, chopped

2 large yellow onions, chopped
4 cloves of garlic, minced
2 star anise pods
2 C. beef stock
3 tbsp. sesame seed oil

Directions:

Place all ingredients except for the sesame oil in the CrockPot. Close the lid and cook on high for 8 hours or on low for 10 hours. Once cooked, drizzle with sesame seed oil or sesame seeds. You can also garnish it with chopped scallions if desired.

Mussaman Curry

Ingredients: Servings: 4   Cooking Time: 5 Hours

16 oz. beef sirloin, cubed
1 tbsp. curry powder

1 tbsp. sesame oil
2 tbsp. peanut butter
¼ C. peanuts,

2 tbsp. coconut aminos
2 tbsp. soy sauce

chopped
1 C. coconut cream

Directions:

Mix curry powder with coconut aminos, soy sauce, sesame oil, and coconut cream. After this, mix the curry mixture with beef and transfer in the Crock Pot. Add all remaining ingredients and mix well. Close the lid and cook the curry on High for 5 hours.

Pork Cobbler

Ingredients: Servings: 4   Cooking Time: 4.5 Hours

½ C. flour
3 tbsp. coconut oil
6 oz. ground pork
1 carrot, grated
½ C. tomato juice

1 tsp. salt
1 tsp. chili flakes
¼ C. Cheddar cheese, shredded

Directions:

In the mixing bowl mix ground pork, carrot, tomato juice, salt, and chili flakes. Then mix flour with coconut oil. Separate the flour mixture into 3 parts. Crumble every flour part. Make the layer of flour crumbs in the Crock Pot. Top it with ground pork mixture. Then top the ground pork mixture with the second part of the crumble flour mixture. Repeat the same steps till you use all ingredients. Top the cobbler with Cheddar cheese. Add tomato juice and close the lid. Cook the cobbler on High for 4.5 hours.

Mole Pork Chops

Ingredients: Servings: 3   Cooking Time: 10 Hours

1 tbsp. butter, melted
3 pork chops, bone in
2 tsp. paprika

½ tsp. cocoa powder, unsweetened
Salt and pepper to taste

Directions:

Place the butter into the crockpot. Season the pork chops with paprika, cocoa powder, salt and pepper. Arrange in the crockpot. Close the lid and cook on low for 10 hours or on high for 8 hours. Halfway through the cooking time, be sure to flip the pork chops.

Bbq Meatballs

Ingredients: Servings: 4   Cooking Time: 7 Hours

3 tbsp. BBQ sauce
10 oz. minced pork
1 garlic clove, diced
1 tsp. chili powder

3 tbsp. water
1 tsp. salt
1 tsp. dried cilantro
4 tbsp. coconut oil

Directions:

In the bowl mix minced pork, garlic, chili powder, water, salt, and dried cilantro. Make the medium size meatballs and arrange them in the Crock Pot in one layer. Add coconut oil and close the lid. Cook the meatballs on low for 7 hours. When the meatballs are cooked, brush them gently with BBW sauce.

Jalapeno Mississippi Roast

Ingredients: Servings: 4   Cooking Time: 8 Hours

3 pepperoncini
1-lb. beef chuck roast
1 tsp. ground black pepper

2 tbsp. flour
½ tsp. salt
2 tbsp. avocado oil
2 C. of water

Directions:

Put all ingredients in the Crock Pot.   Close the lid and cook the meal on Low for 8 hours.   Then open the lid and shred the beef.

Beef And Sprouts

Ingredients: Servings: 2   Cooking Time: 7 Hours

1 tsp. olive oil
1 lb. beef stew meat, roughly cubed
1 C. Brussels sprouts, trimmed and halved

1 red onion, chopped
1 C. tomato passata
A pinch of salt and black pepper
1 tbsp. chives, chopped

Directions:

In your Crock Pot, mix the beef with the sprouts, oil and the other ingredients, toss, put the lid on and cook on Low for 7 hours. Divide the mix between plates and serve.

Pork Roast In Crockpot

Ingredients: Servings: 8   Cooking Time: 12 Hours

3 lb. pork shoulder roast
2 tbsp. herb mix of your choice

1 C. onion, chopped
Salt and pepper to taste
2 C. chicken broth

Directions:

Combine everything in the crockpot.   Close the lid and cook on low for 12 hours or on high for 8 hours.

Beef Chops With Sprouts

Ingredients: Servings: 5   Cooking Time: 7 Hours

1-lb. beef loin
½ C. bean sprouts
1 tbsp. tomato paste

1 C. of water
1 tsp. chili powder
1 tsp. salt

Directions:

Cut the beef loin into 5 beef chops and sprinkle the beef chops with chili powder and salt.   Then place them in the Crock Pot. Add water and tomato paste. Cook the meat on low for 7 hours. Then transfer the cooked beef chops in the plates, sprinkle with tomato gravy from the Crock Pot, and top with bean sprouts.

Short Ribs With Tapioca Sauce

Ingredients: Servings: 6   Cooking Time: 10 Hrs.

3 lbs. beef short ribs
1 fennel bulb, cut into wedges
2 yellow onions, cut into wedges
1 C. carrot, sliced
14 oz. canned tomatoes, chopped

1 C. dry red wine
2 tbsp. tapioca, crushed
2 tbsp. tomato paste
1 tsp. rosemary, dried
Salt and black pepper to the taste
4 garlic cloves, minced

Directions:

Add short ribs, onion, and all other ingredients to the insert of Crock Pot.   Put the cooker's lid on and set the cooking time to 10 hours on Low settings.   Serve warm.

Beef Meatballs Casserole

Ingredients: Servings: 8   Cooking Time: 7 Hours

1/3 C. flour
2 eggs
1 lb. beef sausage, chopped
Salt and black pepper to taste
1 tbsp. parsley, dried
¼ tsp. red pepper flakes
¼ C. parmesan, grated

1 lb. beef, ground
¼ tsp. onion powder
½ tsp. garlic powder
¼ tsp. oregano, dried
1 C. ricotta cheese
2 C. marinara sauce
1 and ½ C. mozzarella cheese, shredded

Directions:

In a bowl, mix sausage with beef, salt, pepper, almond flour, parsley, pepper flakes, onion powder, garlic powder, oregano, parmesan and eggs, stir well and shape meatballs out of this mix. Arrange meatballs in your Crock Pot, add half of the marinara sauce, ricotta cheese and top with the rest of the marinara.   Add mozzarella at the end, cover and cook on Low for 7 hours. Divide between plates and serve.

Lamb Saute

Ingredients: Servings: 5   Cooking Time: 4.5 Hours

1 C. tomatoes, chopped
1 C. bell pepper, chopped
1 chili pepper, chopped
1 C. of water

1 tbsp. avocado oil
12 oz. lamb fillet, chopped
½ C. cremini mushrooms, sliced

Directions:

Heat the avocado oil in the skillet well.   Add chopped lamb and roast it for 5 minutes. Stir the meat from time to time.   After this, transfer the meat in the Crock Pot and add all remaining ingredients.   Close the lid and cook the saute on High for 5 hours.

Beef Burger

Ingredients: Servings: 4   Cooking Time: 6 Hours

1 tsp. ground black pepper
12 oz. ground beef
¼ C. Cheddar cheese, shredded

1 tsp. salt
1 tbsp. sunflower oil
¼ C. cream

Directions:

Mix ground beef with salt, and ground black pepper.   Then add shredded cheese and carefully mix the meat mixture.   Pour sunflower oil in the Crock Pot.   Then make the burgers and place them in the Crock Pot.   Add cream and close the lid. Cook the meal on Low for 6 hours.

Ginger Beef Balls

Ingredients: Servings: 4   Cooking Time: 4 Hours

1 tsp. ground ginger	1 tsp. chili flakes
1 tsp. garlic powder	¼ C. of water
¼ C. butter	12 oz. ground beef
	1 egg, beaten

Directions:

In the mixing bowl mix ground beef, egg, chili flakes, garlic powder, and ground ginger. Make the small balls. After this, melt the butter in the skillet. Add meatballs and roast them for 3 minutes per side. Transfer the meatballs in the Crock Pot. Add water and close the lid. Cook the meatballs on High for 4 hours.

Pork Ragu With Basil

Ingredients: Servings: 4   Cooking Time: 4 Hours

8 oz. pork loin, chopped	½ C. carrot, chopped
1 C. russet potatoes	1 tsp. salt
3 oz. fennel bulb, chopped	3 C. of water
1 tbsp. dried basil	½ C. plain yogurt
	1 tsp. tomato paste

Directions:

In the mixing bowl mix tomato paste with plain yogurt, salt, dried basil, and pork loin. Transfer the mixture in the Crock Pot and close the lid. Cook the meat on high for 2 hours. Then add water and all remaining ingredients. Carefully mix the mixture. Close the lid and cook the ragu on low for 5 hours.

Strip Steak With Poblano Peppers

Ingredients: Servings: 4   Cooking Time: 12 Hours

2 New York strip steaks	1 onion, cut into wedges
¼ tsp. smoked paprika	1 tbsp. sesame oil
2 poblano peppers, sliced	

Directions:

Place all ingredients except for the sesame oil in the crockpot. Add a few tbsp. of water. Give a good stir. Close the lid and cook on low for 12 hours or on high for 10 hours. Pour sesame oil before serving.

Seasoned Beef Stew

Ingredients: Servings: 6   Cooking Time: 8 Hrs.

4 lbs. beef roast	1 yellow onion, chopped
2 C. beef stock	1 tbsp. onion powder
2 sweet potatoes, cubed	1 tbsp. garlic powder
6 carrots, sliced	1 tbsp. sweet paprika
7 celery stalks, chopped	Salt and black pepper to the taste

Directions:

Add sweet potatoes, beef and all other ingredients to the insert of Crock Pot. Put the cooker's lid on and set the cooking time to 8 hours on Low settings. Slice the cooked roast and serve with mixed vegetables. Enjoy.

Herbed Lamb Shanks

Ingredients: Servings: 4   Cooking Time: 8 Hrs. 10 Minutes

4 lamb shanks, trimmed	2 carrots, chopped
3 tbsp. olive oil	2 tbsp. tomato paste
1 onion, chopped	2 C. veggie stock
15 oz. canned tomatoes, chopped	1 tbsp. rosemary, dried
2 garlic cloves, minced	1 tbsp. thyme, dried
2 celery stalks, chopped	1 tbsp. oregano, dried
	Salt and black pepper to the taste

Directions:

Place a suitable pan over medium-high heat and add 2 tbsp. oil. Add lamb shanks to the oil and sear for 5 minutes per side. Transfer the lamb shank to the Crock Pot along with onion and other ingredients. Put the cooker's lid on and set the cooking time to 8 hours on Low settings. Serve warm.

Ground Beef Zucchini Squares

Ingredients: Servings: 4   Cooking Time: 4.5 Hours

2 large zucchinis, trimmed	1 tsp. ground black pepper
2 tbsp. ricotta cheese	½ C. of water
9 oz. ground beef	1 tsp. butter

Directions:

Slice the zucchini into strips. Then put butter in the Crock Pot and melt it. Add ground beef and ground black pepper. Roast the meat mixture for 5 minutes. After this, add ricotta cheese and carefully mix. Make the cross from 2 zucchini strips. Put the small amount of the ground beef mixture in the center of the zucchini cross and wrap it into squares. Repeat the same steps with all remaining zucchini and meat mixture. Put the zucchini squares in the Crock Pot. Add water and close the lid. Cook the meal on High for 4.5 hours.

Braised Pork Knuckle

Ingredients: Servings: 7   Cooking Time: 10 Hours

3-lb. pork knuckles	2 C. of water
1 tbsp. liquid honey	1 tsp. dried mint
1 C. red wine	1 tsp. salt
	1 cinnamon stick

Directions:

Put all ingredients in the Crock Pot. Close the lid and cook the pork knuckle on Low for 10 hours.

Tomatillo Lamb

Ingredients: Servings: 8   Cooking Time: 7 Hrs.

4 tbsp. dried rosemary	18 oz. lamb leg
1 C. tomatillos, chopped	1 tsp. salt
1 tbsp. minced garlic	1 C. cream
	½ tsp. ground black pepper

2 oz. fresh rosemary
1 onion, grated

Directions:

Add tomatillos, garlic, dried and fresh rosemary, black pepper, salt, and onion to a blender jug. Blend the tomatillos mixture until smooth. Add lamb leg to the insert of the Crock Pot and pour the tomatillo mixture on top. Put the cooker's lid on and set the cooking time to 7 hours on Low settings. Serve warm.

Pork And Zucchini Bowl

Ingredients: Servings: 4   Cooking Time: 5 Hours

12 oz. pork stew meat, cubed	1 tsp. dried dill
1 C. zucchini, chopped	1 tsp. salt
1 tsp. white pepper	½ C. sour cream
	1 C. of water
	1 chili pepper, chopped

Directions:

Put meat in the Crock Pot. Add white pepper, dried dill, salt, sour cream, water, and chili pepper. Close the lid and cook the meal on High for 4 hours. Then add zucchini and cook the meal on High for 1 hour more.

Skirt Steak With Red Pepper Sauce

Ingredients: Servings: 4   Cooking Time: 12 Hours

2 red bell peppers, chopped	1-lb. skirt steak, sliced into 1 inch thick
2 tbsp. olive oil	Salt and pepper to taste
1 tsp. thyme leaves	

Directions:

In a food processor, mix together the red bell peppers, olive oil, and thyme leaves. Blend until smooth. Add water to make the mixture slightly runny. Set aside. Season the skirt steak with salt and pepper. Place in the crockpot and pour over the pepper sauce. Add more salt and pepper if desired. Close the lid and cook on low for 12 hours or on high for 10 hours.

Crockpot Gingered Pork Stew

Ingredients: Servings: 9   Cooking Time: 12 Hours

2 tbsp. ground cinnamon	1 ½ tsp. ground cloves
2 tbsp. ground ginger	3 lb. pork shoulder, cut into cubes
1 tbsp. ground allspice	2 C. homemade chicken broth
1 tbsp. ground nutmeg	Salt and pepper to taste
1 tbsp. paprika	

Directions:

Place all ingredients in the CrockPot. Give a good stir. Close the lid and cook on high for 10 hours or on low for 12 hours.

Spicy Beef Curry

Ingredients: Servings: 6   Cooking Time: 10 Hours

2 ½ lb. beef chuck, cubed	1 onion, chopped
2 tbsp. curry powder	½-inch ginger, grated
3 cloves of garlic, minced	2 C. coconut milk, unsweetened
	Salt and pepper to taste

Directions:

Place all ingredients in the CrockPot. Close the lid and cook on high for 8 hours or on low for 10 hours.

Pork Ribs Braised In Wine

Ingredients: Servings: 4   Cooking Time: 6 Hours

1-lb. pork ribs, roughly chopped	1 tsp. brown sugar
½ C. wine	1 tsp. clove
2 garlic cloves, crushed	½ tsp. chili flakes

Directions:

Rub the pork ribs with chili flakes and put in the Crock Pot. Add garlic, brown sugar, and clove. Then add the wine and close the lid. Cook the meal on Low for 6 hours.

Wine-braised Beef Heart

Ingredients: Servings: 4   Cooking Time: 5 Hours

10 oz. beef heart	1 tsp. salt
1/3 C. red wine	1 tsp. peppercorns
½ C. beef broth	1 tsp. brown sugar
½ C. potatoes, chopped	Cooking spray
3 oz. fennel bulb, chopped	

Directions:

Spray the skillet with cooking spray. Then chop the beef heart roughly and put it in the skillet. Roast the beef heart on high heat for 6 minutes (for 3 minutes per side). Transfer the beef heart in the Crock Pot. Add all remaining ingredients and close the lid. Cook the meal on High for 5 hours.

Beef And Artichokes Bowls

Ingredients: Servings: 2   Cooking Time: 7 Hours

6 oz. beef sirloin, chopped	½ tsp. white pepper
½ tsp. cayenne pepper	4 artichoke hearts, chopped
1 C. of water	1 tsp. salt

Directions:

Mix meat with white pepper and cayenne pepper. Transfer it in the Crock Pot bowl. Add salt, artichoke hearts, and water. Close the lid and cook the meal on Low for 7 hours.

Veal Stew

Ingredients: Servings: 12   Cooking Time: 8 Hours

2 tbsp. avocado oil	1 C. water
3 lb. veal, cubed	10 oz. canned tomato paste
1 yellow onion,	

chopped
1 small garlic clove, minced
Salt and black pepper to the taste
1 and ½ C. marsala wine
1 carrot, chopped
7 oz. mushrooms, chopped
3 egg yolks
½ C. heavy cream
2 tsp. oregano, dried

Directions:

Heat up a Crock Pot with the oil over medium-high heat, add veal, stir, brown for a few minutes, transfer to your Crock Pot, add garlic, onion, wine, water, oregano, tomato paste, mushrooms, carrots, salt and pepper, stir, cover and cook on Low for 7 hours and 30 minutes   In a bowl, mix cream with egg yolks and whisk well.   Pour this over the meat, cover and cook on Low for 30 minutes more.   Divide between plates and serve hot.

Ginger Ground Pork

Ingredients: Servings: 3   Cooking Time: 6 Hours

1.5 C. ground pork
1 oz. minced ginger
2 tbsp. coconut oil
1 tbsp. tomato paste
½ tsp. chili powder

Directions:

Mix ground pork with minced ginger, tomato paste, and chili powder.   Put the ground pork in the Crock Pot.   Add coconut oil and close the lid.   Cook the meal on Low for 6 hours.

Smothered Pepper Steak

Ingredients: Servings: 4   Cooking Time: 10 Hours

1 package bell peppers
Salt and pepper to taste
1 can diced tomatoes
1 tbsp. soy sauce
4 sirloin patties

Directions:

Place the diced tomatoes (juices and all) in the crockpot.   Add the bell peppers. Season with salt, pepper, and soy sauce. Arrange the sirloin patties on top.   Close the lid and cook on low for 10 hours or on high for 7 hours.

Pork And Eggplant Mix

Ingredients: Servings: 2   Cooking Time: 7 Hours

1 lb. pork stew meat, cubed
1 eggplant, cubed
2 scallions, chopped
2 garlic cloves, minced
½ C. beef stock
¼ C. tomato sauce
1 tsp. sweet paprika
1 tbsp. chives, chopped

Directions:

In your Crock Pot, mix the pork stew meat with the scallions, eggplant and the other ingredients, toss, put the lid on and cook on Low for 7 hours.   Divide the mix between plates and serve right away.

Beef And Sauce

Ingredients: Servings: 2   Cooking Time: 8 Hours

1 lb. beef stew meat, cubed
1 C. beef stock
1 tsp. garlic, minced

1 tsp. garam masala
½ tsp. turmeric powder
Salt and black pepper to the taste
½ C. sour cream
2 oz. cream cheese, soft
1 tbsp. chives, chopped

Directions:

In your Crock Pot, mix the beef with the turmeric, garam masala and the other ingredients, toss, put the lid on and cook on Low for 8 hours.   Divide everything into bowls and serve.

Beef And Peppers

Ingredients: Servings: 2   Cooking Time: 4 Hours

1 lb. lamb stew meat, cubed
1 red bell pepper, cut into strips
1 green bell pepper, cut into strips
1 orange bell pepper, cut into strips
2 tsp. olive oil
A pinch of salt and black pepper
1 C. beef stock
1 tbsp. chives, chopped
½ tsp. sweet paprika

Directions:

In your Crock Pot, mix the lamb with the peppers and the other ingredients, toss, put the lid on and cook on High for 4 hours. Divide the mix between plate sand serve.

Hot Sloppy Joes

Ingredients: Servings: 4   Cooking Time: 6 Hours

2 C. ground pork
2 tbsp. hot sauce
½ C. bell pepper, chopped
1 C. white onion, diced
1 tbsp. tomato paste
½ C. tomato juice
1 tsp. ground cumin
¼ C. of water

Directions:

Put the ground pork in the Crock Pot.   Add hot sauce, bell pepper, white onion, tomato paste, tomato juice, and ground cumin.   Carefully mix the meat mixture and add water.   Close the lid and cook the meal on Low for 6 hours.   Stir the meal well before serving.

Pork And Olives Mix

Ingredients: Servings: 2   Cooking Time: 8 Hours

1 lb. pork roast, sliced
½ C. tomato passata
1 red onion, sliced
1 C. kalamata olives, pitted and halved
Juice of ½ lime
¼ C. beef stock
Salt and black pepper to the taste
1 tbsp. chives, hopped

Directions:

In your Crock Pot, mix the pork slices with the passata, onion, olives and the other ingredients, toss, put the lid on and cook on Low for 8 hours.   Divide the mix between plates and serve.

Pork Sirloin Salsa Mix

Ingredients: Servings: 4   Cooking Time: 8 Hours

2 lb. pork sirloin
roast, cut into thick
slices
Salt and black pepper
to the taste
2 tsp. garlic powder

2 tsp. cumin, ground
1 tbsp. olive oil
16 oz. green chili
tomatillo salsa

Directions:

In your Crock Pot, mix pork with cumin, salt, pepper and garlic powder and rub well. Add oil and salsa, toss, cover and cook on Low for 8 hours. Divide between plates and serve hot.

Carrot And Pork Cubes

Ingredients: Servings: 2   Cooking Time: 4 Hours

8 oz. pork tenderloin,
cubed
1 C. carrot, cubed
1 tbsp. tomato paste

1 tbsp. avocado oil
1 tsp. salt
1 tsp. white pepper

Directions:

Pour the avocado oil in the skillet and preheat it well. Then put the pork tenderloins in the hot oil and roast on high heat for 3 minutes per side. Transfer the roasted meat in the Crock Pot and add all remaining ingredients. Close the lid and cook the pork on high for 4 hours.

Tarragon Pork Chops

Ingredients: Servings: 2   Cooking Time: 6 Hours

½ lb. pork chops
¼ tbsp. olive oil
2 garlic clove, minced
¼ tsp. chili powder
½ C. beef stock

½ tsp. coriander,
ground
Salt and black pepper
to the taste
¼ tsp. mustard
powder
1 tbsp. tarragon,
chopped

Directions:

Grease your Crock Pot with the oil and mix the pork chops with the garlic, stock and the other ingredients inside. Toss, put the lid on, cook on Low for 6 hours, divide between plates and serve with a side salad.

Parmesan Rosemary Potato

Ingredients: Servings: 5   Cooking Time: 4 Hours

1 lb. small potato,
peeled
½ C. fresh dill,
chopped
7 oz. Parmesan,
shredded

1 tsp. rosemary
1 tsp. thyme
1 C. of water
¼ tsp. chili flakes
3 tbsp. cream
1 tsp. salt

Directions:

Add potatoes, salt, rosemary, chili flakes, thyme, and water to the Crock Pot. Put the cooker's lid on and set the cooking time to 2 hours on High settings. Drizzle the remaining ingredients over the potatoes. Cover again and slow cook for another 2 hours on High. Serve warm.

Sausage Soup

Ingredients: Servings: 6   Cooking Time: 6 Hours

1 tbsp. avocado oil
32 oz. pork sausage
meat, ground
10 oz. canned
tomatoes and
jalapenos, chopped
10 oz. spinach
1 green bell pepper,
chopped
4 C. beef stock

1 tsp. onion powder
Salt and black pepper
to the taste
1 tbsp. cumin
1 tbsp. chili powder
1 tsp. garlic powder
1 tsp. Italian
seasoning

Directions:

Heat up a pan with the oil over medium heat, add sausage, stir, brown for a couple of minutes on all sides and transfer to your Crock Pot. Add green bell pepper, canned tomatoes and jalapenos, stock, onion powder, salt, pepper, cumin, chili powder, garlic powder, Italian seasoning and stock, stir, cover and cook on Low for 5 hours and 30 minutes. Add spinach, cover, cook on Low for 30 minutes more, stir soup, ladle it into bowls and serve.

Lamb And Kale

Ingredients: Servings: 2   Cooking Time: 4 Hours

1 lb. lamb shoulder,
cubed
1 C. baby kale
1 tbsp. olive oil
1 yellow onion,
chopped
½ tsp. coriander,
ground

½ tsp. cumin,
ground
½ tsp. sweet paprika
A pinch of salt and
black pepper
¼ C. beef stock
1 tbsp. chives,
chopped

Directions:

In your Crock Pot, mix the lamb with the kale, oil, onion and the other ingredients, toss, put the lid on and cook on High for 4 hours. Divide everything between plates and serve.

Italian Pork Roast

Ingredients: Servings: 10   Cooking Time: 12 Hours

5 lb. pork shoulder,
bone in
7 cloves of garlic,
slivered
1 tbsp. salt
1 tsp. dried oregano

1 tsp. dried basil
1 tsp. dried rosemary
½ tsp. black pepper

Directions:

Place all ingredients in the CrockPot. Give a good stir. Close the lid and cook on high for 10 hours or on low for 12 hours.

Thyme Pork Belly

Ingredients: Servings: 6   Cooking Time: 10 Hours

10 oz. pork belly
1 tsp. ground thyme
1 tsp. ground black
pepper

1 tsp. salt
1 tsp. garlic powder
½ C. of water

Directions:

In the shallow bowl mix salt, ground thyme, ground black pepper, and garlic powder. Then rub the pork belly with the spice mixture and place it in the Crock Pot. Add water and close the lid. Cook the pork belly on Low for 10 hours. Then slice the cooked pork belly into servings.

Mexican Bubble Pizza

Ingredients: Servings: 6   Cooking Time: 6 Hours

1 ½ lb. ground beef	1 C. mozzarella
1 tbsp. taco seasoning	cheese
2 C. cheddar cheese, shredded	1 can condensed tomato soup

Directions:

Heat skillet over medium flame and brown the ground beef for a few minutes. Stir in taco seasoning. Place the cheddar cheese into the crockpot. Add the sautéed ground beef on top of the cheddar cheese. Pour the tomato sauce. Sprinkle with mozzarella cheese on top. Close the lid and cook on low for 6 hours and on high for 4 hours.

Simple Pork Chop Casserole

Ingredients: Servings: 4   Cooking Time: 10 Hours

4 pork chops, bones removed and cut into bite-sized pieces	½ C. water
3 tbsp. minced onion	Salt and pepper to taste
	1 C. heavy cream

Directions:

Place the pork chop slices, onions, and water in the crockpot. Season with salt and pepper to taste. Close the lid and cook on low for 10 hours or on high for 8 hours. Halfway through the cooking time, pour in the heavy cream.

Walnut And Coconut Beef

Ingredients: Servings: 2   Cooking Time: 7 Hours

1 lb. beef stew meat, cubed	½ tsp. Italian seasoning
2 tbsp. walnuts, chopped	A pinch of salt and black pepper
½ C. coconut cream	1 tbsp. rosemary, chopped
2 scallions, chopped	
1 C. beef stock	

Directions:

In your Crock Pot, mix the beef with the walnuts, scallions and the other ingredients except the cream, toss, put the lid on and cook on Low for 6 hours. Add the cream, toss, cook on Low for 1 more hour, divide everything between plates and serve.

Caribbean Pork Chop

Ingredients: Servings: 4   Cooking Time: 10 Hours

1 tbsp. curry powder	1 tsp. cumin
Salt and pepper to taste	1-lb. pork loin roast, bones removed
	½ C. chicken broth

Directions:

Place all ingredients in the crockpot. Give a good stir. Close the lid and cook on low for 8 to 10 hours or on high for 7 hours.

Cucumber And Pork Cubes Bowl

Ingredients: Servings: 4   Cooking Time: 4 Hours

3 cucumbers, chopped	1 red onion, diced
1 jalapeno pepper, diced	1 tbsp. olive oil
	8 oz. pork tenderloin
3 tbsp. soy sauce	1 C. of water

Directions:

Pour water in the Crock Pot. Add pork tenderloin and cook it on High for 4 hours. Meanwhile, mix the red onion with jalapeno pepper and cucumbers in the salad bowl. In the shallow bowl mix soy sauce and olive oil. When the pork is cooked, chop it roughly and add in the cucumber salad. Sprinkle the salad with oil-soy sauce mixture and shake well.

Lamb With Thyme

Ingredients: Servings: 2   Cooking Time: 10 Hours

2 lamb shoulder chops, bone in	¼ C. thyme sprigs, chopped
1 C. homemade chicken broth	Salt and pepper to taste
1 tsp. garlic paste	

Directions:

Place all ingredients in the CrockPot. Give a good stir. Close the lid and cook on high for 8 hours or on low for 10 hours.

FISH & SEAFOOD RECIPES

Thai Style Flounder

Ingredients: Servings: 6   Cooking Time: 6 Hours

24 oz. flounder, peeled, cleaned	1 lemon, sliced
1 tsp. ground ginger	1 tsp. salt
½ tsp. cayenne pepper	1 tsp. ground turmeric
½ tsp. chili powder	1 tbsp. sesame oil
	1 C. of water

Directions:

Chop the flounder roughly and put in the Crock Pot. Add water and all remaining ingredients. Close the lid and cook the fish on low for 6 hours.

Balsamic-glazed Salmon

Ingredients: Servings: 7   Cooking Time: 1.5 Hrs.

5 tbsp. brown sugar	½ tsp. ground black pepper
2 tbsp. sesame seeds	
1 tbsp. balsamic vinegar	1 tsp. ground paprika
1 tbsp. butter	1 tsp. turmeric
3 tbsp. water	¼ tsp. fresh rosemary
1 tsp. salt	1 tsp. olive oil
	21 oz. salmon fillet

Directions:

Whisk rosemary, black pepper, salt, turmeric, and paprika in a small bowl. Rub the salmon fillet with this spice's mixture. Grease a suitable pan with olive oil and place it over medium-high heat. Place the spiced salmon fillet in the hot pan and sear it for 3 minutes per side. Add butter, sesame seeds, brown sugar, balsamic vinegar, and water to the insert of the Crock Pot. Put the cooker's lid on and set the cooking time to 30 minutes on High settings. Stir this sugar mixture occasionally. Place the salmon fillet in the Crock Pot. Put the cooker's lid on and set the cooking time to 1 hour on Low settings. Serve warm.

Baked Cod

Ingredients: Servings: 2   Cooking Time: 5 Hours

2 cod fillets	1 tsp. salt
2 tsp. cream cheese	½ tsp. cayenne
2 tbsp. bread crumbs	pepper
	2 oz. Mozzarella, shredded

Directions:

Sprinkle the cod fillets with cayenne pepper and salt. Put the fish in the Crock Pot. Then top it with cream cheese, bread crumbs, and Mozzarella. Close the lid and cook the meal for 5 hours on Low.

Tuna And Green Beans

Ingredients: Servings: 2   Cooking Time: 3 Hours

1 lb. tuna fillets, boneless	3 scallions, minced
1 C. green beans, trimmed and halved	½ tsp. ginger, ground
½ C. chicken stock	1 tbsp. olive oil
½ tsp. sweet paprika	1 tbsp. chives, chopped
½ tsp. garam masala	Salt and black pepper to the taste

Directions:

In your Crock Pot, mix the tuna with the green beans, stock and the other ingredients, toss gently, put the lid on and cook on High for 3 hours. Divide the mix between plates and serve.

Poached Cod And Pineapple Mix

Ingredients: Servings: 2   Cooking Time: 4 Hours

1 lb. cod, boneless	1 C. pineapple, chopped
6 garlic cloves, minced	¼ C. white vinegar
1 small ginger pieces, chopped	4 jalapeno peppers, chopped
½ tbsp. black peppercorns	Salt and black pepper to the taste
1 C. pineapple juice	

Directions:

Put the fish in your crock, season with salt and pepper. Add garlic, ginger, peppercorns, pineapple juice, pineapple chunks, vinegar and jalapenos. Stir gently, cover and cook on Low for 4 hours. Divide fish between plates, top with the pineapple mix and serve.

Butter Crab

Ingredients: Servings: 4   Cooking Time: 4.5 Hours

1-lb. crab meat, roughly chopped	1 tbsp. fresh parsley, chopped
3 tbsp. butter	2 tbsp. water

Directions:

Melt butter and pour it in the Crock Pot. Add water, parsley, and crab meat. Cook the meal on Low for 4.5 hours.

Orange Cod

Ingredients: Servings: 4   Cooking Time: 3 Hours

1-lb. cod fillet, chopped	1 C. of water
2 oranges, chopped	1 garlic clove, diced
1 tbsp. maple syrup	1 tsp. ground black pepper

Directions:

Mix cod with ground black pepper and transfer in the Crock Pot. Add garlic, water, maple syrup, and oranges. Close the lid and cook the meal on High for 3 hours.

Crockpot Garlic Shrimps

Ingredients: Servings: 5   Cooking Time: 3 Hours

4 tbsp. butter	¼ tsp. black pepper
¼ C. olive oil	
5 cloves of garlic, minced	1 ½ lb. jumbo shrimps, shelled and deveined.
½ tsp. salt	

Directions:

Place all ingredients in the CrockPot. Give a good stir. Close the lid and cook on high for 2 hours or on low for 3 hours. Garnish with chopped parsley if desired.

Crockpot Shrimp Gambas

Ingredients: Servings: 4   Cooking Time: 3 Hours

1/3 C. extra virgin olive oil	1 ¼ tsp. Spanish paprika
5 cloves of garlic, chopped	Salt and pepper to taste
1 tsp. red pepper flakes	2 tbsp. parsley, chopped
1 ¼ lb. shrimps, peeled and deveined	

Directions:

Place all ingredients in the CrockPot. Give a good stir. Close the lid and cook on high for 2 hours or on low for 3 hours.

Herbed Shrimps

Ingredients: Servings: 4   Cooking Time: 40 Minutes

4 tbsp. fresh dill	1 tsp. ground ginger
¼ C. pineapple juice	½ tsp. lemon juice
2 tbsp. sugar	1 tbsp. tomato juice
3 tbsp. mango puree	1 C. of water
1 tbsp. butter	½ tsp. sage
1 lb. shrimp, peeled	

Directions:

Add shrimp, water, and sage to the insert of Crock Pot. Put the cooker's lid on and set the cooking time to 20 minutes on High settings. Meanwhile, mix melted butter, mango puree, pineapple juice, sugar, lemon juice, ginger ground, dill and tomatoes juice in a bowl. Add this mixture to the shrimp in the Crock Pot. Put the cooker's lid on and set the cooking time to 20 minutes on High settings. Serve warm.

Oregano Shrimp Bowls

Ingredients: Servings: 2   Cooking Time: 1 Hour

1 lb. shrimp, peeled and deveined	½ C. baby spinach
½ C. cherry tomatoes, halved	¼ C. fish stock
1 tbsp. lime juice	½ tsp. sweet paprika
1 tbsp. oregano, chopped	2 garlic cloves, chopped
	A pinch of salt and black pepper

Directions:

In your Crock Pot, mix the shrimp with the cherry tomatoes, spinach and the other ingredients, toss, put the lid on and cook on High for 1 hour. Divide everything between plates and serve.

Mustard Salmon Salad

Ingredients: Servings: 4   Cooking Time: 3 Hours

1 C. lettuce, chopped	1 tbsp. mustard
1 C. spinach, chopped	1 tsp. olive oil
2 tbsp. plain yogurt	8 oz. salmon fillet
	¼ C. of water
	1 tsp. butter

Directions:

Pour water in the Crock Pot. Add butter and salmon. Close the lid and cook it on High for 3 hours. After this, chop the salmon roughly and put it in the salad bowl. Add chopped spinach and lettuce. In the shallow bowl mix mustard, plain yogurt, and olive oil. Whisk the mixture. Shake the salmon salad and sprinkle with mustard dressing.

Hot Salmon

Ingredients: Servings: 4   Cooking Time: 3 Hours

1-lb. salmon fillet, sliced	1 tbsp. olive oil
2 chili peppers, chopped	½ C. cream
1 onion, diced	½ tsp. salt

Directions:

Mix salmon with salt, onion, and olive oil. Transfer the ingredients in the Crock Pot. Add cream and onion. Cook the salmon on high for 3 hours.

Crockpot Tuna Spaghetti

Ingredients: Servings: 3   Cooking Time: 2 Hours

2 stalks of celery, chopped	1 C. full-fat milk
	2 zucchinis,

1/3 C. chicken broth	spiralized or cut into long strips
2 tbsp. parsley flakes	1 tbsp. butter
½ lb. ground tuna, boiled	Salt and pepper to taste

Directions:

Place all ingredients in the CrockPot. Give a good stir. Close the lid and cook on high for 1 hours or on low for 2 hours. Garnish with chopped parsley if desired.

Chili-rubbed Tilapia

Ingredients: Servings: 4   Cooking Time: 4 Hours

2 tbsp. chili powder	2 tbsp. lemon juice
½ tsp. garlic powder	2 tbsp. olive oil
1-lb. tilapia	

Directions:

Place all ingredients in a mixing bowl. Stir to combine everything. Allow to marinate in the fridge for at least 30 minutes. Get a foil and place the fish including the marinade in the middle of the foil. Fold the foil and crimp the edges to seal. Place inside the crockpot. Cook on high for 2 hours or on low for 4 hours.

Shrimp Scampi

Ingredients: Servings: 4   Cooking Time: 4 Hours

1-lb. shrimps, peeled	1 C. of water
2 tbsp. lemon juice	1 tsp. dried parsley
2 tbsp. coconut oil	½ tsp. white pepper

Directions:

Put all ingredients in the Crock Pot and gently mix. Close the lid and cook the scampi on Low for 4 hours.

Bigeye Jack Saute

Ingredients: Servings: 4   Cooking Time: 6 Hours

7 oz. (bigeye jack) tuna fillet, chopped	1 C. tomato, chopped
1 tsp. ground black pepper	1 jalapeno pepper, chopped
	½ C. chicken stock

Directions:

Put all ingredients in the Crock Pot and close the lid. Cook the saute on Low for 6 hours.

Cod With Asparagus

Ingredients: Servings: 4   Cooking Time: 2 Hours

4 cod fillets, boneless	Salt and black pepper to the taste
1 bunch asparagus	
12 tbsp. lemon juice	2 tbsp. olive oil

Directions:

Place the cod fillets in separate foil sheets. Top the fish with asparagus spears, lemon pepper, oil, and lemon juice. Wrap the fish with its foil sheet then place them in Crock Pot. Put the cooker's lid on and set the cooking time to 2 hours on High settings. Unwrap the fish and serve warm.

Vinaigrette Dipped Salmon

Ingredients: Servings: 6   Cooking Time: 2 Hrs.

6 salmon steaks
2 tbsp. olive oil
4 leeks, sliced
2 garlic cloves, minced
2 tbsp. parsley, chopped
1 C. clam juice
2 tbsp. lemon juice

Salt and white pepper to the taste
1 tsp. sherry
1/3 C. dill, chopped
For the raspberry vinegar:
2 pints red raspberries
1-pint cider vinegar

Directions:

Mix raspberries with salmon, and vinegar in a bowl.   Cover the raspberry salmon and refrigerate for 2 hours.   Add the raspberry mixture along with the remaining ingredients to the insert of the Crock Pot.   Put the cooker's lid on and set the cooking time to 2 hours on High settings.   Serve warm.

Mustard Garlic Shrimps

Ingredients: Servings: 4   Cooking Time: 2 Hours And 30 Minutes

1 tsp. olive oil
3 tbsp. garlic, minced
1-lb. shrimp, shelled and deveined

1 tsp. Dijon mustards
Salt and pepper to taste
Parsley for garnish

Directions:

In a skillet, heat the olive oil and sauté the garlic until fragrant and slightly browned.   Transfer to the crockpot and place the shrimps and Dijon mustard. Stir to combine.   Season with salt and pepper to taste.   Close the lid and cook on low for 2 hours or high for 30 minutes.   Once done, sprinkle with parsley.

Fish Mix

Ingredients: Servings: 4   Cooking Time: 2 Hours And 30 Minutes

½ tsp. mustard seeds
Salt and black pepper to the taste
2 green chilies, chopped
1 tsp. ginger, grated
1 tsp. curry powder
¼ tsp. cumin, ground
2 tbsp. olive oil

4 white fish fillets, skinless and boneless
1 small red onion, chopped
1-inch turmeric root, grated
¼ C. cilantro, chopped
1 and ½ C. coconut cream
3 garlic cloves, minced

Directions:

Heat up a Crock Pot with half of the oil over medium heat, add mustard seeds, ginger, onion, garlic, turmeric, chilies, curry powder and cumin, stir and cook for 3-4 minutes.   Add the rest of the oil to your Crock Pot, add spice mix, fish, coconut milk, salt and pepper, cover and cook on High for 2 hours and 30 minutes. Divide into bowls and serve with the cilantro sprinkled on top.

Marinara Salmon

Ingredients: Servings: 4   Cooking Time: 3 Hours

1-lb. salmon fillet, chopped
½ C. marinara sauce

¼ C. fresh cilantro, chopped
¼ C. of water

Directions:

Put the salmon in the Crock Pot.   Add marinara sauce, cilantro, and water.   Close the lid and cook the fish on High for 3 hours.

Paprika Cod

Ingredients: Servings: 2   Cooking Time: 3 Hours

1 tbsp. olive oil
1 lb. cod fillets, boneless
1 tsp. sweet paprika
¼ C. chicken stock

¼ C. white wine
2 scallions, chopped
½ tsp. rosemary, dried
A pinch of salt and black pepper

Directions:

In your Crock Pot, mix the cod with the paprika, oil and the other ingredients, toss gently, put the lid on and cook on High for 3 hours.   Divide everything between plates and serve.

Salmon With Almond Crust

Ingredients: Servings: 2   Cooking Time: 2.5 Hours

8 oz. salmon fillet
2 tbsp. almond flakes
1 tsp. ground black pepper

1 tsp. butter
1 tsp. salt
1 egg, beaten
¼ C. of coconut milk

Directions:

Sprinkle the salmon fillet with ground black pepper and salt. Then dip the fish in egg and coat in the almond flakes.   Put butter and coconut milk in the Crock Pot.   Then add salmon and close the lid.   Cook the salmon on High for 2.5 hours.

Mackerel In Wine Sauce

Ingredients: Servings: 4   Cooking Time: 3.5 Hours

1-lb. mackerel
½ C. white wine
1 tsp. cornflour
1 tsp. cayenne pepper

1 tbsp. olive oil
½ tsp. dried rosemary

Directions:

Mix white wine with cornflour and pour it in the Crock Pot. Then rub the fish with cayenne pepper and dried rosemary. Sprinkle the fish with olive oil and put it in the Crock Pot.   Close the lid and cook the mackerel on High for 3.5 hours.

Garlic Tuna

Ingredients: Servings: 4   Cooking Time: 2 Hours

1-lb. tuna fillet
1 tsp. garlic powder

1 tbsp. olive oil
½ C. of water

Directions:

Sprinkle the tuna fillet with garlic powder. Then pour olive oil in the skillet and heat it well. Add the tuna and roast it for 1 minute per side. Transfer the tuna in the Crock Pot. Add water and cook it on High for 2 hours.

Rice Stuffed Squid

Ingredients: Servings: 4   Cooking Time: 3 Hrs.

3 squids	2 tbsp. sake
Tentacles from 1 squid, chopped	4 tbsp. soy sauce
1 C. sticky rice	1 tbsp. mirin
14 oz. dashi stock	2 tbsp. sugar

Directions:

Toss the chopped tentacles with rice and stuff the 3 squids with rice mixture. Seal the squid using toothpicks then place them in the Crock Pot. Add soy sauce, stock, sugar, sake, and mirin to the squids. Put the cooker's lid on and set the cooking time to 3 hours on High settings. Serve warm.

Calamari Curry

Ingredients: Servings: 2   Cooking Time: 3 Hours

1 lb. calamari rings	2 garlic cloves, minced
½ tbsp. yellow curry paste	½ tbsp. coriander, chopped
1 C. coconut milk	A pinch of salt and black pepper
½ tsp. turmeric powder	2 tbsp. lemon juice
½ C. chicken stock	

Directions:

In your Crock Pot, mix the rings with the curry paste, coconut milk and the other ingredients, toss, put the lid on and cook on High for 3 hours. Divide the curry into bowls and serve.

Trout Capers Piccata

Ingredients: Servings: 4   Cooking Time: 45 Minutes

4 oz. dry white wine	1 tsp. oregano
1 lb. trout fillet	1 tsp. cilantro
2 tbsp. capers	1 tbsp. fresh dill, chopped
3 tbsp. olive oil	1 tsp. ground white pepper
3 tbsp. flour	
1 tsp. garlic powder	1 tsp. butter
1 tsp. dried rosemary	

Directions:

Pour olive oil into the insert of Crock Pot then place the trout in it. Add garlic powder, dried rosemary, white pepper, cilantro, and oregano over the trout. Put the cooker's lid on and set the cooking time to 30 minutes on High settings. Flip the fish when cooked halfway through. Meanwhile, mix dry wine with flour and add to the cooker. Add butter, capers, and dill on top. Put the cooker's lid on and set the cooking time to 15 minutes on High settings. Serve warm.

Mediterranean Octopus

Ingredients: Servings: 6   Cooking Time: 3 Hours

1 octopus, cleaned and prepared	½ lemon
	For the marinade:
2 rosemary springs	¼ C. extra virgin olive oil
2 tsp. oregano, dried	Juice of ½ lemon
½ yellow onion, roughly chopped	4 garlic cloves, minced
4 thyme springs	2 thyme springs
1 tsp. black peppercorns	1 rosemary spring
3 tbsp. extra virgin olive oil	Salt and black pepper to the taste

Directions:

Put the octopus in your Crock Pot, add oregano, 2 rosemary springs, 4 thyme springs, onion, lemon, 3 tbsp. olive oil, peppercorns and salt, stir, cover and cook on High for 2 hours. Transfer octopus on a cutting board, cut tentacles, put them in a bowl, mix with ¼ C. olive oil, lemon juice, garlic, 1 rosemary springs, 2 thyme springs, salt and pepper, toss to coat and leave aside for 1 hour. Transfer octopus and the marinade to your Crock Pot again, cover and cook on High for 1 more hour. Divide octopus on plates, drizzle the marinade all over and serve.

Salmon With Saffron Rice

Ingredients: Servings: 2   Cooking Time: 2 Hrs.

2 wild salmon fillets, boneless	1 C. chicken stock
Salt and black pepper to the taste	¼ C. veggie stock
	1 tbsp. butter
½ C. jasmine rice	A pinch of saffron

Directions:

Add stock, rice, butter, and saffron to the insert of Crock Pot. Mix well, then add salmon, salt, and black pepper to the cooker. Put the cooker's lid on and set the cooking time to 2 hours on High settings. Serve warm.

Dill Cod

Ingredients: Servings: 2   Cooking Time: 3 Hours

1 tbsp. olive oil	½ tsp. cumin, ground
1 lb. cod fillets, boneless and cubed	2 garlic cloves, minced
1 tbsp. dill, chopped	
½ tsp. sweet paprika	1 tsp. lemon juice
1 C. tomato passata	A pinch of salt and black pepper

Directions:

In your Crock Pot, mix the cod with the oil, dill and the other ingredients, toss, put the lid on and cook on Low for 3 hours. Divide the mix between plates and serve.

Chinese Cod

Ingredients: Servings: 4   Cooking Time: 2 Hours

1 lb. cod, cut into medium pieces	3 tbsp. soy sauce
Salt and black pepper to the taste	1 tbsp. balsamic vinegar
2 green onions, chopped	1 tbsp. ginger, grated
3 garlic cloves,	½ tsp. chili pepper, crushed

minced
1 C. fish stock

Directions:

In your Crock Pot, mix fish with salt, pepper green onions, garlic, soy sauce, fish stock, vinegar, ginger and chili pepper, toss, cover and cook on High for 2 hours. Divide everything between plates and serve.

Miso-poached Cod

Ingredients: Servings: 4   Cooking Time: 2.5 Hours

1 tsp. miso paste	½ C. of water
½ tsp. dried lemongrass	4 cod fillets
	1 tsp. olive oil

Directions:

Mix miso paste with water, dried lemongrass, and olive oil. Then pour the liquid in the Crock Pot. Add cod fillets. Cook the cod on High for 2.5 hours.

Mussels, Clams And Chorizo Mix

Ingredients: Servings: 4   Cooking Time: 2 Hours

15 small clams	30 mussels, scrubbed
2 chorizo links, sliced	10 oz. beer
1 lb. baby red potatoes, peeled	2 tbsp. parsley, chopped
1 yellow onion, chopped	1 tsp. olive oil
	Lemon wedges for serving

Directions:

Grease your Crock Pot with the oil, add clams, mussels, chorizo, potatoes, onion, beer and parsley, cover and cook on High for 2 hours. Add parsley, stir, divide into bowls and serve with lemon wedges on the side.

Lamb Bacon Stew

Ingredients: Servings: 6   Cooking Time: 7 Hrs And 10 Minutes

2 tbsp. flour	3 and ½ C. veggie stock
2 oz. bacon, cooked and crumbled	1 C. carrots, chopped
1 and ½ lbs. lamb loin, chopped	1 C. celery, chopped
Salt and black pepper to the taste	2 C. sweet potatoes, chopped
1 garlic clove, minced	1 tbsp. thyme, chopped
1 C. yellow onion, chopped	1 bay leaf
	2 tbsp. olive oil

Directions:

Thoroughly mix lamb meat with salt, black pepper, and flour in a bowl. Take oil in a non-stick skillet and heat over medium-high heat. Stir in lamb meat and sauté for 5 minutes. Transfer the sauteed meat to the Crock Pot along with the rest of the ingredients to the cooker. Put the cooker's lid on and set the cooking time to 7 hours on Low settings. Discard the bay leaf and serve warm.

Fish Pie(2)

Ingredients: Servings: 6   Cooking Time: 7 Hours

7 oz. yeast dough	1 onion, diced
1 tbsp. cream cheese	1 tsp. salt
8 oz. salmon fillet, chopped	1 tbsp. fresh dill
	1 tsp. olive oil

Directions:

Brush the Crock Pot bottom with olive oil. Then roll up the dough and place it in the Crock Pot. Flatten it in the shape of the pie crust. After this, in the mixing bowl mix cream cheese, salmon, onion, salt, and dill. Put the fish mixture over the pie crust and cover with foil. Close the lid and cook the pie on Low for 7 hours.

Sage Shrimps

Ingredients: Servings: 4   Cooking Time: 1 Hour

1-lb. shrimps, peeled	1 tsp. white pepper
1 tsp. dried sage	1 C. tomatoes chopped
1 tsp. minced garlic	½ C. of water

Directions:

Put all ingredients in the Crock Pot and close the lid. Cook the shrimps on High for 1 hour.

Mackerel Stuffed Tacos

Ingredients: Servings: 6   Cooking Time: 2 Hrs.

9 oz. mackerel fillet	1 tsp. paprika
1 tsp. salt	6 corn tortillas
¼ C. fish stock	¼ C. of salsa
1 tsp. butter	1 tsp. minced garlic
½ tsp. ground white pepper	½ tsp. mayo

Directions:

Whisk mayo with butter, garlic, white pepper, salt, and paprika in a small bowl. Rub the mackerel fillet with the mayo garlic mixture. Place this fish in the insert of Crock Pot and pour in fish stock. Put the cooker's lid on and set the cooking time to 2 hours on Low settings. Meanwhile, layer the corn tortilla with salad evenly. Shred the cooked mackerel fillet and mix it with 2 tsp. cooking liquid. Divide the fish shreds on the corn tortillas and wrap them. Serve warm.

Lobster Cheese Soup

Ingredients: Servings: 6   Cooking Time: 3.5 Hrs.

5 C. fish stock	8 oz. lobster tails
1 tbsp. paprika	1/3 C. fresh dill, chopped
½ tsp. powdered chili	
1 tsp. salt	1 tbsp. almond milk
6 oz. Cheddar cheese, shredded	1 garlic clove, peeled
	3 potatoes, peeled and diced
1 tsp. ground white pepper	

Directions:

Add stock, potatoes, paprika, salt, almond milk, garlic cloves, white pepper, powdered chili to the insert of Crock Pot. Put the cooker's lid on and set the cooking time to 2 hours on High settings.   Now add dill, and lobster tails to the cooker.   Put the cooker's lid on and set the cooking time to 1.5 hours on High settings.   Serve warm with shredded cheese on top.

Shrimp, Tomatoes And Kale

Ingredients: Servings: 2   Cooking Time: 1 Hour

1 lb. shrimp, peeled and deveined	Salt and black pepper to the taste
½ C. cherry tomatoes, halved	Juice of 1 lime
1 C. baby kale	½ tsp. sweet paprika
½ C. chicken stock	1 tbsp. cilantro, chopped
1 tbsp. olive oil	

Directions:

In your Crock Pot, mix the shrimp with the cherry tomatoes, kale and the other ingredients, toss, put the lid on and cook on High for 1 hour.   Divide the mix into bowls and serve.

Soy Sauce Catfish

Ingredients: Servings: 4   Cooking Time: 5 Hours

1-lb. catfish fillet, chopped	1 tbsp. olive oil
¼ C. of soy sauce	4 tbsp. fish stock
1 jalapeno pepper, diced	

Directions:

Sprinkle the catfish with olive oil and put in the Crock Pot.   Add soy sauce, jalapeno pepper, and fish stock.   Close the lid and cook the meal on Low for 5 hours.

Orange Marmalade Salmon

Ingredients: Servings: 2   Cooking Time: 2 Hrs.

2 lemons, sliced	¼ C. red-orange juice
1 lb. wild salmon, skinless and cubed	1 tsp. olive oil
¼ C. balsamic vinegar	1/3 C. orange marmalade

Directions:

Mix orange juice, vinegar, and marmalade in a saucepan.   Stir cook this marmalade mixture for 1 minute on a simmer. Transfer this mixture to the insert of the Crock Pot.   Add lemon slices, oil, and salmon to the cooker.   Put the cooker's lid on and set the cooking time to 2 hours on High settings.   Serve warm.

Parsley Cod

Ingredients: Servings: 2   Cooking Time: 2 Hours

1 lb. cod fillets, boneless	Juice of 1 lime
3 scallions, chopped	Salt and black pepper to the taste
2 tsp. olive oil	1 tbsp. parsley, chopped
1 tsp. coriander, ground	

Directions:

In your Crock Pot, mix the cod with the scallions, the oil and the other ingredients, rub gently, put the lid on and cook on High for 1 hour.   Divide everything between plates and serve.

Japanese Shrimp

Ingredients: Servings: 4   Cooking Time: 1 Hour

1 lb. shrimp, peeled and deveined	3 tbsp. vinegar
2 tbsp. soy sauce	¾ C. pineapple juice
½ lb. pea pods	1 C. chicken stock
	3 tbsp. sugar

Directions:

Put shrimp and pea pods in your Crock Pot, add soy sauce, vinegar, pineapple juice, stock and sugar, stir, cover and cook on High for 1 hour,   Divide between plates and serve.

Chili Salmon

Ingredients: Servings: 4   Cooking Time: 5 Hours

1-lb. salmon fillet, chopped	3 oz. chili, chopped, canned
½ C. of water	½ tsp. salt

Directions:

Place all ingredients in the Crock Pot and close the lid.   Cook the meal on Low for 5 hours.

Cod And Mustard Sauce

Ingredients: Servings: 2   Cooking Time: 3 Hours

1 tbsp. olive oil	2 garlic cloves, minced
1 lb. cod fillets, boneless	A pinch of salt and black pepper
2 tbsp. mustard	1 tbsp. chives, chopped
½ C. heavy cream	
¼ C. chicken stock	

Directions:

In your Crock Pot, mix the cod with the oil, mustard and the other ingredients, toss gently, put the lid on and cook on Low for 3 hours.   Divide the mix between plates and serve.

Cod Sticks

Ingredients: Servings: 2   Cooking Time: 1.5 Hour

2 cod fillets	1/3 C. breadcrumbs
1 tsp. ground black pepper	1 tbsp. coconut oil
1 egg, beaten	¼ C. of water

Directions:

Cut the cod fillets into medium sticks and sprinkle with ground black pepper.   Then dip the fish in the beaten egg and coat in the breadcrumbs.   Pour water in the Crock Pot.   Add coconut oil and fish sticks.   Cook the meal on High for 1.5 hours.

Shrimp And Mushrooms

Ingredients: Servings: 2   Cooking Time: 1 Hour

1 lb. shrimp, peeled and deveined	4 scallions, minced
1 C. white	½ C. chicken stock

mushrooms, halved
1 tbsp. avocado oil
½ tbsp. tomato paste

Juice of 1 lime
Salt and black pepper
to the taste
1 tbsp. chives, minced

Directions:
In your Crock Pot, mix the shrimp with the mushrooms, oil and the other ingredients, toss, put the lid on and cook on High for 1 hour. Divide the mix into bowls and serve.

Steamed Clams With Cheddar Cheese

Ingredients: Servings: 6   Cooking Time: 4 Hours 15 Minutes

1/8 C. tea seed oil
2 lb. shell clams
½ C. white wine
½ C. feta cheese

2/3 C. fresh lemon juice
2 tsp. garlic powder

Directions:
Mix together white wine, tea seed oil and lemon juice in a bowl. Microwave for 1 minute and stir well to refrigerate for 1 day. Put the clams in the crock pot and pour in the white wine mixture. Cover and cook on LOW for about 4 hours. Stir in the feta cheese well and dish out to serve hot.

Turmeric Mackerel

Ingredients: Servings: 4   Cooking Time: 2.5 Hours

1-lb. mackerel fillet
1 tbsp. ground turmeric

½ tsp. salt
¼ tsp. chili powder
½ C. of water

Directions:
Rub the mackerel fillet with ground turmeric and chili powder. Then put it in the Crock Pot. Add water and salt. Close the lid and cook the fish on High for 2.5 hours.

Taco Mackerel

Ingredients: Servings: 4   Cooking Time: 1.5 Hours

12 oz. mackerel fillets
1 tbsp. taco seasonings

2 tbsp. coconut oil
3 tbsp. water

Directions:
Melt the coconut oil in the skillet and heat it well. Meanwhile, rub the mackerel fillets with taco seasonings. Put the fish in the hot coconut oil. Roast it for 2 minutes per side. Then put the roasted fish in the Crock Pot. Add water and cook it on High for 1.5 hours.

Fish Potato Cakes

Ingredients: Servings: 12   Cooking Time: 5 Hrs.

1 lb. trout, minced
6 oz. mashed potato
1 carrot, grated
½ C. fresh parsley
1 tsp. salt
½ C. panko bread crumbs

1 egg, beaten
1 tsp. minced garlic
1 onion, grated
1 tsp. olive oil
1 tsp. ground black pepper
¼ tsp. cilantro

Directions:
Mix minced trout with mashed potatoes, carrot, salt, garlic, cilantro, onion, black pepper, and egg in a bowl. Stir in breadcrumbs and olive oil, then mix well. Make 12 balls out of this mixture then flatten the balls. Place these fish cakes in the insert of Crock Pot. Put the cooker's lid on and set the cooking time to 5 hours on Low settings. Flip all the fish cakes when cooked halfway through. Serve warm.

Flavored Squid

Ingredients: Servings: 4   Cooking Time: 3 Hours

17 oz. squids
1 and ½ tbsp. red chili powder
Salt and black pepper to the taste
¼ tsp. turmeric powder
2 C. water
5 pieces coconut, shredded

4 garlic cloves, minced
½ tsp. cumin seeds
3 tbsp. olive oil
¼ tsp. mustard seeds
1-inch ginger pieces, chopped

Directions:
Put squids in your Crock Pot, add chili powder, turmeric, salt, pepper and water, stir, cover and cook on High for 2 hours. In your blender, mix coconut with ginger, oil, garlic and cumin and blend well. Add this over the squids, cover and cook on High for 1 more hour. Divide everything into bowls and serve.

Rosemary Sole

Ingredients: Servings: 2   Cooking Time: 2 Hours

1 tbsp. dried rosemary
1 tbsp. avocado oil

8 oz. sole fillet
1 tbsp. apple cider vinegar
5 tbsp. water

Directions:
Pour water in the Crock Pot. Then rub the sole fillet with dried rosemary and sprinkle with avocado oil and apple cider vinegar. Put the fish fillet in the Crock Pot and cook it on High for 2 hours.

Spicy Cajun Scallops

Ingredients: Servings: 6   Cooking Time: 2 Hours

2 lb. scallops
2 tsp. Cajun seasoning
2 tbsp. unsalted butter

1 tsp. cayenne pepper
Salt and pepper to taste

Directions:
Place everything in the crockpot. Give a stir to combine all ingredients. Close the lid and cook on low for 2 hours or on high for 45 minutes.

Miso Cod

Ingredients: Servings: 4   Cooking Time: 4 Hours

1-lb. cod fillet, sliced
½ tsp. ground ginger

1 tsp. miso paste
2 C. chicken stock

½ tsp. ground
nutmeg

Directions:

In the mixing bowl mix chicken stock, ground nutmeg, ground ginger, and miso paste.   Then pour the liquid in the Crock Pot. Add cod fillet and close the lid.   Cook the fish on Low for 4 hours.

Tuna And Fennel

Ingredients: Servings: 2   Cooking Time: 2 Hours

1 lb. tuna fillets, boneless and cubed
1 fennel bulb, sliced
½ tsp. sweet paprika
½ tsp. chili powder

½ C. chicken stock
1 red onion, chopped
A pinch of salt and black pepper
2 tbsp. cilantro, chopped

Directions:

In your Crock Pot, mix the tuna with the fennel, stock and the other ingredients, toss, put the lid on and cook on High for 2 hour. Divide the mix between plates and serve.

Buttered Bacon And Scallops

Ingredients: Servings: 4   Cooking Time: 2 Hours

2 cloves of garlic, chopped
24 scallops, rinsed and patted dry

1 tbsp. butter
Salt and pepper to taste
1 C. bacon, chopped

Directions:

In a skillet, heat the butter and sauté the garlic until fragrant and lightly browned.   Transfer to a crockpot and add the scallops. Season with salt and pepper to taste.   Close the lid and cook on high for 45 minutes or on low for 2 hours.   Meanwhile, cook the bacon until the fat has rendered and crispy.   Sprinkle the cooked scallops with crispy bacon.

Spicy Creole Shrimp

Ingredients: Servings: 2   Cooking Time: 1 Hour And 30 Minutes

½ lb. big shrimp, peeled and deveined
2 tsp. Worcestershire sauce
2 tsp. olive oil

Juice of 1 lemon
Salt and black pepper to the taste
1 tsp. Creole seasoning

Directions:

In your Crock Pot, mix shrimp with Worcestershire sauce, oil, lemon juice, salt, pepper and Creole seasoning, toss, cover and cook on High for 1 hour and 30 minutes.   Divide into bowls and serve.

Salmon Pudding

Ingredients: Servings: 4   Cooking Time: 6 Hours

1-lb. salmon fillet, chopped
½ C. milk
2 tbsp. breadcrumbs

1 tsp. coconut oil
1 tsp. fish sauce
1 tsp. salt
2 eggs, beaten

Directions:

Mix all ingredients in the Crock Pot and close the lid.   Cook the pudding on Low for 6 hours.

Pesto Salmon

Ingredients: Servings: 4   Cooking Time: 2.5 Hours

1-lb. salmon fillet
3 tbsp. pesto sauce

1 tbsp. butter
¼ C. of water

Directions:

Pour water in the Crock Pot.   Add butter and 1 tbsp. of pesto. Add salmon and cook the fish on High for 2.5 hours.   Chop the cooked salmon and top with remaining pesto sauce.

Garlic Perch

Ingredients: Servings: 4   Cooking Time: 4 Hours

1 tsp. minced garlic
1 tbsp. butter, softened

1-lb. perch
1 tbsp. fish sauce
½ C. of water

Directions:

In the shallow bowl mix minced garlic, butter, and fish sauce. Rub the perch with a garlic butter mixture and arrange it in the Crock Pot.   Add remaining garlic butter mixture and water. Cook the fish on high for 4 hours.

Haddock Chowder

Ingredients: Servings: 5   Cooking Time: 6 Hours

1-lb. haddock, chopped
2 bacon slices, chopped, cooked
½ C. potatoes, chopped

1 tsp. ground coriander
½ C. heavy cream
4 C. of water
1 tsp. salt

Directions:

Put all ingredients in the Crock Pot and close the lid.   Cook the chowder on Low for 6 hours.

Chili Catfish

Ingredients: Servings: 4   Cooking Time: 6 Hours

1 catfish, boneless and cut into 4 pieces
3 red chili peppers, chopped
½ C. sugar
1 tbsp. soy sauce

¼ C. water
1 shallot, minced
A small ginger piece, grated
1 tbsp. coriander, chopped

Directions:

Put catfish pieces in your Crock Pot.   Heat up a pan with the coconut sugar over medium-high heat and stir until it caramelizes.   Add soy sauce, shallot, ginger, water and chili pepper, stir, pour over the fish, add coriander, cover and cook on Low for 6 hours.   Divide fish between plates and serve with the sauce from the Crock Pot drizzled on top.

Tarragon Mahi Mahi

Ingredients: Servings: 4   Cooking Time: 2.5 Hours

1-lb. mahi-mahi fillet	1 tbsp. coconut oil
1 tbsp. dried tarragon	½ C. of water

Directions:

Melt the coconut oil in the skillet. Add mahi-mahi fillet and roast it on high heat for 2 minutes per side. Put the fish fillet in the Crock Pot. Add dried tarragon and water. Close the lid and cook the fish on High for 2.5 hours.

Octopus And Veggies Mix

Ingredients: Servings: 4   Cooking Time: 3 Hours

1 octopus, already prepared	1 tbsp. paprika
1 C. red wine	Salt and black pepper to the taste
1 C. white wine	½ bunch parsley, chopped
1 C. water	2 garlic cloves, minced
1 C. olive oil	1 yellow onion, chopped
2 tsp. pepper sauce	4 potatoes, cut into quarters.
1 tbsp. hot sauce	
1 tbsp. tomato sauce	

Directions:

Put octopus in a bowl, add white wine, red one, water, half of the oil, pepper sauce, hot sauce, paprika, tomato paste, salt, pepper and parsley, toss to coat, cover and keep in a cold place for 1 day. Add the rest of the oil to your Crock Pot and arrange onions and potatoes on the bottom. Add the octopus and the marinade, stir, cover, cook on High for 3 hours, divide everything between plates and serve.

Seafood Bean Chili

Ingredients: Servings: 8   Cooking Time: 3.5 Hrs.

1 lb. salmon, diced	1 C. fish stock
7 oz. shrimps, peeled	1 tsp. cayenne pepper
1 tbsp. salt	1 C. bell pepper, chopped
1 C. tomatoes, canned	1 tbsp. olive oil
1 tsp. ground white pepper	1 tsp. coriander
1 tbsp. tomato sauce	1 C. of water
2 onions, chopped	6 oz. Parmesan, shredded
1 C. carrot, chopped	1 garlic clove, sliced
1 can red beans	
½ C. tomato juice	

Directions:

Add tomatoes, white pepper, tomato sauce, red beans, carrots, tomato juice, bell pepper, fish stock, cayenne pepper, garlic, water and coriander to the insert of Crock Pot. Put the cooker's lid on and set the cooking time to 3 hours on High settings. Add olive oil and seafood to a suitable pan, then sauté for 3 minutes. Transfer the sautéed seafood to the Crock Pot. Put the cooker's lid on and set the cooking time to 30 minutes on High settings. Serve warm.

Crockpot Smoked Trout

Ingredients: Servings: 4   Cooking Time: 2 Hours

2 tbsp. liquid smoke	2 tbsp. olive oil
4 oz. smoked trout, skin removed then flaked	Salt and pepper to taste
	2 tbsp. mustard

Directions:

Place all ingredients in the crockpot. Cook on high for 1 hour or on low for 2 hours until the trout flakes have absorbed the sauce.

Salmon And Raspberry Vinaigrette

Ingredients: Servings: 6   Cooking Time: 2 Hours

6 salmon steaks	1 C. clam juice
2 tbsp. olive oil	Salt and white pepper to the taste
4 leeks, sliced	1 tsp. sherry
2 garlic cloves, minced	1/3 C. dill, chopped
2 tbsp. parsley, chopped	For the raspberry vinegar:
2 tbsp. lemon juice	2 pints red raspberries
	1-pint cider vinegar

Directions:

In a bowl, mix red raspberries with vinegar and salmon, toss, cover and keep in the fridge for 2 hours. In your Crock Pot, mix oil with parsley, leeks, garlic, clam juice, lemon juice, salt, pepper, sherry, dill and salmon, cover and cook on High for 2 hours. Divide everything between plates and serve.

Shrimp And Avocado

Ingredients: Servings: 2   Cooking Time: 1 Hour

1 lb. shrimp, peeled and deveined	1 tbsp. olive oil
1 C. avocado, peeled, pitted and cubed	2 tbsp. chili pepper, minced
½ C. chicken stock	A pinch of salt and black pepper
½ tsp. sweet paprika	1 tbsp. chives, chopped
Juice of 1 lime	

Directions:

In your Crock Pot, mix the shrimp with the avocado, stock and the other ingredients, toss, put the lid on and cook on High for 1 hour. Divide the mix into bowls and serve.

Stuffed Squid

Ingredients: Servings: 4   Cooking Time: 3 Hours

4 squid	4 tbsp. soy sauce
1 C. sticky rice	1 tbsp. mirin
14 oz. dashi stock	2 tbsp. sugar
2 tbsp. sake	

Directions:

Chop tentacles from 1 squid, mix with the rice, stuff each squid with this mix and seal ends with toothpicks. Place squid in your Crock Pot, add stock, soy sauce, sake, sugar and mirin, stir, cover and cook on High for 3 hours. Divide between plates and serve.

Italian Clams

Ingredients: Servings: 6   Cooking Time: 2 Hours

½ C. butter, melted
36 clams, scrubbed
1 tsp. red pepper
flakes, crushed
1 tsp. parsley,
chopped

5 garlic cloves,
minced
1 tbsp. oregano, dried
2 C. white wine

Directions:

In your Crock Pot, mix butter with clams, pepper flakes, parsley, garlic, oregano and wine, stir, cover and cook on High for 2 hours. Divide into bowls and serve.

Semolina Fish Balls

Ingredients: Servings: 11   Cooking Time: 8 Hrs.

1 C. sweet corn
5 tbsp. fresh dill,
chopped
1 tbsp. minced garlic
7 tbsp. bread crumbs
2 eggs, beaten
10 oz. salmon,
salmon
2 tbsp. semolina
2 tbsp. canola oil
1 tsp. salt

1 tsp. ground black
pepper
1 tsp. cumin
1 tsp. lemon zest
¼ tsp. cinnamon
3 tbsp. almond flour
3 tbsp. scallion,
chopped
3 tbsp. water

Directions:

Mix sweet corn, dill, garlic, semolina, eggs, salt, cumin, almond flour, scallion, cinnamon, lemon zest, and black pepper in a large bowl. Stir in chopped salmon and mix well. Make small meatballs out of this fish mixture then roll them in the breadcrumbs. Place the coated fish ball in the insert of the Crock Pot. Add canola oil and water to the fish balls. Put the cooker's lid on and set the cooking time to 8 hours on Low settings. Serve warm.

Cod Bacon Chowder

Ingredients: Servings: 6   Cooking Time: 3 Hours

1 yellow onion,
chopped
10 oz. cod, cubed
3 oz. bacon, sliced
1 tsp. sage
5 oz. potatoes, peeled
and cubed

1 carrot, grated
5 C. of water
1 tbsp. almond milk
1 tsp. ground
coriander
1 tsp. salt

Directions:

Place grated carrots and onion in the Crock Pot. Add almond milk, coriander, water, sage, fish, potatoes, and bacon. Put the cooker's lid on and set the cooking time to 3 hours on High settings. Garnish with chopped parsley. Serve.

Sea Bass And Squash

Ingredients: Servings: 2   Cooking Time: 3 Hours

1 lb. sea bass,
boneless and cubed
1 C. butternut squash,

1 tsp. olive oil
½ tsp. Italian
seasoning

peeled and cubed
½ tsp. turmeric
powder

1 C. chicken stock
1 tbsp. cilantro,
chopped

Directions:

In your Crock Pot, mix the sea bass with the squash, oil, turmeric and the other ingredients, toss, the lid on and cook on Low for 3 hours. Divide everything between plates and serve.

White Fish With Olives Sauce

Ingredients: Servings: 4   Cooking Time: 2 Hrs.

4 white fish fillets,
boneless
1 C. olives, pitted and
chopped
1 lb. cherry tomatoes
halved
A pinch of thyme,
dried

1 garlic clove, minced
A drizzle of olive oil
Salt and black pepper
to the taste
¼ C. chicken stock

Directions:

Pour the stock into the insert of the Crock Pot. Add fish, tomatoes, olives, oil, black pepper, salt, garlic, and thyme to the stock. Put the cooker's lid on and set the cooking time to 2 hours on High settings. Serve warm.

Fish Soufflé(2)

Ingredients: Servings: 4   Cooking Time: 7 Hours

4 eggs, beaten
8 oz. salmon fillet,
chopped

¼ C. of coconut milk
2 oz. Provolone
cheese, grated

Directions:

Mix coconut milk with eggs and pour the liquid in the Crock Pot. Add salmon and cheese. Close the lid and cook soufflé for 7 hours on low.

Cream White Fish

Ingredients: Servings: 6   Cooking Time: 2 Hrs.

17 oz. white fish,
skinless, boneless
and cut into chunks
1 yellow onion,
chopped
13 oz. potatoes,
peeled and cut into
chunks

13 oz. milk
Salt and black pepper
to the taste
14 oz. chicken stock
14 oz. water
14 oz. half and half
cream

Directions:

Add onion, fish, potatoes, water, stock, and milk to the insert of Crock Pot. Put the cooker's lid on and set the cooking time to 2 hours on High settings. Add half and half cream, black pepper, and salt to the fish. Mix gently, then serve warm.

Seafood Casserole

Ingredients: Servings: 8   Cooking Time: 4 Hours 30 Minutes

5 C. milk
3 C. celery, chopped

6 tbsp. butter
½ lb. lobster meat

2 C. onions, chopped
12 tbsp. all-purpose flour
8 oz. Cheddar cheese, sliced

½ lb. crabmeat
1 tsp. black pepper
½ lb. scallops
1 tsp. salt
½ lb. medium shrimp

Directions:
Melt half butter in a skillet and add the onions and celery. Sauté for about 3 minutes and dish out. Put the milk in a saucepan over medium heat and add flour and remaining butter. Blend the cheese into the mixture and sprinkle with salt and black pepper. Combine the cheese sauce mixture with onions mixture in a bowl and add crabmeat, lobster, shrimp and scallops. Put this mixture into the crock pot and cover the lid. Cook on LOW for about 4 hours and dish out to serve.

SOUPS & STEWS RECIPES

Bacon Stew

Ingredients: Servings: 4   Cooking Time: 5 Hours

3 oz. bacon, chopped, cooked
1/3 tsp. ground black pepper
½ tsp. garlic powder
½ C. carrot, chopped

2 C. vegetable stock
1 tbsp. cornstarch
1 C. turnip, peeled, chopped

Directions:
Mix cornstarch with vegetable stock and whisk until smooth. Pour the liquid in the Crock Pot. Add all remaining ingredients and close the lid. Cook the stew on low for 5 hours.

Thai Chicken Soup

Ingredients: Servings: 8   Cooking Time: 6 1/2 Hours

8 chicken thighs
2 celery stalks, sliced
1 sweet onion, chopped
1 tsp. grated ginger
2 tbsp. soy sauce
1 tbsp. brown sugar

1 tsp. fish sauce
1 lime, juiced
2 C. coconut milk
2 C. chicken stock
4 C. water
1 lemongrass stalk, crushed
1 C. green peas
Salt and pepper to taste

Directions:
Combine the chicken, celery, onion, ginger, fish sauce, soy sauce, sugar and lime juice in your Crock Pot. Add the remaining ingredients and season with salt and pepper if needed. Cook the soup on low settings for 6 hours. Serve the soup warm and fresh.

Sweet Potato & Sausage Soup

Ingredients: Servings: 6 (12.4 oz. Per Serving)   Cooking Time: 7 Hours And 35 Minutes

1 lb. sausage links, pork or chicken
8 large sweet

3 C. water
Salt and pepper to taste and other

potatoes, cubed
1 onion, chopped
1 glass red wine
4 tbsp. tomato sauce
Olive oil

seasonings
1 C. of bacon, cooked, cubed
1 C. smoked ham, cooked, cubed
1 red pepper, diced

Directions:
Chop the onion into cubes. Grease a frying pan and sauté onion until golden in color, for about six minutes. Add the cubed ham and bacon. Add cubed potatoes and salt and pepper to taste. Pour in wine and stir. Place all ingredients in Crock Pot. Add the water and cover and cook on LOW for 6-7 hours. Add the chopped pepper and tomato sauce and cook on LOW for an additional 30 minutes more. Serve hot.

Vegetable Chickpea Soup

Ingredients: Servings: 6   Cooking Time: 6 1/2 Hours

2/3 C. dried chickpeas, rinsed
2 C. chicken stock
4 C. water
1 celery stalk, sliced
1 carrot, diced
2 ripe tomatoes, peeled and diced

1 shallot, chopped
1 red bell pepper, cored and diced
1 potato, peeled and diced
1 tbsp. lemon juice
Salt and pepper to taste

Directions:
Combine all the ingredients in your Crock Pot. Add salt and pepper to taste and cook on low settings for 6 hours. Serve the soup warm and fresh.

Light Zucchini Soup

Ingredients: Servings: 4   Cooking Time: 30 Minutes

1 large zucchini
1 white onion, diced
1 tsp. dried thyme

4 C. beef broth
½ tsp. dried rosemary

Directions:
Pour the beef broth in the Crock Pot. Add onion, dried thyme, and dried rosemary. After this, make the spirals from the zucchini with the help of the spiralizer and transfer them in the Crock Pot. Close the lid and cook the sou on High for 30 minutes.

Bean And Bacon Soup

Ingredients: Servings: 8   Cooking Time: 6 1/2 Hours

1 1/2 C. diced bacon
1 large sweet onion, chopped
2 carrots, diced
1 celery stalk, diced
2 ripe tomatoes, peeled and diced

2 C. dried white beans, rinsed
6 C. water
2 C. chicken stock
1 thyme sprig
Salt and pepper to taste

Directions:
Heat a skillet over medium flame and add the bacon. Cook on all sides until golden then transfer in your Crock Pot. Add the remaining ingredients and cook over low settings for 6 hours. Serve the soup warm.

93

Chicken, Corn And Bean Stew

Ingredients: Servings: 10   Cooking Time: 5 Hours 15 Minutes

3 lb. chicken tenders	1 can seasoned diced
1 C. Parmesan cheese, shredded	tomatoes
	1 can chili beans
	1 can corn, drained

Directions:

Arrange chicken at the bottom of a crockpot and stir in the remaining ingredients.   Cover and cook on HIGH for about 5 hours.   Sprinkle with Parmesan cheese and dish out to serve.

Beef Liver Stew

Ingredients: Servings: 3   Cooking Time: 7 Hours

6 oz. beef liver, cut into strips	½ C. sour cream
2 tbsp. all-purpose flour	½ C. of water
1 tbsp. olive oil	1 onion, roughly chopped
	1 tsp. ground black pepper

Directions:

Mix beef liver with flour and roast it in the olive oil on high heat for 2 minutes per side.   Then transfer the liver in the Crock Pot. Add all remaining ingredients and close the lid.   Cook the stew on low for 7 hours.

Paprika Hominy Stew

Ingredients: Servings: 4   Cooking Time: 4 Hours

2 C. hominy, canned	½ C. full-fat cream
1 tbsp. smoked paprika	½ C. ground chicken
1 tsp. hot sauce	1 C. of water

Directions:

Carefully mix all ingredients in the Crock Pot and close the lid. Cook the stew on high for 4 hours.

Beef Vegetable Soup

Ingredients: Servings: 8   Cooking Time: 7 1/4 Hours

1 lb. beef roast, cubed	1/2 head cauliflower, cut into florets
2 tbsp. canola oil	2 large potatoes, peeled and cubed
1 celery stalk, sliced	1 C. diced tomatoes
1 sweet onion, chopped	1/2 tsp. dried basil
1 carrot, sliced	2 C. beef stock
1 garlic clove, chopped	4 C. water
	Salt and pepper to taste

Directions:

Heat the oil in a skillet and add the beef. Cook on all sides for a few minutes then transfer the beef in your Crock Pot.   Add the remaining ingredients and season with salt and pepper.   Cover and cook on low settings for 7 hours.   The soup is delicious either warm or chilled.

Zucchini Soup

Ingredients: Servings: 6   Cooking Time: 2 1/4 Hours

1 lb. Italian sausages, sliced	2 C. vegetable stock
2 celery stalks, sliced	1/2 tsp. dried oregano
2 zucchinis, cubed	1/2 tsp. dried basil
2 large potatoes, peeled and cubed	1/4 tsp. garlic powder
2 yellow bell peppers, cored and diced	Salt and pepper to taste
2 carrots, sliced	2 tbsp. chopped parsley
1 shallot, chopped	
3 C. water	

Directions:

Combine the sausages, celery stalks, zucchinis, potatoes, bell peppers, carrots, shallot, water, stock and seasoning in your Crock Pot.   Add salt and pepper to taste and cook on high settings for 2 hours.   When done, stir in the parsley and serve the soup warm.

Okra Vegetable Soup

Ingredients: Servings: 8   Cooking Time: 7 1/4 Hours

1 lb. ground beef	2 potatoes, peeled and cubed
2 tbsp. canola oil	1/2 C. sweet corn, drained
2 shallots, chopped	Salt and pepper to taste
1 carrot, sliced	
1 can fire roasted tomatoes, chopped	
2 C. chopped okra	2 C. water
1/2 C. green peas	2 C. chicken stock
	1 lemon, juiced

Directions:

Heat the oil in a skillet and stir in the beef. Cook for a few minutes then transfer the meat in your Crock Pot.   Add the shallots, carrot, tomatoes, okra, peas, potatoes, corn, water and stock, as well as lemon juice, salt and pepper.   Cook the soup on low settings for 7 hours.   Serve the soup warm and fresh.

Lasagna Soup

Ingredients: Servings: 8   Cooking Time: 8 1/2 Hours

2 tbsp. olive oil	1 lb. ground beef
1 large sweet onion, chopped	1 C. diced tomatoes
2 garlic cloves, chopped	2 C. beef stock
	6 C. water
1 tsp. dried oregano	1 1/2 C. uncooked pasta shells
1 1/2 C. tomato sauce	Salt and pepper to taste
	Grated Cheddar for serving

Directions:

Heat the oil in a skillet and add the ground beef. Cook for 5 minutes then transfer in your Crock Pot.   Add the remaining ingredients and season with salt and pepper.   Cook on low settings for 8 hours.   When done, pour into serving bowls and top with cheese.   Serve the soup warm and fresh.

Coconut Squash Soup

Ingredients: Servings: 6   Cooking Time: 2 1/4 Hours

1 tbsp. olive oil
1 shallot, chopped
1/2 tsp. grated ginger
2 garlic cloves, minced
1 tbsp. curry paste
1 tsp. brown sugar

1 tsp. Worcestershire sauce
3 C. butternut squash cubes
2 C. chicken stock
2 C. water
1 C. coconut milk
1 tbsp. tomato paste
Salt and pepper to taste

Directions:

Heat the oil in a skillet and stir in the shallot, garlic, ginger and curry paste. Sauté for 1 minute then transfer the mixture in your Crock Pot. Add the remaining ingredients and season with salt and pepper. Cover with its lid and cook on high settings for 2 hours. When done, puree the soup with an immersion blender until smooth. Pour the soup into serving bowls and serve it warm.

Black Bean Mushroom Soup

Ingredients: Servings: 8   Cooking Time: 6 1/2 Hours

2 garlic cloves, chopped
1 can (15 oz.) black beans, drained
1/2 lb. mushrooms, sliced
1 can fire roasted tomatoes
2 C. vegetable stock

1 shallot, chopped
4 C. water
1/2 tsp. mustard seeds
1/2 tsp. cumin seeds
Salt and pepper to taste
2 tbsp. chopped parsley

Directions:

Combine the shallot, garlic and black beans with the mushrooms, tomatoes, stock, water and seeds in your Crock Pot. Add salt and pepper to taste and cook on low settings for 6 hours. When done, add the parsley and serve the soup warm.

Quick Lentil Ham Soup

Ingredients: Servings: 6   Cooking Time: 1 3/4 Hours

1 tbsp. olive oil
4 oz. ham, diced
1 carrot, diced
1 celery stalk, sliced
1/2 tsp. dried oregano
1/2 tsp. dried basil

1 shallot, chopped
1 C. dried lentils, rinsed
2 C. water
1/2 C. tomato sauce
1 1/2 C. chicken stock
Salt and pepper to taste

Directions:

Combine the olive oil, ham, carrot, celery, shallot, oregano, basil, lentils, water, tomato sauce and stock. Add salt and pepper to taste and cook on high settings for 1 1/2 hours. The soup can be served both warm and chilled.

Chunky Pumpkin And Kale Soup

Ingredients: Servings: 6   Cooking Time: 6 1/2 Hours

1 sweet onion, chopped
1 red bell pepper, cored and diced
1/2 red chili, chopped
2 tbsp. olive oil
2 C. pumpkin cubes

2 C. vegetable stock
2 C. water
1 bunch kale, shredded
1/2 tsp. cumin seeds
Salt and pepper to taste

Directions:

Combine the onion, bell pepper, chili and olive oil in your Crock Pot. Add the remaining ingredients and adjust the taste with salt and pepper. Mix gently just to evenly distribute the ingredients then cook on low settings for 6 hours. Serve the soup warm or chilled.

Hearty Turkey Chili

Ingredients: Servings: 5   Cooking Time: 8 Hours 15 Minutes

1/4 C. olive oil
1 lb. ground turkey breast
1/2 tsp. salt
1 can white beans, drained and rinsed
2 tsp. dried marjoram
1 large onion, chopped

1 green pepper, chopped
1 can diced tomatoes
2 tbsp. chili powder
4 garlic cloves, minced
1 can no-salt-added tomatoes

Directions:

Put olive oil, green peppers, onions and garlic in the crock pot and sauté for about 3 minutes. Add rest of the ingredients and cover the lid. Cook on LOW for about 8 hours and dish out in a bowl to serve hot.

Chicken And Noodles Soup

Ingredients: Servings: 8   Cooking Time: 7 Hours

1-lb. chicken breast, skinless, boneless, chopped
1 tsp. salt
1 tsp. chili flakes

1 tsp. coriander
1 C. bell pepper, chopped
4 oz. egg noodles
8 C. chicken stock

Directions:

Mix chicken breast with salt, chili flakes, coriander, and place in the Crock Pot. Add chicken stock and close the lid. Cook the ingredients on Low for 6 hours. Then add egg noodles and bell pepper and cook the soup for 1 hour on High.

Indian Cauliflower Creamy Soup

Ingredients: Servings: 8   Cooking Time: 6 1/2 Hours

2 tbsp. olive oil
1 sweet onion, chopped
1 celery stalk, sliced
2 garlic cloves, chopped
1 tbsp. red curry paste
1 cauliflower head, cut into florets

2 medium size potatoes, peeled and cubed
2 C. vegetable stock
2 C. water
1/4 tsp. cumin powder
1 pinch red pepper flakes
Salt and pepper to taste

Directions:

Heat the oil in a skillet and stir in the onion, celery and garlic. Sauté for 2 minutes until softened. Transfer the mix in your Crock Pot. Add the remaining ingredients and cook on low settings for 6 hours. When done, puree the soup with an immersion blender and serve it warm.

Green Peas Chowder

Ingredients: Servings: 6   Cooking Time: 8 Hours

1-lb. chicken breast, skinless, boneless, chopped	1 tbsp. dried basil
	1 tsp. ground black pepper
6 C. of water	½ tsp. salt
1 C. green peas	
¼ C. Greek Yogurt	

Directions:

Mix salt, chicken breast, ground black pepper, and dried basil. Transfer the ingredients in the Crock Pot. Add water, green peas, yogurt, and close the lid. Cook the chowder on Low for 8 hours.

Ginger Fish Stew

Ingredients: Servings: 5   Cooking Time: 6 Hours

1 oz. fresh ginger, peeled, chopped	1 tsp. fish sauce
1 C. baby carrot	½ tsp. ground nutmeg
1-lb. salmon fillet, chopped	½ C. green peas
	3 C. of water

Directions:

Put all ingredients in the Crock Pot bowl. Gently stir the stew ingredients and close the lid. Cook the stew on low for 6 hours.

Chunky Potato Ham Soup

Ingredients: Servings: 8   Cooking Time: 8 1/2 Hours

2 C. diced ham	2 carrots, sliced
1 sweet onion, chopped	1/2 tsp. dried oregano
1 garlic clove, chopped	1/2 tsp. dried basil
1 leek, sliced	2 C. chicken stock
1 celery stalk, sliced	3 C. water
2 lb. potatoes, peeled and cubed	Salt and pepper to taste

Directions:

Combine all the ingredients in your Crock Pot. Add salt and pepper to taste and cook on low settings for 8 hours. Serve the soup warm or chilled.

Beef Taco Soup

Ingredients: Servings: 8   Cooking Time: 7 1/4 Hours

1 lb. beef stock, cubed	1 onion, chopped
1 tbsp. olive oil	1 C. tomato sauce
1 garlic clove, chopped	1 C. dark beer
1 can (15 oz.) black	2 tbsp. taco seasoning
	1 jalapeno pepper,

beans, drained	chopped
1 can (15 oz.) cannellini beans, drained	Salt and pepper to taste
1 C. canned corn, drained	3 C. water
	2 C. beef stock
	1 avocado, sliced
	1/2 C. sour cream

Directions:

Heat the oil in a skillet and add the onion and beef, garlic. Sauté for 2 minutes then transfer in your Crock Pot. Stir in the beans, corn, tomato sauce, beer, taco seasoning and jalapeno. Add salt and pepper to taste and cook on low settings for 7 hours. To serve, pour the soup into serving bowls and top with sour cream and avocado slices.

Lobster Soup

Ingredients: Servings: 4   Cooking Time: 2 Hours

4 C. of water	1 C. coconut cream
1-lb. lobster tail, chopped	1 tsp. ground coriander
½ C. fresh cilantro, chopped	1 garlic clove, diced

Directions:

Pour water and coconut cream in the Crock Pot. Add a lobster tail, cilantro, and ground coriander. Then add the garlic clove and close the lid. Cook the lobster soup on High for 2 hours.

Rabbit Stew

Ingredients: Servings: 5   Cooking Time: 8 Hours 15 Minutes

½ C. celery, diced	1 piece of bacon
1 sausage, cubed	½ C. apple cider vinegar
1 bay leaf	
1 garlic clove, diced	3 C. chicken broth
1 C. Swiss chards, stalks	½ C. olive oil
½ can water chestnuts, diced	1 lb. rabbit, cubed
	Salt and black pepper, to taste

Directions:

Marinate rabbit in olive oil and apple cider vinegar and keep aside overnight. Put chicken broth in the crock pot and warm it up. Meanwhile, sear bacon and sausage in a pan and transfer it to the crock pot. Stir in rest of the ingredients and cover the lid. Cook on LOW for about 8 hours and dish out to serve hot.

Meatball Soup

Ingredients: Servings: 8   Cooking Time: 6 1/2 Hours

1 lb. ground pork	2 celery stalk, sliced
1/4 C. white rice	1 carrot, sliced
1/2 tsp. dried oregano	1 fennel bulb, sliced
1/2 tsp. dried basil	1 C. diced tomatoes
Salt and pepper to taste	2 C. chicken stock
	4 C. water
1 sweet onion, chopped	Salt and pepper to taste

Directions:

Mix the pork, rice, oregano, basil, salt and pepper in a bowl. Combine the onion, celery stalk, carrot, fennel, tomatoes, stock and water in your Crock Pot. Adjust the taste with salt and pepper then form small meatballs and place them in the Crock Pot. Cook on low settings for 6 hours. Serve the soup warm.

Salmon Fennel Soup

Ingredients: Servings: 6   Cooking Time: 5 1/4 Hours

1 shallot, chopped	3 salmon fillets,
1 garlic clove, sliced	cubed
1 fennel bulb, sliced	1 lemon, juiced
1 carrot, diced	1 bay leaf
1 celery stalk, sliced	Salt and pepper to
	taste

Directions:

Combine the shallot, garlic, fennel, carrot, celery, fish, lemon juice and bay leaf in your Crock Pot. Add salt and pepper to taste and cook on low settings for 5 hours. Serve the soup warm.

Moroccan Lentil Soup

Ingredients: Servings: 6   Cooking Time: 6 1/4 Hours

1 large sweet onion, chopped	1 parsnip, diced
2 garlic cloves, chopped	1/2 tsp. ground coriander
2 tbsp. olive oil	2 C. water
2 carrots, diced	3 C. chicken stock
1 C. chopped cauliflower	1 C. red lentils
1/2 tsp. cumin powder	2 tbsp. tomato paste
1/4 tsp. turmeric powder	2 tbsp. lemon juice
	Salt and pepper to taste

Directions:

Heat the oil in a skillet and stir in the onion, garlic, carrots and parsnip. Cook for 5 minutes then transfer in your Crock Pot. Stir in the cauliflower, cumin powder, turmeric and coriander, as well as water, stock, lentils and tomato paste. Add the lemon juice, salt and pepper and cook on low settings for 6 hours. Serve the soup warm or chilled.

Creamy White Bean Soup

Ingredients: Servings: 6   Cooking Time: 4 1/4 Hours

1 tbsp. olive oil	1 can (15 oz.) white
1 sweet onion, chopped	beans, drained
2 garlic cloves, chopped	2 C. chicken stock
1/2 celery root, peeled and cubed	3 C. water
1 parsnip, diced	1/2 tsp. dried thyme
	Salt and pepper to taste

Directions:

Heat the oil in a skillet and stir in the onion, garlic, celery and parsnip. Cook for 5 minutes until softened then transfer the mix in your Crock Pot. Add the rest of the ingredients and cook on low settings for 4 hours. When done, puree the soup with an immersion blender and pulse until smooth and creamy. Serve the soup warm and fresh.

White Mushroom Soup

Ingredients: Servings: 6   Cooking Time: 8 Hours

9 oz. white mushrooms, chopped	6 chicken stock
1 tsp. dried cilantro	1 tsp. butter
1/2 tsp. ground black pepper	1 C. potatoes, chopped
	1/2 carrot, diced

Directions:

Melt butter in the skillet. Add white mushrooms and roast them for 5 minutes on high heat. Stir the mushrooms constantly. Transfer them in the Crock Pot. Add chicken stock, cilantro, ground black pepper, and potato. Add carrot and close the lid. Cook the soup on low for 8 hours.

Smoky Sweet Corn Soup

Ingredients: Servings: 6   Cooking Time: 5 1/2 Hours

1 shallot, chopped	3 C. frozen corn
1 garlic clove, chopped	2 C. chicken stock
2 tbsp. olive oil	2 C. water
2 bacon slices, chopped	1/4 tsp. chili powder
	Salt and pepper to taste

Directions:

Heat the oil in a skillet and add the garlic, shallot and bacon. Cook on all sides until golden then transfer in your Crock Pot. Add the corn, stock, water and chili powder and season with salt and pepper. Cook on low settings for 5 hours. When done, puree the soup with an immersion blender and serve it warm.

Spinach Sweet Potato Soup

Ingredients: Servings: 6   Cooking Time: 3 1/2 Hours

1 shallot, chopped	4 C. water
1 garlic clove, chopped	Salt and pepper to taste
1/2 lb. ground chicken	4 C. fresh spinach, shredded
2 tbsp. olive oil	1/2 tsp. dried oregano
2 medium size sweet potatoes, peeled and cubed	1/2 tsp. dried basil
2 C. chicken stock	1 tbsp. chopped parsley

Directions:

Heat the oil in a skillet and add the ground chicken, shallot and garlic. Cook for about 5 minutes, stirring often. Transfer the meat mix in your Crock Pot and add the potatoes, stock, water, salt and pepper. Cook on high settings for 2 hours then stir in the spinach, oregano, basil and parsley and cook one additional hour on high. Serve the soup warm.

Two-fish Soup

Ingredients: Servings: 8   Cooking Time: 6 1/4 Hours

1 tbsp. canola oil	1 C. diced tomatoes
1 sweet onion, chopped	1 lemon, juiced
1 red bell pepper, cored and diced	3 salmon fillets, cubed
	3 cod fillets, cubed

1 chipotle pepper, chopped	2 tbsp. chopped parsley
1 carrot, diced	Salt and pepper to taste
1 celery stalk, diced	

Directions:

Heat the canola oil in a skillet and add the onion. Sauté for 2 minutes until softened. Transfer the onion in a Crock Pot and stir in the remaining ingredients. Add salt and pepper to taste and cook on low settings for 6 hours. Serve the soup warm.

Lamb Stew

Ingredients: Servings: 5   Cooking Time: 5 Hours

1 lb. lamb meat, cubed	1 red onion, sliced
1 tsp. cayenne pepper	½ tsp. dried thyme
1 tsp. dried rosemary	1 C. potatoes, chopped
	4 C. of water

Directions:

Sprinkle the lamb meat with cayenne pepper, dried rosemary, and dried thyme. Transfer the meat in the Crock Pot. Add water, onion, and potatoes. Close the lid and cook the stew on high for 5 hours.

Red Chili Quinoa Soup

Ingredients: Servings: 8   Cooking Time: 3 1/4 Hours

2 shallots, chopped	2 C. chicken stock
1 carrot, diced	Salt and pepper to taste
1/2 celery root, peeled and diced	1/2 tsp. chili powder
1 can diced tomatoes	2 tbsp. chopped cilantro for serving
1/2 C. quinoa, rinsed	
1 can (15 oz.) red beans, drained	Sour cream for serving
2 C. water	

Directions:

Combine the shallots, carrot, celery and diced tomatoes in your Crock Pot. Add the quinoa, water, stock and chili powder and season with salt and pepper. Cook on high settings for 3 hours. Serve the soup warm, topped with cilantro and sour cream.

German Style Soup

Ingredients: Servings: 6   Cooking Time: 8.5 Hours

1-lb. beef loin, chopped	1 onion, diced
6 C. of water	1 tsp. cayenne pepper
1 C. sauerkraut	½ C. greek yogurt

Directions:

Put beef and onion in the Crock Pot. Add yogurt, water, and cayenne pepper. Cook the mixture on low for 8 hours. When the beef is cooked, add sauerkraut and stir the soup carefully. Cook the soup on high for 30 minutes.

Sweet Corn Chowder

Ingredients: Servings: 8   Cooking Time: 6 1/4 Hours

2 shallots, chopped	1 can (15 oz.) sweet corn, drained
4 medium size potatoes, peeled and cubed1	2 C. chicken stock
	2 C. water
1 celery stalk, sliced	Salt and pepper to taste

Directions:

Combine the shallot, potatoes, celery, corn, stock and water in a Crock Pot. Add salt and pepper to taste and cook on low settings for 6 hours. When done, remove a few tbsp. of corn from the pot then puree the remaining soup in the pot. Pour the soup into serving bowls and top with the reserved corn. Serve warm.

Grits Potato Soup

Ingredients: Servings: 6   Cooking Time: 6 1/4 Hours

4 bacon slices, chopped	1 carrot, diced
1/2 C. grits	1 parsnip, diced
2 C. chicken stock	1 C. diced tomatoes
4 C. water	1/2 tsp. dried thyme
1 1/2 lb. potatoes, peeled and cubed	1/2 tsp. dried oregano
1/2 celery stalk, sliced	Salt and pepper to taste

Directions:

Cook the bacon until crisp in a skillet or pan. Transfer in your Crock Pot and add the remaining ingredients. Cook the soup on low settings, adjusting the taste with salt and pepper as needed. The soup is done in about 6 hours. Serve warm.

Tender Mushroom Stew

Ingredients: Servings: 6   Cooking Time: 8 Hours

1-lb. cremini mushrooms, chopped	1 yellow onion, diced
1 C. carrot, grated	½ C. greek yogurt
2 tsp. dried basil	½ C. rutabaga, chopped
	5 C. beef broth

Directions:

Put all ingredients in the Crock Pot. Close the lid and cook the stew on Low for 8 hours.

Taco Soup

Ingredients: Servings: 3   Cooking Time: 8 Hours

1 C. ground chicken	1 tbsp. taco seasoning
3 C. chicken stock	¼ C. black olives, sliced
1 tomato, chopped	
¼ C. corn kernels	
1 jalapeno pepper, sliced	3 corn tortillas, chopped

Directions:

Put the ground chicken in the Crock Pot. Add chicken stock, tomato, corn kernels, jalapeno pepper, taco seasoning, and black olives. Close the lid and cook the soup on low for 8 hours. When the soup is cooked, ladle it in the bowls and top with chopped tortillas.

Paprika Noddle Soup

Ingredients: Servings: 4   Cooking Time: 4 Hours

3 oz. egg noodles
3 C. chicken stock
1 tsp. ground paprika

1 tsp. butter
½ tsp. salt
2 tbsp. fresh parsley, chopped

Directions:

Put egg noodles in the Crock Pot. Add chicken stock, butter, ground paprika, and salt. Close the lid and cook the soup on High for 4 hours. Then open the lid, add parsley, and stir the soup.

Crab Stew

Ingredients: Servings: 4   Cooking Time: 5 Hours

8 oz. crab meat, chopped
1 tsp. dried lemongrass
1 tsp. ground turmeric

½ C. mango, chopped
1 potato, peeled chopped
1 C. of water
½ C. of coconut milk

Directions:

Put all ingredients in the Crock Pot. Gently stir them with the help of the spoon and close the lid. Cook the stew on low for 5 hours. Then leave the cooked stew for 10-15 minutes to rest.

Smoked Sausage Stew

Ingredients: Servings: 5   Cooking Time: 3.5 Hours

1-lb. smoked sausages, chopped
1 C. broccoli, chopped
1 C. tomato juice
1 C. of water

1 tsp. butter
1 tsp. dried thyme
¼ C. Cheddar cheese, shredded

Directions:

Grease the Crock Pot bowl with butter from inside. Put the smoked sausages in one layer in the Crock Pot. Add the layer of broccoli and Cheddar cheese. Then mix water with tomato juice and dried thyme. Pour the liquid over the sausage mixture and close the lid. Cook the stew on high for 3.5 hours.

Butternut Squash Soup

Ingredients: Servings: 5   Cooking Time: 7 Hours

2 C. butternut squash, chopped
1 C. carrot, chopped
3 C. chicken stock
1 C. heavy cream

1 tsp. ground cardamom
1 tsp. ground cinnamon

Directions:

Put the butternut squash in the Crock Pot. Sprinkle it with ground cardamom and ground cinnamon. Then add carrot and chicken stock. Close the lid and cook the soup on High for 5 hours. Then blend the soup until smooth with the help of the immersion blender and add heavy cream. Cook the soup on high for 2 hours more.

Mixed Bean Vegetarian Soup

Ingredients: Servings: 8   Cooking Time: 4 1/4 Hours

1 tbsp. olive oil
1 sweet onion, chopped
1 garlic clove, chopped
1 celery stalk, sliced
1 red bell pepper, cored and diced
1/2 tsp. chili powder
1/2 tsp. cumin powder
2 C. vegetable stock

1 carrot, diced
1 can (15 oz.) white bean, drained
1 can (15 oz.) cannellini beans, drained
1 C. diced tomatoes
2 C. water
Salt and pepper to taste
2 tbsp. chopped cilantro
1 lime, juiced
1 avocado, peeled and sliced

Directions:

Heat the oil in a skillet and add the onion, carrot, garlic and celery. Cook for 5 minutes until softened. Transfer in your Crock Pot and stir in the remaining ingredients, except the cilantro, lime and avocado. Adjust the taste with salt and pepper and cook on low settings for 4 hours. When done, pour the soup into serving bowls and top with cilantro and avocado. Drizzle with lime juice and serve right away.

Creamy Cauliflower Soup

Ingredients: Servings: 6   Cooking Time: 3 1/4 Hours

1 tbsp. canola oil
1 sweet onion, chopped
2 garlic cloves, chopped
2 medium size potatoes, peeled and cubed

1 head cauliflower, cut into florets
1 can condensed cream of chicken soup
Salt and pepper to taste
1/2 C. water
1/2 C. grated Parmesan cheese

Directions:

Heat the oil in a skillet and add the onion. Cook for 2 minutes then transfer the onion in your Crock Pot. Add the remaining ingredients, except the cheese, and season with salt and pepper. Cook on high settings for 3 hours. When done, puree the soup with an immersion blender. Serve the soup warm.

Minestrone Soup

Ingredients: Servings: 6   Cooking Time: 6 1/2 Hours

1 shallot, chopped
1 garlic clove, chopped
1 celery stalk, sliced
1 red bell pepper, cored and diced
1 carrot, diced
2 potatoes, peeled and diced

1 C. diced tomatoes
1 tsp. Italian herbs
2 C. chicken stock
4 C. water
1 C. short pasta of your choice
Salt and pepper to taste

Directions:

Combine all the ingredients in your Crock Pot. Add salt and pepper to taste and cook on low settings for 6 hours. Serve the soup warm or chilled.

Cream Of Broccoli Soup

Ingredients: Servings: 6   Cooking Time: 2 1/4 Hours

2 shallots, chopped	1 C. chicken stock
2 garlic cloves, chopped	2 C. water
2 tbsp. olive oil	Salt and pepper to taste
1 head broccoli, cut into florets	1/2 tsp. dried basil
2 potatoes, peeled and cubed	1/2 tsp. dried oregano

Directions:

Heat the oil in a skillet and stir in the shallots and garlic. Sauté for a few minutes until softened then transfer in your Crock Pot. Add the broccoli, potatoes, chicken stock and water, as well as dried herbs, salt and pepper. Cook on high settings for 2 hours then puree the soup in a blender until creamy and rich. Pour the soup into bowls in order to serve.

Southwestern Turkey Stew

Ingredients: Servings: 6   Cooking Time: 7 Hours 15 Minutes

½ C. red kidney beans	½ medium onion, diced
½ C. corn	
2 C. diced canned tomatoes	½ C. sour cream
15 oz. ground turkey	½ C. cheddar cheese, shredded
1 C. red bell peppers, sliced	1 garlic clove, minced
	1½ medium red potatoes, cubed

Directions:

Put all the ingredients in a bowl except sour cream and cheddar cheese. Transfer into the crock pot and cook on LOW for about 7 hours. Stir in the sour cream and cheddar cheese. Dish out in a bowl and serve hot.

Cream Of Chicken Soup

Ingredients: Servings: 6   Cooking Time: 7 1/2 Hours

6 chicken thighs	1/4 tsp. garlic powder
6 C. water	1 pinch chili flakes
1/4 C. all-purpose flour	Salt and pepper to taste
1 C. chicken stock	

Directions:

Combine the chicken with water and cook on low settings for 6 hours. When done, remove the meat from the liquid and shred it off the bone. Combine the flour with stock and mix well. Add the garlic powder and chili flakes and give it a good mix. Pour this mixture over the liquid in the crock pot. Add the meat and cook for 1 additional hour on high settings. Serve the soup warm and fresh.

Jamaican Stew

Ingredients: Servings: 8   Cooking Time: 1 Hour

1 tbsp. coconut oil	1-lb. salmon fillet, chopped
1 tsp. garlic powder	
½ C. bell pepper, sliced	1 tsp. ground coriander
½ C. heavy cream	½ tsp. ground cumin

Directions:

Put the coconut oil in the Crock Pot. Then mix the salmon with ground cumin and ground coriander and put in the Crock Pot. Add the layer of bell pepper and sprinkle with garlic powder. Add heavy cream and close the lid. Cook the stew on High for 1 hour.

Sweet Potato Black Bean Chili

Ingredients: Servings: 6 (3/4 C. Per Serving)   Cooking Time: 6 Hours 35 Minutes

1 medium yellow onion, diced (+coconut or olive oil)	Chili: Optional Spices:
	1 tbsp. chili powder
3 medium sweet potatoes, scrubbed and rinsed, in bite-size pieces, 4 cups	2 tsp. cumin, ground
	½ tsp. cinnamon, ground
1 16-ounce jar salsa, chunky	1-2 tsp. hot sauce
	For Toppings (optional):
1 15-ounce can black beans with salt	Fresh cilantro
	Chopped red onion
2 C. vegetable stock, + 2 C. of water	Avocado
	Lime juice

Directions:

In a large pan, heat 1 tbsp. of oil on medium heat; add sweet onions, along with salt and pepper. Stir and cook until translucent, about 15 minutes. Add sweet potatoes and cook until potatoes begin to soften, about 20 minutes. Add all ingredients to Crock-Pot and stir; cover and cook on LOW for 6 hours. Serve hot.

Snow Peas Soup

Ingredients: Servings: 4   Cooking Time: 3.5 Hours

1 tbsp. chives, chopped	5 oz. bamboo shoots, canned, chopped
1 tsp. ground ginger	2 C. snow peas
8 oz. salmon fillet, chopped	1 tsp. hot sauce
	5 C. of water

Directions:

Put bamboo shoots in the Crock Pot. Add ground ginger, salmon, snow peas, and water. Close the lid and cook the soup for 3 hours on high. Then add hot sauce and chives. Stir the soup carefully and cook for 30 minutes on high.

Leek Potato Soup

Ingredients: Servings: 8   Cooking Time: 6 1/2 Hours

4 leeks, sliced	3 C. water
1 tbsp. olive oil	1 bay leaf

4 bacon slices, chopped
1 celery stalk, sliced
4 large potatoes, peeled and cubed
2 C. chicken stock
Salt and pepper to taste
1/4 tsp. cayenne pepper
1/4 tsp. smoked paprika
1 thyme sprig
1 rosemary sprig

Directions:

Heat the oil in a skillet and add the bacon. Cook until crisp then stir in the leeks. Sauté for 5 minutes until softened then transfer in your Crock Pot. Add the remaining ingredients and cook on low settings for about 6 hours. Serve the soup warm.

Creamy Bacon Soup

Ingredients: Servings: 6   Cooking Time: 1 3/4 Hours

1 tbsp. olive oil
6 bacon slices, chopped
1 1/2 lb. potatoes, peeled and cubed
1 parsnip, diced
1 sweet onion, chopped
1/2 celery root, cubed
2 C. chicken stock
3 C. water
Salt and pepper to taste

Directions:

Heat the oil in a skillet and add the bacon. Cook until crisp then remove the bacon on a plate. Pour the fat of the bacon in your Crock Pot and add the remaining ingredients. Adjust the taste with salt and pepper and cook on high settings for 1 1/2 hours. When done, puree the soup with an immersion blender until smooth. Pour the soup in a bowl and top with bacon. Serve right away.

Ham Potato Chowder

Ingredients: Servings: 8   Cooking Time: 4 1/4 Hours

1 tbsp. olive oil
1 sweet onion, chopped
1 can condensed chicken soup
2 C. water
4 potatoes, peeled and cubed
1 C. diced ham
1 C. sweet corn, drained
1/2 tsp. celery seeds
1/2 tsp. cumin seeds
Salt and pepper to taste

Directions:

Mix the olive oil, onion, chicken soup, water, potatoes, ham and corn in your Crock Pot. Add the celery seeds and cumin seeds and season with salt and pepper. Cook on high settings for 4 hours. Serve the soup warm.

Crock-pot Veggie Tortilla Soup

Ingredients: Servings: 6   Cooking Time: 8 Hours

1 tbsp. olive oil
2 medium cloves, garlic, minced
½ medium jalapeno pepper, seeded and diced
1 (14.5-ounce) can black beans, drained
1 medium onion, diced
1 bay leaf
½ tsp. sea salt
½ tsp. black pepper
½ tsp. coriander,

and rinsed
1 C. fresh or frozen corn kernels
6 C. vegetable broth
2 tsp. chili powder
1 tsp. cumin, ground
ground
Crispy Tortilla Strips: Preheat oven to 400° Fahrenheit. Using a pizza cutter, cut corn tortillas into ½-inch strips. Spread the strips in a single layer on cookie sheet and bake for 12 minutes.

Directions:

In a pan, cook onion and garlic in oil for about 7 minutes over medium heat, then add them to Crock-Pot. Add tomatoes, jalapeno peppers, black beans, corn, broth, cumin, chili powder, bay leaf, salt and pepper to Crock-Pot. Cover and cook on LOW for 8 hours.

Crock-pot Chicken Parmesan Soup

Ingredients: Servings: 4   Cooking Time: 7 Hours

1 green bell pepper, chopped
4 garlic cloves, minced
½ medium white onion, chopped
1 can (14.5-ounces) crushed tomatoes
½ lb. chicken breasts, raw, boneless, skinless
½ C. Parmesan cheese, shredded
2 tbsp. basil, fresh, chopped
5 C. chicken broth
2 tsp. oregano, fresh, chopped
1 tsp. sea salt
½ tsp. black pepper
¼ tsp. red pepper flakes
4-ounces (uncooked) dry penne pasta
2 tbsp. unsalted butter
Chopped parsley for garnish

Directions:

In a Crock-Pot, stir together bell pepper, onion, tomatoes, garlic, chicken, broth, ½ C. cheese, basil, oregano, salt, black pepper, and red pepper flakes. Cover and cook on LOW for 7 hours. Remove chicken about six hours into cooking time and shred it up on a cutting board, then add it back to Crock-Pot, along with penne pasta. Resume cooking. Serve garnished with parsley and Parmesan cheese.

Chicken Parmesan Soup

Ingredients: Servings: 8   Cooking Time: 8 1/4 Hours

8 chicken thighs
1 sweet onion, chopped
1 celery stalk, sliced
1 carrot, sliced
1 celery root, peeled and cubed
2 large potatoes, peeled and cubed
1 can diced tomatoes
2 C. chicken stock
6 C. water
Salt and pepper to taste
2 tbsp. chopped parsley
Parmesan shavings for serving

Directions:

Combine the chicken thighs, onion, celery, carrot, celery root, potatoes and tomatoes in your Crock Pot. Add the stock, water, salt and pepper and cook on low settings for 8 hours. When done, stir in the chopped parsley. Serve the soup topped with Parmesan shavings.

Lentil Stew

Ingredients: Servings: 4   Cooking Time: 6 Hours

2 C. chicken stock	1 eggplant, chopped
½ C. red lentils	1 C. of water
1 tbsp. tomato paste	1 tsp. Italian seasonings

Directions:

Mix chicken stock with red lentils and tomato paste. Pour the mixture in the Crock Pot. Add eggplants and Italian seasonings. Cook the stew on low for 6 hours.

Ham Bone Cabbage Soup

Ingredients: Servings: 8   Cooking Time: 7 1/4 Hours

1 ham bone	1 can diced tomatoes
1 sweet onion, chopped	2 C. beef stock
1 mediums size cabbage head, shredded	Salt and pepper to taste
2 tbsp. tomato paste	1 bay leaf
	1 thyme sprig
	1 lemon, juiced

Directions:

Combine the ham bone, onion, cabbage, tomato paste, tomatoes, stock, bay leaf and thyme sprig in your Crock Pot. Add salt and pepper to taste and cook on low settings for 7 hours. When done, stir in the lemon juice and serve the soup warm.

Chicken Sweet Potato Soup

Ingredients: Servings: 6   Cooking Time: 6 1/4 Hours

2 chicken breasts, cubed	2 shallots, chopped
2 tbsp. olive oil	1 C. chicken stock
1 celery stalk, sliced	4 C. water
1 can fire roasted tomatoes	Salt and pepper to taste
1 1/2 lb. sweet potatoes, peeled and cubed	1/2 tsp. cumin seeds
	1/4 tsp. caraway seeds
	1 thyme sprig

Directions:

Heat the oil in a skillet and stir in the chicken, shallots and celery. Sauté for a few minutes until softened then transfer in your Crock Pot. Add the remaining ingredients and season with salt and pepper. Cook on low settings for 6 hours. The soup is best served warm.

Kale Potato Soup

Ingredients: Servings: 6   Cooking Time: 2 1/4 Hours

1 shallot, chopped	1/4 lb. kale, chopped
1 garlic clove, chopped	2 C. chicken stock
1 celery stalk, sliced	4 C. water
2 carrots, sliced	Salt and pepper to taste
1 1/2 lb. potatoes,	1/4 tsp. chili flakes
	2 tbsp. lemon juice

peeled and cubed
1/2 C. diced tomatoes

Directions:

Combine the shallot, garlic, celery, carrots, potatoes and tomatoes in your Crock Pot. Add the kale, chili flakes, lemon juice, water and stock and season with salt and pepper. Cook on high settings for 2 hours. Serve the soup warm.

Hot Lentil Soup

Ingredients: Servings: 4   Cooking Time: 24.5 Hours

1 potato, peeled, diced	1 onion, diced
1 C. lentils	1 tsp. cayenne pepper
5 C. chicken stock	1 tsp. olive oil
1 tsp. chili powder	1 tbsp. tomato paste

Directions:

Roast the onion in the olive oil until light brown and transfer in the Crock Pot. Add lentils, chicken stock, potato, chili powder, cayenne pepper, and tomato paste. Carefully stir the soup mixture until the tomato paste is dissolved. Close the lid and cook the soup on High for 5 hours.

Chicken Sausage Soup

Ingredients: Servings: 8   Cooking Time: 6 1/2 Hours

1 lb. Italian sausages, sliced	1 can diced tomatoes
1 sweet onion, chopped	1 can cannellini beans
2 garlic cloves, chopped	1/4 C. dry white wine
1 red bell pepper, cored and diced	2 C. chicken stock
1 carrot, diced	3 C. water
1/2 tsp. dried oregano	1/2 C. short pasta
1/2 tsp. dried basil	Salt and pepper to taste
	2 tbsp. chopped parsley

Directions:

Combine the sausages, onion, garlic, bell pepper, carrot, oregano, basil, tomatoes, beans, wine, stock and water in a Crock Pot. Cook on high settings for 1 hour then add the pasta and continue cooking for 5 hours. Serve the soup warm, topped with freshly chopped parsley.

Chicken Chili

Ingredients: Servings: 4   Cooking Time: 5 Hours

1 chili pepper, chopped	2 C. ground chicken
1 yellow onion, chopped	1 tsp. dried basil
2 tbsp. tomato paste	½ tsp. ground coriander
	3 C. of water

Directions:

Mix ground chicken with dried basil and ground coriander. Then transfer the chicken in the Crock Pot. Add onion, chili pepper, tomato paste, and water. Carefully stir the mixture and close the lid. Cook the chili on high for 5 hours.

Moroccan Lamb Soup

Ingredients: Servings: 6   Cooking Time: 7 1/2 Hours

1 lb. lamb shoulder
1 tsp. turmeric powder
1/2 tsp. cumin powder
1/2 tsp. chili powder
2 tbsp. canola oil
2 C. chicken stock
1 C. fire roasted tomatoes

3 C. water
1 C. canned chickpeas, drained
1 thyme sprig
1/2 tsp. dried sage
1/2 tsp. dried oregano
Salt and pepper to taste
1 lemon, juiced

Directions:

Sprinkle the lamb with salt, pepper, turmeric, cumin powder and chili powder.   Heat the oil in a skillet and add the lamb. Cook on all sides for a few minutes then transfer it in a Crock Pot. Add the remaining ingredients and season with salt and pepper. Cook the soup on low settings for 7 hours.   Serve the soup warm.

Three Bean Soup

Ingredients: Servings: 10   Cooking Time: 4 1/2 Hours

2 tbsp. olive oil
2 sweet onions, chopped
2 garlic cloves, minced
2 red bell peppers, cored and diced
1 can (15 oz.) black beans, drained
1 can (15 oz.) kidney beans, drained

2 carrots, diced
1 can (15 oz.) pinto beans, drained
2 C. chicken stock
4 C. water
1 C. diced tomatoes
Salt and pepper to taste
1 lime, juiced
1/2 C. sour cream
2 tbsp. chopped parsley

Directions:

Heat the oil in a skillet and stir in the onions, garlic, peppers and carrot. Sauté for 5 minutes.   Transfer the mixture in your Crock Pot and stir in the beans, stock, water, tomatoes, salt and pepper. Cook on low settings for 4 hours.   When done, add the lime juice. Pour the soup in serving bowls and top with sour cream and parsley.   The soup is best served warm or cold.

Creamy Noodle Soup

Ingredients: Servings: 8   Cooking Time: 8 1/4 Hours

2 chicken breasts, cubed
2 tbsp. all-purpose flour
1 celery stalk, sliced
1 can condensed chicken soup

2 shallots, chopped
2 C. water
2 C. chicken stock
Salt and pepper to taste
1 C. green peas
6 oz. egg noodles

Directions:

Sprinkle the chicken with salt, pepper and flour and place it in your Crock Pot.   Add the remaining ingredients and season with salt and pepper.   Cover and cook on low settings for 8 hours. This soup is best served warm.

Cheddar Garlic Soup

Ingredients: Servings: 6   Cooking Time: 2 1/4 Hours

8 garlic cloves, chopped
2 tbsp. olive oil
1 tsp. cumin seeds
1 tsp. mustard seeds

2 tbsp. all-purpose flour
2 C. chicken stock
1/4 C. white wine
4 C. water
3 C. grated Cheddar
Salt and pepper to taste

Directions:

Heat the oil in a skillet and add the garlic. Sauté on low heat for 2 minutes then add the seeds and cook for 1 minute to release flavor.   Add the flour and cook for 1 hour then transfer the mix in your Crock Pot.   Add the remaining ingredients and season with salt and pepper.   Cook on high settings for 2 hours.   The soup is best served warm.

Pumpkin Stew With Chicken

Ingredients: Servings: 2   Cooking Time: 4 Hours

½ C. pumpkin, chopped
6 oz. chicken fillet, cut into strips
¼ C. coconut cream

1 tbsp. curry powder
½ tsp. ground cinnamon
1 onion, chopped

Directions:

Mix pumpkin with chicken fillet strips in the mixing bowl.   Add curry powder, coconut cream, ground cinnamon, and onion. Mix the stew ingredients and transfer them in the Crock Pot. Cook the meal on high for 4 hours.

Shrimp Chowder

Ingredients: Servings: 4   Cooking Time: 1 Hour

1-lb. shrimps
½ C. fennel bulb, chopped
1 bay leaf
½ tsp. peppercorn

1 C. of coconut milk
3 C. of water
1 tsp. ground coriander

Directions:

Put all ingredients in the Crock Pot.   Close the lid and cook the chowder on High for 1 hour.

Split Pea Sausage Soup

Ingredients: Servings: 8   Cooking Time: 6 1/4 Hours

2 C. split peas, rinsed
8 C. water
4 Italian sausages, sliced
1 sweet onion, chopped
2 carrots, diced
1 celery stalk, diced
1 garlic clove, chopped

1 red chili, chopped
1/2 tsp. dried oregano
2 tbsp. tomato paste
Salt and pepper to taste
1 lemon, juiced
2 tbsp. chopped parsley

Directions:

Combine the split peas, water, sausages, onion, carrots, celery, garlic, red chili, oregano and tomato paste in your Crock Pot. Add salt and pepper to taste and cook on low settings for 6 hours. When done, stir in the lemon juice and parsley and serve the soup warm.

Vegan Grain-free Cream Of Mushroom Soup

Ingredients: Servings: 2   Cooking Time: 4 Hours

2 C. cauliflower florets	1 2/3 C. unsweetened almond milk
1 tsp. onion powder	¼ tsp. Himalayan rock salt
1 ½ C. white mushrooms, diced	½ yellow onion, diced

Directions:

Place onion powder, milk, cauliflower, salt, and pepper in a pan, cover and bring to a boil over medium heat. Reduce heat to low and simmer for 8 minutes or until cauliflower is softened. Then, puree mixture in food processor. In a pan, add oil, mushrooms, and onions, heat over high heat for about 8 minutes. Add mushrooms and onion mix to cauliflower mixture in Crock-Pot. Cover and cook on LOW for 4 hours. Serve hot.

Hungarian Goulash Soup

Ingredients: Servings: 8   Cooking Time: 8 1/2 Hours

2 sweet onions, chopped	2 carrots, diced
1 lb. beef roast, cubed	2 tbsp. tomato paste
2 tbsp. canola oil	1 C. diced tomatoes
1/2 celery stalk, diced	1/2 C. beef stock
2 red bell peppers, cored and diced	5 C. water
1 1/2 lb. potatoes, peeled and cubed	1/2 tsp. cumin seeds
	1/2 tsp. smoked paprika
	Salt and pepper to taste

Directions:

Heat the oil in a skillet and stir in the beef. Cook for 5 minutes on all sides then stir in the onion. Sauté for 2 additional minutes then transfer in your Crock Pot. Add the remaining ingredients and season with salt and pepper. Cook on low settings for 8 hours. Serve the soup warm.

Bacon Cheeseburger Soup

Ingredients: Servings: 8   Cooking Time: 6 1/2 Hours

4 bacon slices, chopped	1/2 tsp. dried thyme
1 lb. ground beef	1/2 tsp. dried oregano
1 large sweet onion, chopped	1 C. cream cheese
2 carrots, diced	2 C. beef stock
1 celery stalk, sliced	5 C. water
2 potatoes, peeled and cubed	Salt and pepper to taste
1 C. diced tomatoes	Processed cheese for serving

Directions:

Heat the bacon in a skillet and cook until crisp. Add the beef and cook for a few minutes, stirring often. Add the remaining

ingredients and season with salt and pepper. Cook on low settings for 6 hours. The soup is best served warm, topped with shredded processed cheese.

Broccoli Cheese Soup

Ingredients: Servings: 6   Cooking Time: 6 Hours 20 Minutes

1½ C. heavy cream	¾ tsp. salt
2½ C. water	2 tbsp. butter
½ C. red bell pepper, chopped	½ tsp. dry mustard
2 C. broccoli, chopped, thawed and drained	8 oz. cheddar cheese, shredded
2 tbsp. chives, chopped	4 C. chicken broth
	¼ tsp. cayenne pepper

Directions:

Put all the ingredients in a crockpot except chives and cheese and mix well. Cover and cook on LOW for about 6 hours. Sprinkle with cheese and cook on LOW for about 30 minutes. Garnish with chives and serve hot.

Roasted Garlic Soup

Ingredients: Servings: 6   Cooking Time: 3 ½ Hours

1 tbsp. extra-virgin olive oil	1 large head of cauliflower, chopped, about 5 cups
2 bulbs of garlic	
3 shallots, chopped	Fresh ground pepper to taste
6 C. gluten-free vegetable broth	Sea salt to taste

Directions:

Preheat oven to 400° Fahrenheit. Peel the outer layers off garlic bulbs. Cut about 1/4 inch off the top of the bulbs, place into foil pan. Coat bulbs with olive oil, and cook in oven for 35 minutes. Once cooked, allow them to cool. Squeeze the garlic out of the bulbs into your food processor. Meanwhile, in a pan, sauté remaining olive oil and chopped shallots over medium-high heat for about 6 minutes. Add other ingredients to saucepan, cover and reduce heat to a simmer for 20 minutes or until the cauliflower is softened. Add the mixture to food processor and puree until smooth. Add mix to Crock Pot, cover with lid, and cook on LOW for 3 ½ hours. Serve hot.

Winter Veggie Soup

Ingredients: Servings: 8   Cooking Time: 6 1/2 Hours

1 sweet onion, chopped	Salt and pepper to taste
2 carrots, sliced	2 C. vegetable stock
1 celery stalk, sliced	3 C. water
1/2 head cabbage, shredded	1 C. diced tomatoes
1 parsnip, sliced	1/4 C. white rice, rinsed
1 celery root, peeled and cubed	1 lemon, juiced

Directions:

Combine the onion, carrots, celery, cabbage, parsnip, celery, stock, water, tomatoes and rice in your Crock Pot. Add salt and pepper to taste, as well as the rice and cook on low settings for 6 hours.   The soup is best served warm.

Spicy White Chicken Soup

Ingredients: Servings: 8   Cooking Time: 6 1/4 Hours

2 chicken breasts, cubed	1/4 tsp. cayenne pepper
2 tbsp. olive oil	1/2 tsp. dried oregano
1 large onion, chopped	1/2 tsp. dried basil
2 garlic cloves, chopped	2 cans (15 oz.) white beans, drained
2 C. chicken stock	5 C. water
1 parsnip, diced	1 bay leaf
1/2 tsp. cumin seeds	Salt and pepper to taste

Directions:
Heat the oil in a skillet and add the chicken. Cook on all sides until golden then transfer in your Crock Pot.   Add the onion, garlic, stock, parsnip, cumin seeds, cayenne pepper, oregano, basil, beans, water and bay leaf.   Adjust the taste with salt and pepper and cook on low settings for 6 hours.   Serve the soup warm and fresh.

Comforting Chicken Soup

Ingredients: Servings: 8   Cooking Time: 8 1/2 Hours

1 whole chicken, cut into pieces	8 C. water
2 carrots, cut into sticks	6 oz. egg noodles
1 celery stalk, sliced	2 garlic cloves, chopped
4 potatoes, peeled and cubed	Salt and pepper to taste
	1 whole onion
	1 bay leaf

Directions:
Combine all the ingredients in your Crock Pot.   Add salt and pepper to taste and cook on low settings for 8 hours.   Serve the soup warm.

Butternut Squash Chili

Ingredients: Servings: 4   Cooking Time: 3.5 Hours

1 C. butternut squash, chopped	1 tsp. smoked paprika
2 tbsp. pumpkin puree	½ tsp. chili flakes
½ C. red kidney beans, canned	1 tbsp. cocoa powder
½ tsp. salt	2 C. chicken stock

Directions:
Mix cocoa powder with chicken stock and stir it until smooth. Then pour the liquid in the Crock Pot.   Add all remaining ingredients and carefully mix the chili.   Close the lid and cook the chili on high for 3.5 hours.

Curried Turkey Soup

Ingredients: Servings: 8   Cooking Time: 6 1/2 Hours

2 tbsp. olive oil	2 carrots, diced
1 1/2 lb. turkey	1 tsp. grated ginger
breast, cubed	1 C. coconut milk
1 sweet onion, chopped	3 C. chicken stock
1 celery stalk, sliced	1 C. water
2 garlic cloves, chopped	1 tbsp. curry powder
	Salt and pepper to taste

Directions:
Heat the oil in a skillet and stir in the turkey. Cook on all sides for a few minutes until golden then transfer in your Crock Pot. Add the carrots, onion, celery, garlic, ginger, coconut milk, stock, water and curry powder.   Season with salt and pepper and cook on low settings for 6 hours.   Serve the soup warm.

Smoked Sausage Lentil Soup

Ingredients: Servings: 6   Cooking Time: 6 1/4 Hours

2 links smoked sausages, sliced	1/2 tsp. smoked paprika
1 sweet onion, chopped	1 bay leaf
2 carrots, diced	1 thyme sprig
1 C. red lentils	1 lemon, juiced
1/2 C. green lentils	1 C. fire roasted tomatoes
2 C. chicken stock	Salt and pepper to taste
2 C. water	

Directions:
Combine the sausages with the remaining ingredients in your Crock Pot.   Add salt and pepper to taste and cover with a lid. Cook on low settings for 6 hours.   The soup can be served both warm and chilled.

Orange Soup

Ingredients: Servings: 6   Cooking Time: 4 Hours

1 C. sweet potato, chopped	1 tsp. curry powder
1 C. carrot, chopped	1 C. heavy cream
1 tsp. ground turmeric	4 C. of water

Directions:
Put sweet potato and carrot in the Crock Pot.   Add ground turmeric and water.   Then mix the curry powder and heavy cream and pour the liquid over the vegetables.   Close the lid and cook the soup for 4 hours on High.   Blend the soup with the help of the immersion blender if desired.

Provencal Beef Soup

Ingredients: Servings: 8   Cooking Time: 7 1/4 Hours

2 tbsp. olive oil	2 carrots, sliced
1 lb. beef roast, cubed	1 can diced tomatoes
1 sweet onion, chopped	1 C. beef stock
1 garlic clove, chopped	1 C. red wine
1 celery stalk, sliced	4 C. water
	1/2 tsp. dried thyme
	1 bay leaf
	Salt and pepper to taste

Directions:

Heat the oil in a skillet and stir in the beef roast. Cook on all sides for a few minutes then transfer the beef in a Crock Pot.   Add the remaining ingredients and adjust the taste with salt and pepper. Cook on low settings for 7 hours.   Serve the soup warm or chilled.

Meat Baby Carrot Stew

Ingredients: Servings: 3   Cooking Time: 8 Hours

1 C. baby carrot	1 tsp. peppercorns
6 oz. lamb loin, chopped	3 C. of water
1 tbsp. tomato paste	1 bay leaf

Directions:

Put all ingredients in the Crock Pot.   Close the lid and cook the stew on Low for 8 hours.   Carefully stir the stew and cool it to the room temperature.

Quinoa Soup With Parmesan Topping

Ingredients: Servings: 6   Cooking Time: 3 1/2 Hours

2 chicken breasts, cubed	1 sweet onion, chopped
2 tbsp. olive oil	1 garlic clove, chopped
2/3 C. quinoa, rinsed	2 C. chicken stock
1/2 tsp. dried oregano	4 C. water
1/2 tsp. dried basil	Salt and pepper to taste
1 C. diced tomatoes	1 C. grated Parmesan for serving

Directions:

Heat the oil in a skillet and add the chicken. Cook on all sides until golden brown then transfer the chicken in your Crock Pot. Add the remaining ingredients, except the Parmesan, and cook on high settings for 3 hours.   When done, pour the soup into serving bowls and top with grated Parmesan before serving.

Light Minestrone Soup

Ingredients: Servings: 4   Cooking Time: 4 Hours

1 C. green beans, chopped	1 tsp. curry powder
1 small zucchini, chopped	2 tbsp. tomato paste
¼ C. garbanzo beans	½ C. ground pork
5 C. chicken stock	

Directions:

Put all ingredients in the Crock Pot bowl.   Close the lid and cook the soup on High for 4 hours.

SIDE DISH RECIPES

Eggplant And Kale Mix

Ingredients: Servings: 6   Cooking Time: 2 Hours

14 oz. canned roasted tomatoes and garlic	2 tbsp. olive oil
4 C. eggplant, cubed	1 tsp. mustard
1 yellow bell pepper, chopped	3 tbsp. red vinegar
1 red onion, cut into medium wedges	1 garlic clove, minced
4 C. kale leaves	Salt and black pepper to the taste
	½ C. basil, chopped

Directions:

In your Crock Pot, mix the eggplant with tomatoes, bell pepper and onion, toss, cover and cook on High for 2 hours.   Add kale, toss, cover Crock Pot and leave aside for now.   In a bowl, mix oil with vinegar, mustard, garlic, salt and pepper and whisk well. Add this over eggplant mix, also add basil, toss, divide between plates and serve as a side dish.

Mustard Brussels Sprouts(1)

Ingredients: Servings: 2   Cooking Time: 3 Hours

1 lb. Brussels sprouts, trimmed and halved	Salt and black pepper to the taste
1 tbsp. olive oil	¼ C. veggie stock
1 tbsp. mustard	A pinch of red pepper, crushed
1 tbsp. balsamic vinegar	2 tbsp. chives, chopped

Directions:

In your Crock Pot, mix the Brussels sprouts with the oil, mustard and the other ingredients, toss, put the lid on and cook on High for 3 hours.   Divide the mix between plates and serve as a side dish.

Butter Green Beans

Ingredients: Servings: 2   Cooking Time: 2 Hours

1 lb. green beans, trimmed and halved	½ C. veggie stock
2 tbsp. butter, melted	1 tbsp. chives, chopped
1 tsp. rosemary, dried	Salt and black pepper to the taste
	¼ tsp. soy sauce

Directions:

In your Crock Pot, combine the green beans with the melted butter, stock and the other ingredients, toss, put the lid on and cook on Low for 2 hours.   Divide between plates and serve as a side dish.

Lemon Kale Mix

Ingredients: Servings: 2   Cooking Time: 2 Hours

1 yellow bell pepper, chopped	1 tbsp. lemon juice
1 red bell pepper, chopped	½ C. veggie stock
1 tbsp. olive oil	1 garlic clove, minced
1 red onion, sliced	A pinch of salt and black pepper
4 C. baby kale	1 tbsp. basil, chopped
1 tsp. lemon zest, grated	

Directions:

In your Crock Pot, mix the kale with the oil, onion, bell peppers and the other ingredients, toss, put the lid on and cook on Low for 2 hours.   Divide the mix between plates and serve as a side dish.

Millet With Dill

Ingredients: Servings: 6   Cooking Time: 5 Hours

2 tbsp. butter
½ C. half and half
1 tsp. salt
½ C. fresh dill

1 tsp. basil
4 C. of water
4 C. millet
1 tsp. olive oil

Directions:
Add water, millet, olive oil, half and half cream, salt, and basil to the Crock Pot.   Put the cooker's lid on and set the cooking time to 5 hours on Low settings.   Garnish with dill and serve.

Cauliflower And Carrot Gratin

Ingredients: Servings: 12   Cooking Time: 7 Hours

16 oz. baby carrots
6 tbsp. butter, soft
1 cauliflower head, florets separated
Salt and black pepper to the taste

1 yellow onion, chopped
1 tsp. mustard powder
1 and ½ C. milk
6 oz. cheddar cheese, grated
½ C. breadcrumbs

Directions:
Put the butter in your Crock Pot, add carrots, cauliflower, onion, salt, pepper, mustard powder and milk and toss.   Sprinkle cheese and breadcrumbs all over, cover and cook on Low for 7 hours.   Divide between plates and serve as a side dish.

Okra And Corn

Ingredients: Servings: 4   Cooking Time: 8 Hours

3 garlic cloves, minced
1 small green bell pepper, chopped
1 small yellow onion, chopped
1 C. water
16 oz. okra, sliced
2 C. corn
1 and ½ tsp. smoked paprika

28 oz. canned tomatoes, crushed
1 tsp. oregano, dried
1 tsp. thyme, dried
1 tsp. marjoram, dried
A pinch of cayenne pepper
Salt and black pepper to the taste

Directions:
In your Crock Pot, mix garlic with bell pepper, onion, water, okra, corn, paprika, tomatoes, oregano, thyme, marjoram, cayenne, salt and pepper, cover, cook on Low for 8 hours, divide between plates and serve as a side dish.

Blueberry And Spinach Salad

Ingredients: Servings: 3   Cooking Time: 1 Hour

¼ C. pecans, chopped
2 tsp. maple syrup
1 tbsp. white vinegar
2 tbsp. orange juice

½ tsp. sugar
1 tbsp. olive oil
4 C. spinach
2 oranges, peeled and

cut into segments
1 C. blueberries

Directions:
In your Crock Pot, mix pecans with sugar, maple syrup, vinegar, orange juice, oil, spinach, oranges and blueberries, toss, cover and cook on High for 1 hour.   Divide between plates and serve as a side dish.

Carrot Beet Salad

Ingredients: Servings: 6   Cooking Time: 7 Hours

½ C. walnuts, chopped
¼ C. lemon juice
½ C. olive oil
1 shallot, chopped
1 tsp. Dijon mustard
Salt and black pepper to the taste

1 tbsp. brown sugar
2 beets, peeled and cut into wedges
2 carrots, peeled and sliced
1 C. parsley
5 oz. arugula

Directions:
Add beets, carrots, and rest of the ingredients to the Crock Pot. Put the cooker's lid on and set the cooking time to 7 hours on Low settings.   Serve warm.

Cauliflower And Potatoes Mix

Ingredients: Servings: 2   Cooking Time: 4 Hours

1 C. cauliflower florets
½ lb. sweet potatoes, peeled and cubed
1 C. veggie stock
½ C. tomato sauce

1 tbsp. chives, chopped
Salt and black pepper to the taste
1 tsp. sweet paprika

Directions:
In your Crock Pot, mix the cauliflower with the potatoes, stock and the other ingredients, toss, put the lid on and cook on High for 4 hours.   Divide between plates and serve as a side dish.

Creamy Risotto

Ingredients: Servings: 4   Cooking Time: 1 Hour

4 oz. mushrooms, sliced
½ quart veggie stock
2 tbsp. porcini mushrooms

1 tsp. olive oil
2 C. white rice
A small bunch of parsley, chopped

Directions:
In your Crock Pot, mix mushrooms with stock, oil, porcini mushrooms and rice, stir, cover and cook on High for 1 hour. Add parsley, stir, divide between plates and serve as a side dish.

Cauliflower Carrot Gratin

Ingredients: Servings: 12   Cooking Time: 7 Hours

16 oz. baby carrots
1 cauliflower head, florets separated
Salt and black pepper to the taste

6 tbsp. butter, soft
1 tsp. mustard powder
1 and ½ C. of milk
6 oz. cheddar cheese,

1 yellow onion, chopped	grated
	½ C. breadcrumbs

Directions:
Add carrots, cauliflower, and rest of the ingredients to the Crock Pot. Put the cooker's lid on and set the cooking time to 7 hours on Low settings. Serve warm.

Orange Squash

Ingredients: Servings: 6   Cooking Time: 5 Hours

1 lb. butternut squash, peeled and diced	1 tsp. ground cinnamon
1 Poblano pepper,chopped	1 tbsp. salt
	1 C. heavy cream
1 tsp. brown sugar	1 orange, sliced
	¼ tsp. ground cardamom

Directions:
Toss the butternut squash with poblano pepper, salt, cream, cardamom, sugar, and cardamom. Spread the orange slices in the insert of the Crock Pot. Spread the butternut squash-poblano pepper mixture over the orange slices. Put the cooker's lid on and set the cooking time to 5 hours on Low settings. Serve warm.

Italian Black Beans Mix

Ingredients: Servings: 2   Cooking Time: 5 Hours

2 tbsp. tomato paste Cooking spray	½ celery rib, chopped
2 C. black beans	
¼ C. veggie stock	½ sweet red pepper, chopped
1 red onion, sliced Cooking spray	
1 tsp. Italian seasoning	¼ tsp. mustard seeds
	Salt and black pepper to the taste
½ red bell pepper, chopped	2 oz. canned corn, drained
	1 tbsp. cilantro, chopped

Directions:
Grease the Crock Pot with the cooking spray, and mix the beans with the stock, onion and the other ingredients inside. Put the lid on, cook on Low for 5 hours, divide between plates and serve as a side dish.

Maple Brussels Sprouts

Ingredients: Servings: 12   Cooking Time: 3 Hours

1 C. red onion, chopped	¼ C. apple juice
2 lb. Brussels sprouts, trimmed and halved	3 tbsp. olive oil
	¼ C. maple syrup
Salt and black pepper to the taste	1 tbsp. thyme, chopped

Directions:
In your Crock Pot, mix Brussels sprouts with onion, salt, pepper and apple juice, toss, cover and cook on Low for 3 hours. In a bowl, mix maple syrup with oil and thyme, whisk really well, add

over Brussels sprouts, toss well, divide between plates and serve as a side dish.

Veggies Rice Pilaf

Ingredients: Servings: 4   Cooking Time: 5 Hours

2 C. basmati rice	2 tbsp. butter
1 C. mixed carrots, peas, corn, and green beans	1 cinnamon stick
	1 tbsp. cumin seeds
	2 bay leaves
2 C. of water	3 whole cloves
½ tsp. green chili, minced	5 black peppercorns
	2 whole cardamoms
½ tsp. ginger, grated	1 tbsp. sugar
3 garlic cloves, minced	Salt to the taste

Directions:
Add water, rice, veggies and all other ingredients to the Crock Pot. Put the cooker's lid on and set the cooking time to 5 hours on Low settings. Discard the cinnamon and serve warm.

Butternut Squash And Eggplant Mix

Ingredients: Servings: 2   Cooking Time: 4 Hours

1 butternut squash, peeled and roughly cubed	¼ C. tomato paste
	½ tbsp. parsley, chopped
1 eggplant, roughly cubed	
	Salt and black pepper to the taste
1 red onion, chopped	
Cooking spray	2 garlic cloves, minced
½ C. veggie stock	

Directions:
Grease the Crock Pot with the cooking spray and mix the squash with the eggplant, onion and the other ingredients inside. Put the lid on and cook on Low for 4 hours. Divide between plates and serve as a side dish.

Mint Farro Pilaf

Ingredients: Servings: 2   Cooking Time: 4 Hours

½ tbsp. balsamic vinegar	½ tbsp. olive oil
½ C. whole grain farro	1 tbsp. green onions, chopped
A pinch of salt and black pepper	1 tbsp. mint, chopped
1 C. chicken stock	

Directions:
In your Crock Pot, mix the farro with the vinegar and the other ingredients, toss, put the lid on and cook on Low for 4 hours. Divide between plates and serve.

Bean Medley

Ingredients: Servings: 12   Cooking Time: 5 Hours

2 celery ribs, chopped	16 oz. kidney beans, drained
1 and ½ C. ketchup	
1 green bell pepper, chopped	Salt and black pepper to the taste
1 yellow onion,	15 oz. canned black-

chopped
1 sweet red pepper, chopped
½ C. brown sugar
½ C. Italian dressing
½ C. water
1 tbsp. cider vinegar
2 bay leaves

eyed peas, drained
15 oz. canned northern beans, drained
15 oz. canned corn, drained
15 oz. canned lima beans, drained
15 oz. canned black beans, drained

Directions:

In your Crock Pot, mix celery with ketchup, red and green bell pepper, onion, sugar, Italian dressing, water, vinegar, bay leaves, kidney beans, black-eyed peas, northern beans, corn, lima beans and black beans, stir, cover and cook on Low for 5 hours. Divide between plates and serve as a side dish.

Mango Rice

Ingredients: Servings: 2   Cooking Time: 2 Hours

1 C. rice
2 C. chicken stock
½ C. mango, peeled and cubed

Salt and black pepper to the taste
1 tsp. olive oil

Directions:

In your Crock Pot, mix the rice with the stock and the other ingredients, toss, put the lid on and cook on High for 2 hours. Divide between plates and serve as a side dish.

Okra Side Dish(2)

Ingredients: Servings: 4   Cooking Time: 4 Hours

1 lb. okra, sliced
1 tomato, chopped
6 oz. tomato sauce
Salt and black pepper to the taste

1 C. water
1 yellow onion, chopped
2 garlic cloves, minced

Directions:

In your Crock Pot, mix okra with tomato, tomato sauce, water, salt, pepper, onion and garlic, stir, cover and cook on Low for 4 hours. Divide between plates and serve as a side dish.

Bbq Beans

Ingredients: Servings: 2   Cooking Time: 8 Hours

¼ lb. navy beans, soaked overnight and drained
1 C. bbq sauce
1 tbsp. sugar
1 tbsp. ketchup
1 tbsp. water

1 tbsp. apple cider vinegar
1 tbsp. olive oil
1 tbsp. soy sauce

Directions:

In your Crock Pot, mix the beans with the sauce, sugar and the other ingredients, toss, put the lid on and cook on Low for 8 hours. Divide between plates and serve as a side dish.

Herbed Eggplant Cubes

Ingredients: Servings: 8   Cooking Time: 4 Hours

17 oz. eggplants, peeled and cubed
1 tbsp. salt
1 tsp. ground black pepper
1 tsp. cilantro

4 C. of water
7 tbsp. mayo
1 tsp. onion powder
1 tsp. garlic powder
1 tbsp. nutmeg
3 tbsp. butter

Directions:

Add eggplant, salt, and water to the Crock Pot. Put the cooker's lid on and set the cooking time to 1 hour on High settings. Meanwhile, mix remaining spices, butter, and mayo in a bowl. Drain the cooked eggplants and return them to the Crock Pot. Now add the butter-mayo mixture to the eggplants. Put the cooker's lid on and set the cooking time to 3 hours on Low settings. Serve warm.

Creamy Red Cabbage

Ingredients: Servings: 9   Cooking Time: 8 Hours

17 oz. red cabbage, sliced
1 C. fresh cilantro, chopped
3 red onions, diced
1 tbsp. sliced almonds
1 C. sour cream
½ C. chicken stock

1 tsp. salt
1 tbsp. tomato paste
1 tsp. ground black pepper
1 tsp. cumin
½ tsp. thyme
2 tbsp. butter
1 C. green peas

Directions:

Add cabbage, onion and all other ingredients to the Crock Pot. Put the cooker's lid on and set the cooking time to 8 hours on Low settings. Serve warm.

Spinach Mix

Ingredients: Servings: 2   Cooking Time: 1 Hour

1 lb. baby spinach
½ C. cherry tomatoes, halved
½ tbsp. olive oil
1 small yellow onion, chopped
¼ tsp. coriander, ground

½ C. veggie stock
¼ tsp. cumin, ground
¼ tsp. garam masala
¼ tsp. chili powder
Salt and black pepper to the taste

Directions:

In your Crock Pot, mix the spinach with the tomatoes, oil and the other ingredients, toss, put the lid on and cook on High for 1 hour. Divide between plates and serve as a side dish.,

Rice And Beans

Ingredients: Servings: 6   Cooking Time: 5 Hours

1 lb. red kidney beans, soaked overnight and drained
Salt to the taste
1 tsp. olive oil
1 lb. smoked sausage, roughly chopped
1 yellow onion,

1 green bell pepper, chopped
1 tsp. thyme, dried
2 bay leaves
5 C. water
Long grain rice, already cooked
2 green onions, minced

chopped
1 celery stalk,
chopped
4 garlic cloves,
chopped

2 tbsp. parsley,
minced
Hot sauce for serving

Directions:

In your Crock Pot, mix red beans with salt, oil, sausage, onion, celery, garlic, bell pepper, thyme, bay leaves and water, cover and cook on Low for 5 hours. Divide the rice between plates, add beans, sausage and veggies on top, sprinkle green onions and parsley and serve as a side dish with hot sauce drizzled all over.

Lemony Pumpkin Wedges

Ingredients: Servings: 4   Cooking Time: 6 Hours

15 oz. pumpkin,
peeled and cut into
wedges
1 tbsp. lemon juice

1 tsp. salt
1 tsp. honey
½ tsp. ground
cardamom
1 tsp. lime juice

Directions:

Add pumpkin, lemon juice, honey, lime juice, cardamom, and salt to the Crock Pot. Put the cooker's lid on and set the cooking time to 6 hours on Low settings. Serve fresh.

Corn And Bacon

Ingredients: Servings: 20   Cooking Time: 4 Hours

10 C. corn
24 oz. cream cheese,
cubed
½ C. milk
½ C. melted butter
½ C. heavy cream
¼ C. sugar

A pinch of salt and
black pepper
4 bacon strips,
cooked and crumbled
2 tbsp. green onions,
chopped

Directions:

In your Crock Pot, mix corn with cream cheese, milk, butter, cream, sugar, salt, pepper, bacon and green onions, cover and cook on Low for 4 hours. Stir the corn, divide between plates and serve as a side dish.

Mashed Potatoes(2)

Ingredients: Servings: 2   Cooking Time: 6 Hours

1 lb. gold potatoes,
peeled and cubed
2 garlic cloves,
chopped

1 C. milk
1 C. water
2 tbsp. butter
A pinch of salt and
white pepper

Directions:

In your Crock Pot, mix the potatoes with the water, salt and pepper, put the lid on and cook on Low for 6 hours. Mash the potatoes, add the rest of the ingredients, whisk and serve.

Nut Berry Salad

Ingredients: Servings: 4   Cooking Time: 1 Hour

2 C. strawberries,
halved

1 tbsp. canola oil
4 C. spinach, torn

2 tbsp. mint, chopped
1/3 C. raspberry
vinegar
2 tbsp. honey
Salt and black pepper
to the taste

½ C. blueberries
¼ C. walnuts,
chopped
1 oz. goat cheese,
crumbled

Directions:

Toss strawberries with walnuts, spinach, honey, oil, salt, black pepper, blueberries, vinegar, and mint in the Crock Pot. Put the cooker's lid on and set the cooking time to 1 hour on High settings. Serve warm with cheese on top.

Mashed Potatoes(1)

Ingredients: Servings: 12   Cooking Time: 4 Hours

3 lb. gold potatoes,
peeled and cubed
1 bay leaf
6 garlic cloves,
minced

28 oz. chicken stock
1 C. milk
¼ C. butter
Salt and black pepper
to the taste

Directions:

In your Crock Pot, mix potatoes with bay leaf, garlic, salt, pepper and stock, cover and cook on Low for 4 hours. Drain potatoes, mash them, mix with butter and milk, blend really, divide between plates and serve as a side dish.

Brussels Sprouts And Cauliflower

Ingredients: Servings: 2   Cooking Time: 4 Hours

1 C. Brussels sprouts,
trimmed and halved
1 C. cauliflower
florets
1 tbsp. olive oil
2 tbsp. tomato paste

1 C. veggie stock
1 tsp. chili powder
½ tsp. ginger powder
A pinch of salt and
black pepper
1 tbsp. thyme,
chopped

Directions:

In your Crock Pot, mix the Brussels sprouts with the cauliflower, oil, stock and the other ingredients, toss, put the lid on and cook on Low for 4 hours. Divide the mix between plates and serve as a side dish.

Coconut Bok Choy

Ingredients: Servings: 2   Cooking Time: 1 Hour

1 lb. bok choy, torn
½ tsp. chili powder
1 garlic clove, minced

½ C. chicken stock
1 tsp. ginger, grated
1 tbsp. coconut oil
Salt to the taste

Directions:

In your Crock Pot, mix the bok choy with the stock and the other ingredients, toss, put the lid on and cook on High for 1 hour. Divide between plates and serve as a side dish.

Wild Rice Mix

Ingredients: Servings: 16   Cooking Time: 6 Hours

45 oz. chicken stock
1 C. carrots, sliced
2 and ½ C. wild rice
4 oz. mushrooms, sliced
2 tbsp. butter, soft

Salt and black pepper to the taste
2 tsp. marjoram, dried
2/3 C. dried cherries
2/3 C. green onions, chopped
½ C. pecans, chopped

Directions:

In your Crock Pot, mix stock with carrots, rice, mushrooms, butter, salt, pepper and marjoram, cover and cook on Low for 6 hours. Add cherries, green onions and pecans, toss, divide between plates and serve as a side dish.

Scalloped Cheese Potatoes

Ingredients: Servings: 12   Cooking Time: 7 Hours

2 lbs. potato, peeled and sliced
1 lb. sweet potato, peel
1 tsp. ground black pepper
1/3 C. butter, unsalted

1 tbsp. salt
4 tbsp. flour
1 tbsp. minced garlic
4 C. of milk
¼ tsp. nutmeg
4 oz. Parmesan
5 oz. Cheddar cheese

Directions:

Toss potatoes with salt and black pepper to season them. Spread the potatoes and sweet potatoes in the Crock Pot in layers. Whisk butter with flour, nutmeg, milk, garlic, parmesan, and cheddar cheese in a suitable bowl. Pour this milk-flour mixture over the potatoes. Put the cooker's lid on and set the cooking time to 7 hours on Low settings. Serve warm.

Potatoes And Leeks Mix

Ingredients: Servings: 2   Cooking Time: 4 Hours

2 leeks, sliced
½ lb. sweet potatoes, cut into medium wedges
½ tbsp. balsamic vinegar

½ C. veggie stock
1 tbsp. chives, chopped
½ tsp. pumpkin pie spice

Directions:

In your Crock Pot, mix the leeks with the potatoes and the other ingredients, toss, put the lid on and cook on High for 4 hours. Divide between plates and serve as a side dish.

Corn Cucumber Salad

Ingredients: Servings: 6   Cooking Time: 5 Hours

1 C. corn kernels
5 oz. dried tomatoes, cut into strips
1 tsp. salt
1 C. heavy cream
2 cucumbers, diced

1 red onion, diced
1 tsp. ground paprika
1 C. fresh parsley
1 carrot, grated
1 tsp. olive oil

Directions:

Add corn kernels, dried tomatoes, cream, paprika, onion, and salt to the Crock Pot. Put the cooker's lid on and set the cooking

time to 5 hours on Low settings. Transfer this corn mixture to a salad bowl. Toss in parsley, carrot, and cucumbers. Serve fresh.

Cheesy Rice

Ingredients: Servings: 6   Cooking Time: 4 Hrs.

2 garlic cloves, minced
2 tbsp. olive oil
¾ C. yellow onion, chopped
1 and ½ C. Arborio rice
½ C. white wine
12 oz. spinach, chopped

3 and ½ C. hot veggie stock
Salt and black pepper to the taste
4 oz. goat cheese, soft and crumbled
2 tbsp. lemon juice
1/3 C. pecans, toasted and chopped

Directions:

Add spinach, garlic, oil, onion, rice, salt, black, stock, and wine to the Crock Pot. Put the cooker's lid on and set the cooking time to 4 hours on Low settings. Stir in goat cheese and lemon juice. Serve warm.

Cider Dipped Farro

Ingredients: Servings: 6   Cooking Time: 5 Hours

1 tbsp. apple cider vinegar
1 C. whole-grain farro
1 tsp. lemon juice
Salt to the taste
3 C. of water
1 tbsp. olive oil

½ C. cherries, dried and chopped
¼ C. green onions, chopped
10 mint leaves, chopped
2 C. cherries, pitted and halved

Directions:

Add water and farro to the Crock Pot. Put the cooker's lid on and set the cooking time to 5 hours on Low settings. Toss the cooker farro with salt, cherries, mint, green onion, lemon juice, and oil in a bowl. Serve fresh.

Balsamic Cauliflower

Ingredients: Servings: 2   Cooking Time: 5 Hours

2 C. cauliflower florets
1 tbsp. balsamic vinegar
1 tbsp. lemon zest, grated
2 spring onions, chopped

½ C. veggie stock
¼ tsp. sweet paprika
Salt and black pepper to the taste
1 tbsp. dill, chopped

Directions:

In your Crock Pot, mix the cauliflower with the stock, vinegar and the other ingredients, toss, put the lid on and cook on Low for 5 hours. Divide the cauliflower mix between plates and serve.

Hot Lentils

Ingredients: Servings: 2   Cooking Time: 6 Hours

1 tbsp. thyme, chopped
½ tbsp. olive oil
1 C. canned lentils, drained
2 garlic cloves, minced
½ C. veggie stock
1 tbsp. cider vinegar
2 tbsp. tomato paste
1 tbsp. rosemary, chopped

Directions:

In your Crock Pot, mix the lentils with the thyme and the other ingredients, toss, put the lid on and cook on Low for 6 hours. Divide between plates and serve as a side dish.

Stewed Okra

Ingredients: Servings: 4   Cooking Time: 3 Hours

2 C. okra, sliced
2 garlic cloves, minced
6 oz. tomato sauce
A pinch of cayenne peppers
1 red onion, chopped
1 tsp. liquid smoke
Salt and black pepper to the taste

Directions:

In your Crock Pot, mix okra with garlic, onion, cayenne, tomato sauce, liquid smoke, salt and pepper, cover, cook on Low for 3 hours. Divide between plates and serve as a side dish.

Parmesan Spinach Mix

Ingredients: Servings: 2   Cooking Time: 2 Hours

2 garlic cloves, minced
1 lb. baby spinach
A drizzle of olive oil
Salt and black pepper to the taste
¼ C. veggie stock
4 tbsp. heavy cream
2 tbsp. parmesan cheese, grated

Directions:

Grease your Crockpot with the oil, and mix the spinach with the garlic and the other ingredients inside. Toss, put the lid on and cook on Low for 2 hours. Divide the mix between plates and serve as a side dish.

Okra Mix

Ingredients: Servings: 4   Cooking Time: 8 Hours

2 garlic cloves, minced
1 yellow onion, chopped
14 oz. tomato sauce
1 tsp. sweet paprika
2 C. okra, sliced
Salt and black pepper to the taste

Directions:

In your Crock Pot, mix garlic with the onion, tomato sauce, paprika, okra, salt and pepper, cover and cook on Low for 8 hours. Divide between plates and serve as a side dish.

Italian Eggplant

Ingredients: Servings: 2   Cooking Time: 2 Hours

2 small eggplants, roughly cubed
Salt and black pepper
½ C. heavy cream
A pinch of hot pepper

to the taste
1 tbsp. olive oil
flakes
2 tbsp. oregano, chopped

Directions:

In your Crock Pot, mix the eggplants with the cream and the other ingredients, toss, put the lid on and cook on High for 2 hours. Divide between plates and serve as a side dish.

Refried Black Beans

Ingredients: Servings: 10   Cooking Time: 9 Hours

5 oz. white onion, peeled and chopped
4 C. black beans
1 chili pepper, chopped
1 oz. minced garlic
10 C. water
1 tsp. salt
½ tsp. ground black pepper
¼ tsp. cilantro, chopped

Directions:

Add onion, black beans and all other ingredients to the Crock Pot. Put the cooker's lid on and set the cooking time to 9 hours on Low settings. Strain all the excess liquid out of the beans while leaving only ¼ C. of the liquid. Transfer the beans-onion mixture to a food processor and blend until smooth. Serve fresh.

Sweet Potatoes With Bacon

Ingredients: Servings: 6   Cooking Time: 5 Hours

4 lb. sweet potatoes, peeled and sliced
3 tbsp. brown sugar
½ tsp. sage, dried
½ C. orange juice
½ tsp. thyme, dried
4 bacon slices, cooked and crumbled
2 tbsp. soft butter

Directions:

Arrange sweet potato slices in your Crock Pot, add sugar, orange juice, sage, thyme, butter and bacon, cover and cook on Low for 5 hours. Divide between plates and serve them as a side dish.

Squash And Peppers Mix

Ingredients: Servings: 4   Cooking Time: 1 Hr 30 Minutes

2 red bell peppers, cut into wedges
2 green bell peppers, cut into wedges
1/3 C. Italian dressing
1 red onion, cut into wedges
12 small squash, peeled and cut into wedges
Salt and black pepper to the taste
1 tbsp. parsley, chopped

Directions:

Add squash, peppers, and rest of the ingredients to the Crock Pot. Put the cooker's lid on and set the cooking time to 1.5 hours on High settings. Garnish with parsley. Serve warm.

Asparagus Mix(1)

Ingredients: Servings: 2   Cooking Time: 2 Hours

1 lb. asparagus,
trimmed and halved
1 red onion, sliced
2 garlic cloves,
minced
1 C. veggie stock

1 tbsp. lemon juice
A pinch of salt and
black pepper
¼ C. parsley,
chopped

Directions:

In your Crock Pot, mix the asparagus with the onion, garlic and the other ingredients, toss, put the lid on and cook on High for 2 hours. Divide between plates and serve as a side dish.

Cabbage And Kale Mix

Ingredients: Servings: 2   Cooking Time: 2 Hours

1 red onion, sliced
1 C. green cabbage,
shredded
½ C. canned
tomatoes, crushed
½ tsp. hot paprika

1 C. baby kale
½ tsp. Italian
seasoning
A pinch of salt and
black pepper
1 tbsp. dill, chopped

Directions:

In your Crock Pot, mix the cabbage with the kale, onion and the other ingredients, toss, put the lid on and cook on High for 2 hours. Divide between plates and serve right away as a side dish.

Cornbread Cream Pudding

Ingredients: Servings: 8   Cooking Time: 8 Hours

11 oz. cornbread mix
1 C. corn kernels
3 C. heavy cream
1 C. sour cream
3 eggs
1 chili pepper
1 tsp. salt

1 tsp. ground black
pepper
2 oz. pickled jalapeno
¼ tbsp. sugar
1 tsp. butter

Directions:

Whisk eggs in a suitable bowl and add cream and cornbread mix. Mix it well then add salt, chili pepper, sour cream, sugar, butter, and black pepper. Add corn kernels and pickled jalapeno then mix well to make a smooth dough. Spread this dough in the insert of a Crock Pot. Put the cooker's lid on and set the cooking time to 8 hours on Low settings. Slice and serve.

Cauliflower And Broccoli Mix

Ingredients: Servings: 10   Cooking Time: 7 Hours

4 C. broccoli florets
4 C. cauliflower
florets
7 oz. Swiss cheese,
torn
14 oz. Alfredo sauce

1 yellow onion,
chopped
Salt and black pepper
to the taste
1 tsp. thyme, dried
½ C. almonds, sliced

Directions:

In your Crock Pot, mix broccoli with cauliflower, cheese, sauce, onion, salt, pepper and thyme, stir, cover and cook on Low for 7 hours. Add almonds, divide between plates and serve as a side dish.

Creamy Hash Brown Mix

Ingredients: Servings: 12   Cooking Time: 3 Hours

2 lb. hash browns
1 and ½ C. milk
10 oz. cream of
chicken soup
1 C. cheddar cheese,
shredded

½ C. butter, melted
Salt and black pepper
to the taste
¾ C. cornflakes,
crushed

Directions:

In a bowl, mix hash browns with milk, cream of chicken, cheese, butter, salt and pepper, stir, transfer to your Crock Pot, cover and cook on Low for 3 hours. Add cornflakes, divide between plates and serve as a side dish.

Scalloped Potatoes

Ingredients: Servings: 6   Cooking Time: 6 Hours

Cooking spray
2 and ½ lb. gold
potatoes, sliced
10 oz. canned cream
of potato soup
1 yellow onion,
roughly chopped
8 oz. sour cream
1 C. Gouda cheese,
shredded

½ C. blue cheese,
crumbled
½ C. parmesan,
grated
½ C. chicken stock
Salt and black pepper
to the taste
1 tbsp. chives,
chopped

Directions:

Grease your Crock Pot with cooking spray and arrange potato slices on the bottom. Add cream of potato soup, onion, sour cream, Gouda cheese, blue cheese, parmesan, stock, salt and pepper, cover and cook on Low for 6 hours. Add chives, divide between plates and serve as a side dish.

Curry Broccoli Mix

Ingredients: Servings: 2   Cooking Time: 3 Hours

1 lb. broccoli florets
1 C. tomato paste
1 tbsp. red curry
paste
½ tsp. Italian
seasoning

1 red onion, sliced
1 tsp. thyme, dried
Salt and black pepper
to the taste
½ tbsp. cilantro,
chopped

Directions:

In your Crock Pot, mix the broccoli with the curry paste, tomato paste and the other ingredients, toss, put the lid on and cook on Low for 3 hours. Divide the mix between plates and serve as a side dish.

Spinach Rice

Ingredients: Servings: 2   Cooking Time: 2 Hours

2 scallions, chopped
1 tbsp. olive oil
1 C. Arborio rice
6 oz. spinach,
chopped

1 C. chicken stock
Salt and black pepper
to the taste
2 oz. goat cheese,
crumbled

Directions:

In your Crock Pot, mix the rice with the stock and the other ingredients, toss, put the lid on and cook on High for 2 hours. Divide between plates and serve as a side dish.

Pumpkin Nutmeg Rice

Ingredients: Servings: 4   Cooking Time: 5 Hours

2 oz. olive oil
1 small yellow onion, chopped
2 garlic cloves, minced
12 oz. risotto rice
4 C. chicken stock
6 oz. pumpkin puree

½ tsp. nutmeg, ground
1 tsp. thyme, chopped
½ tsp. ginger, grated
½ tsp. cinnamon powder
½ tsp. allspice, ground
4 oz. heavy cream

Directions:
Add rice, pumpkin puree, and all other ingredients except the cream to the Crock Pot.   Put the cooker's lid on and set the cooking time to 4 hours 30 minutes on Low settings.   Stir in cream and cover again to the cook for 30 minutes on the low setting.   Serve warm.

Ramen Noodles

Ingredients: Servings: 5   Cooking Time: 25 Minutes

1 tbsp. ramen seasoning
10 oz. ramen noodles
4 C. chicken stock

1 tsp. salt
3 tbsp. soy sauce
1 tsp. paprika
1 tbsp. butter

Directions:
Add chicken stock, butter, ramen, paprika, noodles and all other ingredients to the Crock Pot.   Put the cooker's lid on and set the cooking time to 25 minutes on High settings.   Serve warm.

Pink Salt Rice

Ingredients: Servings: 8   Cooking Time: 5 Hours

1 tsp. salt
2 and ½ C. of water

2 C. pink rice

Directions:
Add rice, salt, and water to the Crock Pot.   Put the cooker's lid on and set the cooking time to 5 hours on Low settings.   Serve warm.

White Beans Mix

Ingredients: Servings: 4   Cooking Time: 6 Hours

1 celery stalk, chopped
2 garlic cloves, minced
1 carrot, chopped
1 C. veggie stock
½ C. canned tomatoes, crushed

½ tsp. chili powder
½ tbsp. Italian seasoning
15 oz. canned white beans, drained
1 tbsp. parsley, chopped

Directions:

In your Crock Pot, mix the beans with the celery, garlic and the other ingredients, toss, put the lid on and cook on Low for 6 hours.   Divide the mix between plates and serve.

Beans And Red Peppers

Ingredients: Servings: 2   Cooking Time: 2 Hrs.

2 C. green beans, halved
1 red bell pepper, cut into strips
1 tbsp. olive oil

Salt and black pepper to the taste
1 and ½ tbsp. honey mustard

Directions:
Add green beans, honey mustard, red bell pepper, oil, salt, and black to Crock Pot.   Put the cooker's lid on and set the cooking time to 2 hours on High settings.   Serve warm.

Tangy Red Potatoes

Ingredients: Servings: 4   Cooking Time: 8 Hours

1 lb. red potato
2 tbsp. olive oil
1 garlic clove
1 tsp. sage
4 tbsp. mayo

1 tsp. minced garlic
3 tbsp. fresh dill, chopped
1 tsp. paprika

Directions:
Add potatoes, olive oil, garlic cloves, garlic, and sage to the Crock Pot.   Put the cooker's lid on and set the cooking time to 8 hours on Low settings.   Whisk mayo and minced garlic in a suitable bowl.   Transfer the slow-cooked potatoes to a bowl and mash them using a fork.   Stir in the mayo-garlic mixture then mix well. Serve fresh.

Italian Veggie Mix

Ingredients: Servings: 8   Cooking Time: 6 Hours

38 oz. canned cannellini beans, drained
1 yellow onion, chopped
¼ C. basil pesto
19 oz. canned fava beans, drained
4 garlic cloves, minced

1 and ½ tsp. Italian seasoning, dried and crushed
1 tomato, chopped
15 oz. already cooked polenta, cut into medium pieces
2 C. spinach
1 C. radicchio, torn

Directions:
In your Crock Pot, mix cannellini beans with fava beans, basil pesto, onion, garlic, Italian seasoning, polenta, tomato, spinach and radicchio, toss, cover and cook on Low for 6 hours.   Divide between plates and serve as a side dish.

Creamy Chipotle Sweet Potatoes

Ingredients: Servings: 10   Cooking Time: 4 Hours

1 sweet onion, chopped
2 tbsp. olive oil
¼ C. parsley, chopped
2 shallots, chopped

4 big sweet potatoes, shredded
8 oz. coconut cream
16 oz. bacon, cooked and chopped

2 tsp. chipotle pepper, crushed
Salt and black pepper
½ tsp. sweet paprika
Cooking spray

Directions:

Heat up a pan with the oil over medium-high heat, add shallots and onion, stir, cook for 6 minutes and transfer to a bowl. Add parsley, chipotle pepper, salt, pepper, sweet potatoes, coconut cream, paprika and bacon, stir, pour everything in your Crock Pot after you've greased it with some cooking spray, cover, cook on Low for 4 hours, leave aside to cool down a bit, divide between plates and serve as a side dish.

Squash Side Salad

Ingredients: Servings: 8   Cooking Time: 4 Hours

1 tbsp. olive oil
1 C. carrots, chopped
1 yellow onion, chopped
1 tsp. sugar
1 and ½ tsp. curry powder
1 garlic clove, minced
1 big butternut squash, peeled and cubed
A pinch of sea salt and black pepper
¼ tsp. ginger, grated
½ tsp. cinnamon powder
3 C. coconut milk

Directions:

In your Crock Pot, mix oil with carrots, onion, sugar, curry powder, garlic, squash, salt, pepper, ginger, cinnamon and coconut milk, stir well, cover and cook on Low for 4 hours. Stir, divide between plates and serve as a side dish.

Carrot Shallots Medley

Ingredients: Servings: 7   Cooking Time: 6 Minutes

1 large carrot, cut into strips
1 lb. shallots, chopped
1 C. heavy cream
1 tbsp. sugar
1 tsp. salt
1 tsp. ground black pepper
1 tsp. cilantro
1 tbsp. butter, unsalted
1 tbsp. minced garlic

Directions:

Add carrot and shallots to the Crock Pot. Whisk cream with sugar, salt, black pepper, cilantro, butter, and garlic. Pour this mixture over the veggies. Put the cooker's lid on and set the cooking time to 6 hours on Low settings. Serve warm.

Jalapeno Meal

Ingredients: Servings: 6   Cooking Time: 6 Hrs.

12 oz. jalapeno pepper, cut in half and deseeded
2 tbsp. olive oil
1 tbsp. balsamic vinegar
1 onion, sliced
1 garlic clove, sliced
1 tsp. ground coriander
4 tbsp. water

Directions:

Place the jalapeno peppers in the Crock Pot. Top the pepper with olive oil, balsamic vinegar, onion, garlic, coriander, and

water. Put the cooker's lid on and set the cooking time to 6 hours on Low settings. Serve warm.

Sweet Potato And Cauliflower Mix

Ingredients: Servings: 2   Cooking Time: 4 Hours

2 sweet potatoes, peeled and cubed
1 C. cauliflower florets
½ C. coconut milk
1 tsp. sriracha sauce
A pinch of salt and black pepper
½ tbsp. sugar
1 tbsp. red curry paste
3 oz. white mushrooms, roughly chopped
2 tbsp. cilantro, chopped

Directions:

In your Crock Pot, mix the sweet potatoes with the cauliflower and the other ingredients, toss, put the lid on and cook on Low for 4 hours. Divide between plates and serve as a side dish.

Marjoram Rice Mix

Ingredients: Servings: 2   Cooking Time: 6 Hours

1 C. wild rice
2 C. chicken stock
1 carrot, peeled and grated
2 tbsp. marjoram, chopped
1 tbsp. olive oil
A pinch of salt and black pepper
1 tbsp. green onions, chopped

Directions:

In your Crock Pot, mix the rice with the stock and the other ingredients, toss, put the lid on and cook on Low for 6 hours. Divide between plates and serve.

Garlic Butter Green Beans

Ingredients: Servings: 6   Cooking Time: 2 Hours

22 oz. green beans
2 garlic cloves, minced
¼ C. butter, soft
2 tbsp. parmesan, grated

Directions:

In your Crock Pot, mix green beans with garlic, butter and parmesan, toss, cover and cook on High for 2 hours. Divide between plates, sprinkle parmesan all over and serve as a side dish.

Spinach And Squash Side Salad

Ingredients: Servings: 12   Cooking Time: 4 Hours

3 lb. butternut squash, peeled and cubed
1 yellow onion, chopped
2 tsp. thyme, chopped
3 garlic cloves, minced
A pinch of salt and black pepper
10 oz. veggie stock
6 oz. baby spinach

Directions:

In your Crock Pot, mix squash cubes with onion, thyme, salt, pepper and stock, stir, cover and cook on Low for 4 hours.

Transfer squash mix to a bowl, add spinach, toss, divide between plates and serve as a side dish.

Chorizo And Cauliflower Mix

Ingredients: Servings: 4   Cooking Time: 5 Hours

1 lb. chorizo, chopped	12 oz. canned green
1 yellow onion,	chilies, chopped
chopped	1 cauliflower head,
½ tsp. garlic powder	riced
Salt and black pepper	2 tbsp. green onions,
to the taste	chopped

Directions:

Heat up a pan over medium heat, add chorizo and onion, stir, brown for a few minutes and transfer to your Crock Pot. Add chilies, garlic powder, salt, pepper, cauliflower and green onions, toss, cover and cook on Low for 5 hours.   Divide between plates and serve as a side dish.

Asparagus And Mushroom Mix

Ingredients: Servings: 4   Cooking Time: 5 Hours

2 lb. asparagus	Salt and black pepper
spears, cut into	to the taste
medium pieces	2 C. coconut milk
1 C. mushrooms,	1 tsp. Worcestershire
sliced	sauce
A drizzle of olive oil	5 eggs, whisked

Directions:

Grease your Crock Pot with the oil and spread asparagus and mushrooms on the bottom.   In a bowl, mix the eggs with milk, salt, pepper and Worcestershire sauce, whisk, pour into the Crock Pot, toss everything, cover and cook on Low for 6 hours. Divide between plates and serve as a side dish.

Peas And Carrots

Ingredients: Servings: 12   Cooking Time: 5 Hours

1 yellow onion,	¼ C. honey
chopped	4 garlic cloves,
1 lb. carrots, sliced	minced
16 oz. peas	A pinch of salt and
¼ C. melted butter	black pepper
¼ C. water	1 tsp. marjoram,
	dried

Directions:

In your Crock Pot, mix onion with carrots, peas, butter, water, honey, garlic, salt, pepper and marjoram, cover and cook on Low for 5 hours.   Stir peas and carrots mix, divide between plates and serve as a side dish.

Green Beans And Mushrooms

Ingredients: Servings: 4   Cooking Time: 3 Hours

1 lb. fresh green	1 C. chicken stock
beans, trimmed	8 oz. mushrooms,
1 small yellow onion,	sliced
chopped	Salt and black pepper
6 oz. bacon, chopped	to the taste
1 garlic clove, minced	

A splash of balsamic vinegar

Directions:

In your Crock Pot, mix beans with onion, bacon, garlic, stock, mushrooms, salt, pepper and vinegar, stir, cover and cook on Low for 3 hours.   Divide between plates and serve as a side dish.

Rice And Farro Pilaf

Ingredients: Servings: 12   Cooking Time: 5 Hours

1 shallot, chopped	6 C. chicken stock
1 tsp. garlic, minced	Salt and black pepper
A drizzle of olive oil	to the taste
1 and ½ C. whole	1 tbsp. parsley and
grain farro	sage, chopped
¾ C. wild rice	½ C. hazelnuts,
	toasted and chopped
	¾ C. cherries, dried

Directions:

In your Crock Pot, mix oil with garlic, shallot, farro, rice, stock, salt, pepper, sage and parsley, hazelnuts and cherries, toss, cover and cook on Low for 5 hours.   Divide between plates and serve as a side dish.

Cinnamon Squash

Ingredients: Servings: 2   Cooking Time: 4 Hours

1 acorn squash,	A pinch of cinnamon
peeled and cut into	powder
medium wedges	A pinch of salt and
1 C. coconut cream	black pepper

Directions:

In your Crock Pot, mix the squash with the cream and the other ingredients, toss, put the lid on and cook on Low for 4 hours. Divide between plates and serve as a side dish.

Thyme Beets

Ingredients: Servings: 8   Cooking Time: 6 Hours

12 small beets, peeled	1 tsp. thyme, dried
and sliced	Salt and black pepper
¼ C. water	to the taste
4 garlic cloves,	1 tbsp. fresh thyme,
minced	chopped
2 tbsp. olive oil	

Directions:

In your Crock Pot, mix beets with water, garlic, oil, dried thyme, salt and pepper, cover and cook on Low for 6 hours.   Divide beets on plates, sprinkle fresh thyme all over and serve as a side dish.

Cumin Quinoa Pilaf

Ingredients: Servings: 2   Cooking Time: 2 Hours

1 C. quinoa	1 tsp. turmeric
2 tsp. butter, melted	powder
Salt and black pepper	2 C. chicken stock
to the taste	1 tsp. cumin, ground

Directions:

Grease your Crock Pot with the butter, add the quinoa and the other ingredients, toss, put the lid on and cook on High for 2 hours   Divide between plates and serve as a side dish.

Asian Sesame Asparagus

Ingredients: Servings: 4   Cooking Time: 4 Hrs.

1 tbsp. sesame seeds	1 tsp. salt
1 tsp. miso paste	1 tsp. chili flakes
¼ C. of soy sauce	1 tsp. oregano
1 C. fish stock	1 C. of water
8 oz. asparagus	

Directions:

Fill the insert of the Crock Pot with water and add asparagus. Put the cooker's lid on and set the cooking time to 3 hours on High settings.   During this time, mix miso paste with soy sauce, fish stock, and sesame seeds in a suitable bowl.   Stir in oregano, chili flakes, and salt, then mix well.   Drain the slow-cooked asparagus then return it to the Crock Pot.   Pour the miso-stock mixture over the asparagus.   Put the cooker's lid on and set the cooking time to 1 hour on High settings.   Serve warm.

Kale Mix

Ingredients: Servings: 2   Cooking Time: 2 Hours

1 lb. baby kale	½ C. chicken stock
½ tbsp. tomato paste	1 tbsp. olive oil
½ tsp. chili powder	1 small yellow onion, chopped
A pinch of salt and black pepper	1 tbsp. apple cider vinegar

Directions:

In your Crock Pot, mix the kale with the tomato paste, stock and the other ingredients, toss, put the lid on and cook on Low for 2 hours.   Divide between plates and serve as a side dish.

Garlicky Black Beans

Ingredients: Servings: 8   Cooking Time: 7 Hours

1 C. black beans, soaked overnight, drained and rinsed	1 spring onion, chopped
1 C. of water	2 garlic cloves, minced
Salt and black pepper to the taste	½ tsp. cumin seeds

Directions:

Add beans, salt, black pepper, cumin seeds, garlic, and onion to the Crock Pot.   Put the cooker's lid on and set the cooking time to 7 hours on Low settings.   Serve warm.

Berry Wild Rice

Ingredients: Servings: 4   Cooking Time: 5 Hours 30 Minutes

2 C. wild rice	1 tbsp. chives
4 C. of water	1 tbsp. butter
1 tsp. salt	2 tbsp. heavy cream
6 oz. cherries, dried	

Directions:

Add wild rice, salt, water, and dried cherries to the Crock Pot. Put the cooker's lid on and set the cooking time to 5 hours on High settings.   Stir in cream and butter, then cover again to cook for 30 minutes on the low setting.   Serve.

Veggie And Garbanzo Mix

Ingredients: Servings: 4   Cooking Time: 6 Hours

15 oz. canned garbanzo beans, drained	1 C. carrot, sliced
	½ C. onion, chopped
3 C. cauliflower florets	2 tsp. curry powder
1 C. green beans	¼ C. basil, chopped
14 oz. veggie stock	14 oz. coconut milk

Directions:

In your Crock Pot, mix beans with cauliflower, green beans, carrot, onion, stock, curry powder, basil and milk, stir, cover and cook on Low for 6 hours.   Stir veggie mix again, divide between plates and serve as a side dish.

Apples And Potatoes

Ingredients: Servings: 10   Cooking Time: 7 Hours

2 green apples, cored and cut into wedges	1 C. coconut cream
	½ C. dried cherries
3 lb. sweet potatoes, peeled and cut into medium wedges	1 C. apple butter
	1 and ½ tsp. pumpkin pie spice

Directions:

In your Crock Pot, mix sweet potatoes with green apples, cream, cherries, apple butter and spice, toss, cover and cook on Low for 7 hours.   Toss, divide between plates and serve as a side dish.

Zucchini Onion Pate

Ingredients: Servings: 6   Cooking Time: 6 Hours

3 medium zucchinis, peeled and chopped	1 tsp. butter
	1 tbsp. brown sugar
2 red onions, grated	½ tsp. ground black pepper
6 tbsp. tomato paste	
½ C. fresh dill	1 tsp. paprika
1 tsp. salt	¼ chili pepper

Directions:

Add zucchini to the food processor and blend for 3 minutes until smooth.   Transfer the zucchini blend to the Crock Pot.   Stir in onions and all other ingredients.   Put the cooker's lid on and set the cooking time to 6 hours on Low settings.   Serve warm.

Broccoli Mix

Ingredients: Servings: 10   Cooking Time: 2 Hours

6 C. broccoli florets	¼ C. yellow onion, chopped
1 and ½ C. cheddar cheese, shredded	
10 oz. canned cream of celery soup	Salt and black pepper to the taste
½ tsp. Worcestershire sauce	1 C. crackers, crushed
	2 tbsp. soft butter

Directions:

In a bowl, mix broccoli with cream of celery soup, cheese, salt, pepper, onion and Worcestershire sauce, toss and transfer to your Crock Pot. Add butter, toss again, sprinkle crackers, cover and cook on High for 2 hours. Serve as a side dish.

Farro Mix

Ingredients: Servings: 2   Cooking Time: 4 Hours

2 scallions, chopped	2 C. chicken stock
2 garlic cloves, minced	Salt and black pepper to the taste
1 tbsp. olive oil	½ tbsp. parsley, chopped
1 C. whole grain farro	1 tbsp. cherries, dried

Directions:

In your Crock Pot, mix the farro with the scallions, garlic and the other ingredients, toss, put the lid on and cook on Low for 4 hours. Divide between plates and serve as a side dish.

Saffron Risotto

Ingredients: Servings: 2   Cooking Time: 2 Hours

½ tbsp. olive oil	A pinch of salt and black pepper
¼ tsp. saffron powder	A pinch of cinnamon powder
1 C. Arborio rice	1 tbsp. almonds, chopped
2 C. veggie stock	

Directions:

In your Crock Pot, mix the rice with the stock and the other ingredients, toss, put the lid on and cook on High for 2 hours. Divide between plates and serve as a side dish.

Lemony Honey Beets

Ingredients: Servings: 6   Cooking Time: 8 Hours

6 beets, peeled and cut into medium wedges	Salt and black pepper to the taste
2 tbsp. honey	1 tbsp. white vinegar
2 tbsp. olive oil	½ tsp. lemon peel, grated
2 tbsp. lemon juice	

Directions:

Add beets, honey, oil, salt, black pepper, lemon peel, vinegar, and lemon juice to the Crock Pot. Put the cooker's lid on and set the cooking time to 8 hours on Low settings. Serve warm.

SNACK RECIPES

Blue Cheese Parsley Dip

Ingredients: Servings: 7   Cooking Time: 7 Hours

1 C. parsley, chopped	6 oz. cream
8 oz. celery stalk, chopped	1 tsp. minced garlic
6 oz. Blue cheese, chopped	1 tsp. paprika
	¼ tsp. ground red pepper

1 tbsp. apple cider vinegar	1 onion, peeled and grated

Directions:

Whisk the cream with cream cheese in a bowl and add to the Crock Pot. Toss in parsley, celery stalk, garlic, onion, apple cider vinegar, and red pepper ground. Put the cooker's lid on and set the cooking time to 7 hours on Low settings. Mix the dip after 4 hours of cooking then resume cooked. Serve.

Artichoke Dip(1)

Ingredients: Servings: 2   Cooking Time: 2 Hours

2 oz. canned artichoke hearts, drained and chopped	2 oz. heavy cream
	2 green onions, chopped
2 tbsp. mayonnaise	½ tsp. garam masala
¼ C. mozzarella, shredded	Cooking spray

Directions:

Grease your Crock Pot with the cooking spray, and mix the artichokes with the cream, mayo and the other ingredients inside. Stir, cover, cook on Low for 2 hours, divide into bowls and serve as a party dip.

Almond Spread

Ingredients: Servings: 2   Cooking Time: 8 Hours

¼ C. almonds	1 C. heavy cream
½ tsp. nutritional yeast flakes	A pinch of salt and black pepper

Directions:

In your Crock Pot, mix the almonds with the cream and the other ingredients, toss, put the lid on and cook on Low for 8 hours. Transfer to a blender, pulse well, divide into bowls and serve.

Bacon Fingerling Potatoes

Ingredients: Servings: 15   Cooking Time: 8 Hours

2 lb. fingerling potatoes	1 tsp. garlic powder
	1 tsp. paprika
8 oz. bacon	3 tbsp. butter
1 tsp. onion powder	1 tsp. dried dill
1 tsp. chili powder	1 tbsp. rosemary

Directions:

Grease the base of your Crock Pot with butter. Spread the fingerling potatoes in the buttered cooker. Mix all the spices, herbs, and bacon in a bowl. Spread bacon-spice mixture over the lingering potatoes. Put the cooker's lid on and set the cooking time to 8 hours on Low settings. Serve warm.

Ginger Chili Peppers

Ingredients: Servings: 7   Cooking Time: 3 Hours

2 tbsp. balsamic vinegar	3 tbsp. water
	1 tsp. oregano
10 oz. red chili pepper, chopped	1 tsp. ground black pepper
4 garlic cloves, peeled and sliced	4 tbsp. olive oil

| 1 white onion, chopped | 1 tsp. ground nutmeg |
| | ½ tsp. ground ginger |

Directions:

Spread the red chili peppers in the Crock Pot. Mix onion and garlic with remaining ingredients and spread on top of chili peppers. Put the cooker's lid on and set the cooking time to 3 hours on High settings. Serve.

Mushroom Dip(1)

Ingredients: Servings: 2   Cooking Time: 5 Hours

4 oz. white mushrooms, chopped	A pinch of salt and black pepper
1 eggplant, cubed	1 tbsp. balsamic vinegar
½ C. heavy cream	½ tbsp. basil, chopped
½ tbsp. tahini paste	
2 garlic cloves, minced	½ tbsp. oregano, chopped

Directions:

In your Crock Pot, mix the mushrooms with the eggplant, cream and the other ingredients, toss, put the lid on and cook on High for 5 hours. Divide the mushroom mix into bowls and serve as a dip.

Spinach Dip(1)

Ingredients: Servings: 2   Cooking Time: 1 Hour

1 C. coconut cream	½ tsp. garam masala
10 oz. spinach, torn	1 garlic clove, minced
2 spring onions, chopped	A pinch of salt and black pepper
1 tsp. rosemary, dried	

Directions:

In your Crock Pot, mix the spinach with the cream, spring onions and the other ingredients, toss, put the lid on and cook on High for 1 hour. Blend using an immersion blender, divide into bowls and serve as a party dip.

Broccoli Dip

Ingredients: Servings: 2   Cooking Time: 2 Hours

1 green chili pepper, minced	2 tbsp. cream cheese, cubed
2 tbsp. heavy cream	A pinch of salt and black pepper
1 C. broccoli florets	
1 tbsp. mayonnaise	1 tbsp. chives, chopped

Directions:

In your Crock Pot, mix the broccoli with the chili pepper, mayo and the other ingredients, toss, put the lid on and cook on Low for 2 hours. Blend using an immersion blender, divide into bowls and serve as a party dip.

Salsa Snack

Ingredients: Servings: 6   Cooking Time: 3 Hours

10 roma tomatoes, chopped	3 garlic cloves, minced
2 jalapenos, chopped	1 bunch cilantro, chopped
1 sweet onion, chopped	
28 oz. canned plum tomatoes	Salt and black pepper to the taste

Directions:

In your Crock Pot, mix roma tomatoes with jalapenos, onion, plum tomatoes and garlic, stir, cover and cook on High for 3 hours. Add salt, pepper and cilantro, stir, divide into bowls and serve cold.

Herbed Pecans Snack

Ingredients: Servings: 5   Cooking Time: 2 Hrs 15 Minutes

1 lb. pecans halved	¼ tsp. garlic powder
2 tbsp. olive oil	1 tsp. thyme, dried
1 tsp. basil, dried	½ tsp. onion powder
1 tbsp. chili powder	A pinch of cayenne pepper
1 tsp. oregano, dried	

Directions:

Add pecans, basil, and all other ingredients to the Crock Pot. Put the cooker's lid on and set the cooking time to 2 hours on Low settings. Mix well and serve.

Apple Wedges With Peanuts

Ingredients: Servings: 5   Cooking Time: 2 Hours

1 tbsp. peanut butter	½ tsp. cinnamon
3 tbsp. peanut, crushed	1 tbsp. butter
	2 tsp. water
6 green apples, cut into wedges	1 tsp. lemon zest
	1 tsp. lemon juice

Directions:

Toss the peanuts with peanut butter, butter, lemon zest, cinnamon, and lemon juice in a bowl. Stir in apple wedges and mix well to coat them. Transfer the apple to the Crock Pot along with 2 tsp. water. Put the cooker's lid on and set the cooking time to 2 hours on High settings. Serve.

Piquant Mushrooms

Ingredients: Servings: 3 (13.2 oz. Per Serving)   Cooking Time: Low Setting-4 Hours Or High-2 Hours

2 tbsp. ghee/butter	1 tsp. chili powder
1 lb. mushrooms, fresh	Basil, oregano, parsley, and thyme, to taste
Ginger, grated	
1 onion, chopped	2 C. water
2 cloves garlic, chopped	Salt and pepper to taste
1 tbsp. olive oil	1 tbsp. fresh lemon juice

Directions:

Rinse and slice mushrooms. Peel and grate ginger. Place mushrooms and all remaining ingredients in Crock-Pot. Stir in the water. Cover with lid and cook on LOW for 3-4 hours or on

HIGH for 1-2 hours. Just before serving, sprinkle with fresh lemon juice and parsley. Serve with steak bites.

Curried Meatballs

Ingredients: Servings: 40   Cooking Time: 4 Hours

12 oz. pineapple preserves	½ C. brown sugar
8 oz. pineapple tidbits in juice	1 tsp. curry powder
8 oz. Dijon mustard	2 and ½ lb. frozen meatballs

Directions:

In your Crock Pot, mix pineapple preserves with pineapple tidbits, mustard, sugar and curry powder and whisk well. Add meatballs, toss, cover and cook on High for 4 hours. Serve them hot.

Pesto Pitta Pockets

Ingredients: Servings: 6   Cooking Time: 4 Hours

6 pita bread	1 tsp. salt
2 sweet peppers, deseeded and chopped	2 tbsp. vinegar
	1 tbsp. olive oil
1 chili pepper, chopped	1 tbsp. garlic, sliced
1 red onion, chopped	2 tbsp. pesto

Directions:

Add sweet peppers and all other ingredients, except for pesto and pita bread to the Crock Pot. Put the cooker's lid on and set the cooking time to 4 hours on Low settings. Layer the pocket of each pita bread with pesto. Mix the cooked sweet peppers filling and divide in the pita bread pockets. Serve.

Bbq Chicken Dip

Ingredients: Servings: 10   Cooking Time: 1 Hour And 30 Minutes

1 and ½ C. bbq sauce	3 bacon slices, cooked and crumbled
1 small red onion, chopped	1 plum tomato, chopped
24 oz. cream cheese, cubed	½ C. cheddar cheese, shredded
2 C. rotisserie chicken, shredded	1 tbsp. green onions, chopped

Directions:

In your Crock Pot, mix bbq sauce with onion, cream cheese, rotisserie chicken, bacon, tomato, cheddar and green onions, stir, cover and cook on Low for 1 hour and 30 minutes. Divide into bowls and serve.

Crab Dip(2)

Ingredients: Servings: 6   Cooking Time: 2 Hours

12 oz. cream cheese	½ C. mayonnaise
½ C. parmesan, grated	Juice of 1 lemon
½ C. green onions, chopped	1 and ½ tbsp. Worcestershire sauce
2 garlic cloves, minced	1 and ½ tsp. old bay seasoning
	12 oz. crabmeat

Directions:

In your Crock Pot, mix cream cheese with parmesan, mayo, green onions, garlic, lemon juice, Worcestershire sauce, old bay seasoning and crabmeat, stir, cover and cook on Low for 2 hours. Divide into bowls and serve as a dip.

Candied Pecans

Ingredients: Servings: 4   Cooking Time: 3 Hours

1 C. white sugar	4 C. pecans
1 and ½ tbsp. cinnamon powder	2 tsp. vanilla extract
½ C. brown sugar	¼ C. water
1 egg white, whisked	

Directions:

In a bowl, mix white sugar with cinnamon, brown sugar and vanilla and stir. Dip pecans in egg white, then in sugar mix and put them in your Crock Pot, also add the water, cover and cook on Low for 3 hours. Divide into bowls and serve as a snack.

Beef Dip(2)

Ingredients: Servings: 2   Cooking Time: 7 Hours And 10 Minutes

½ lb. beef, minced	2 garlic cloves, minced
3 spring onions, minced	1 tbsp. hives, chopped
1 tbsp. olive oil	½ tsp. coriander, ground
1 C. mild salsa	
2 oz. white mushrooms, chopped	½ tsp. rosemary, dried
¼ C. pine nuts, toasted	A pinch of salt and black pepper

Directions:

Heat up a pan with the oil over medium heat, add the spring onions, mushrooms, garlic and the meat, stir, brown for 10 minutes and transfer to your Crock Pot. Add the rest of the ingredients, toss, put the lid on and cook on Low for 7 hours. Divide the dip into bowls and serve.

Veggie Spread

Ingredients: Servings: 4   Cooking Time: 7 Hours

1 C. carrots, sliced	1 C. almond milk
1 and ½ C. cauliflower florets	Salt and black pepper to the taste
1/3 C. cashews	¼ tsp. smoked paprika
½ C. turnips, chopped	
2 and ½ C. water	¼ tsp. mustard powder
1 tsp. garlic powder	A pinch of salt

Directions:

In your Crock Pot, mix carrots with cauliflower, cashews, turnips and water, stir, cover and cook on Low for 7 hours. Drain, transfer to a blender, add almond milk, garlic powder, paprika, mustard powder, salt and pepper, blend well, divide into bowls and serve as a snack.

Butter Stuffed Chicken Balls

Ingredients: Servings: 9   Cooking Time: 3.5 Hours

3 oz. butter, cubed	2 oz. white bread
1 tbsp. mayonnaise	4 tbsp. milk
1 tsp. cayenne pepper	1 tsp. olive oil
1 tsp. ground black pepper	1 tbsp. almond flour
1 tsp. salt	1 tsp. dried dill
1 egg	14 oz. ground chicken
	½ tsp. olive oil

Directions:

Whisk mayonnaise with black pepper, dill, chicken, salt, and cayenne pepper in a bowl.   Stir in egg, milk, and white bread then mix well.   Grease the base of the Crock Pot with cooking oil.   Make small meatballs our of this mixture and insert one butter cubes into each ball.   Dust the meatballs with almond then place them in the Crock Pot.   Put the cooker's lid on and set the cooking time to 3.5 hours on High settings.   Serve warm.

Caramel Corn

Ingredients: Servings: 13   Cooking Time: 2 Hours

½ C. butter	1 tsp. baking soda
1 tsp. vanilla extract	12 C. plain popcorn
¼ C. corn syrup	1 C. mixed nuts
1 C. brown sugar	Cooking spray

Directions:

Grease your Crock Pot with cooking spray, add butter, vanilla, corn syrup, brown sugar and baking soda, cover and cook on High for 1 hour, stirring after 30 minutes.   Add popcorn, toss, cover and cook on Low for 1 hour more.   Add nuts, toss, divide into bowls and serve as a snack.

Macadamia Nuts Snack

Ingredients: Servings: 2   Cooking Time: 2 Hours

½ lb. macadamia nuts	¼ C. water
1 tbsp. avocado oil	½ tsp. oregano, dried
½ tbsp. chili powder	½ tsp. onion powder

Directions:

In your Crock Pot, mix the macadamia nuts with the oil and the other ingredients, toss, put the lid on, cook on Low for 2 hours, divide into bowls and serve as a snack.

Lemon Peel Snack

Ingredients: Servings: 80 Pieces   Cooking Time: 4 Hours

5 big lemons, sliced halves, pulp removed and peel cut into strips	2 and ¼ C. white sugar
	5 C. water

Directions:

Put strips in your instant Crock Pot, add water and sugar, stir cover and cook on Low for 4 hours.   Drain lemon peel and keep in jars until serving.

Bean Dip

Ingredients: Servings: 56   Cooking Time: 3 Hours

16 oz. Mexican cheese	16 oz. canned refried beans
5 oz. canned green chilies	2 lb. tortilla chips
Cooking spray	

Directions:

Grease your Crock Pot with cooking spray, line it, add Mexican cheese, green chilies and refried beans, stir, cover and cook on Low for 3 hours.   Divide into bowls and serve with tortilla chips on the side.

Wild Rice Almond Cream

Ingredients: Servings: 4 (7.2 oz. Per Serving)   Cooking Time: 3 Hours And 5 Minutes

3 C. of almond milk	1 C. water
¾ C. wild rice	1 tsp. butter
4 tbsp. sweetener	1 tbsp. vanilla extract

Directions:

Rinse the rice a few times with tap water and drain.   Pour all ingredients into Crock-Pot.   Close the lid and boil on HIGH for 2 ½ to 3 hours.   Stir every 30 minutes.   Ladle rice into serving dishes and allow it to cool before serving.

Artichoke & Spinach Mash

Ingredients: Servings: 8 (5.6 oz. Per Serving)   Cooking Time: 2 Hours And 25 Minutes

1 ½ C. frozen spinach, thawed	½ C. Feta cheese, crumbled
2 cans artichoke hearts, drained and chopped	1 C. cream cheese
1 C. sour cream	2 green onions, diced
¾ C. Parmesan cheese, freshly grated	2 cloves garlic, minced
	¼ tsp. ground pepper

Directions:

Add artichoke hearts, spinach, and other ingredients to Crock-Pot.   Stir until all ingredients are well combined.   Top with cream cheese.   Cover and cook on LOW for 2 hours and 15 minutes.   Before serving, give dish a good stir.

Sweet Potato Dip

Ingredients: Servings: 2   Cooking Time: 4 Hours

2 sweet potatoes, peeled and cubed	½ C. veggie stock
½ C. coconut cream	1 C. basil leaves
½ tsp. turmeric powder	2 tbsp. olive oil
½ tsp. garam masala	1 tbsp. lemon juice
2 garlic cloves, minced	A pinch of salt and black pepper

Directions:

In your Crock Pot, mix the sweet potatoes with the cream, turmeric and the other ingredients, toss, put the lid on and cook on High for 4 hours. Blend using an immersion blender, divide into bowls and serve as a party dip.

Slow-cooked Lemon Peel

Ingredients: Servings: 80 Pieces   Cooking Time: 4 Hours

5 big lemons, peel cut into strips
5 C. of water

2 and ¼ C. white sugar

Directions:

Spread the lemon peel in the Crock Pot and top it with sugar and water. Put the cooker's lid on and set the cooking time to 4 hours on Low settings. Drain the cooked peel and serve.

Mussels Salad

Ingredients: Servings: 4   Cooking Time: 1 Hour

2 lb. mussels, cleaned and scrubbed
1 radicchio, cut into thin strips
1 white onion, chopped
1 lb. baby spinach

½ C. dry white wine
1 garlic clove, crushed
½ C. water
A drizzle of olive oil

Directions:

Divide baby spinach and radicchio in salad bowls and leave aside for now. In your Crock Pot, mix mussels with onion, wine, garlic, water and oil, toss, cover and cook on High for 1 hour. Divide mussels on top of spinach and radicchio, add cooking liquid all over and serve.

Peanut Snack

Ingredients: Servings: 4   Cooking Time: 1 Hour And 30 Minutes

1 C. chocolate peanut butter
12 oz. dark chocolate chips

1 C. peanuts
12 oz. white chocolate chips

Directions:

In your Crock Pot, mix peanuts with peanut butter, dark and white chocolate chips, cover and cook on Low for 1 hour and 30 minutes. Divide this mix into small muffin cups, leave aside to cool down and serve as a snack.

Salsa Beans Dip

Ingredients: Servings: 2   Cooking Time: 1 Hour

¼ C. salsa
1 C. canned red kidney beans, drained and rinsed

½ C. mozzarella, shredded
1 tbsp. green onions, chopped

Directions:

In your Crock Pot, mix the salsa with the beans and the other ingredients, toss, put the lid on cook on High for 1 hour. Divide into bowls and serve as a party dip

Queso Dip

Ingredients: Servings: 10   Cooking Time: 1 Hour

16 oz. Velveeta
1 C. whole milk
½ C. cotija
2 jalapenos, chopped
2 tsp. sweet paprika

2 garlic cloves, minced
A pinch of cayenne pepper
1 tbsp. cilantro, chopped

Directions:

In your Crock Pot, mix Velveeta with milk, cotija, jalapenos, paprika, garlic and cayenne, stir, cover and cook on High for 1 hour. Stir the dip, add cilantro, divide into bowls and serve as a dip.

Chicken Meatballs

Ingredients: Servings: 2   Cooking Time: 7 Hours

A pinch of red pepper flakes, crushed
½ lb. chicken breast, skinless, boneless, ground
1 egg, whisked
½ C. salsa Verde
1 tsp. oregano, dried

½ tsp. chili powder
½ tsp. rosemary, dried
1 tbsp. parsley, chopped
A pinch of salt and black pepper

Directions:

In a bowl, mix the chicken with the egg and the other ingredients except the salsa, stir well and shape medium meatballs out of this mix. Put the meatballs in the Crock Pot, add the salsa Verde, toss gently, put the lid on and cook on Low for 7 hours. Arrange the meatballs on a platter and serve.

Spaghetti Squash

Ingredients: Servings: 6 (6.8 Ounces)   Cooking Time: 6 Hours

1 spaghetti squash (vegetable spaghetti)
1 ¾ C. water

4 tbsp. olive oil
Sea salt

Directions:

Slice the squash in half lengthwise and scoop out the seeds. Drizzle the halves with olive oil and season with sea salt. Place the squash in Crock-Pot and add the water. Close the lid and cook on LOW for 4-6 hours. Remove the squash and allow it to cool for about 30 minutes. Use a fork to scrape out spaghetti squash.

Eggplant Salsa(1)

Ingredients: Servings: 2   Cooking Time: 7 Hours

2 C. eggplant, chopped
1 tsp. capers, drained
1 C. black olives, pitted and halved
2 garlic cloves, minced

½ C. mild salsa
½ tbsp. basil, chopped
1 tsp. balsamic vinegar
A pinch of salt and black pepper

Directions:

In your Crock Pot, mix the eggplant with the capers and the other ingredients, toss, put the lid on and cook on Low for 7 hours. Divide into bowls and serve as an appetizer.

Cheese Onion Dip

Ingredients: Servings: 6   Cooking Time: 1 Hour

8 oz. cream cheese, soft
¾ C. sour cream
1 C. cheddar cheese, shredded
10 bacon slices, cooked and chopped
2 yellow onions, chopped

Directions:

Add cream cheese, bacon and all other ingredients to the Crock Pot. Put the cooker's lid on and set the cooking time to 1 hour on High settings. Serve.

Walnuts And Almond Muffins

Ingredients: Servings: 8 (2.5 oz. Per Serving)   Cooking Time: 1 Hour And 10 Minutes

½ C. flaxseed
1 C. almond flour
¾ C. walnuts, chopped
2 eggs
½ C. coconut oil
¼ C. sweetener
2 tsp. vanilla extract
½ tsp. baking soda
¼ tsp. liquid Stevia

Directions:

Add all ingredients to a mixing bowl and beat until well mixed. Spoon batter into silicone muffin pans. Sprinkle with finely chopped walnuts. Place inside the Crock-Pot, right on the ceramic bottom. Close the lid and cook for about 1 hour on HIGH. Serve hot or cold.

Zucchini Sticks

Ingredients: Servings: 13   Cooking Time: 2 Hours

9 oz. green zucchini, cut into thick sticks
4 oz. Parmesan, grated
1 egg
1 tsp. salt
1 tsp. ground white pepper
1 tsp. olive oil
2 tbsp. milk

Directions:

Grease of the base of your Crock Pot with olive oil. Whisk egg with milk, white pepper, and salt in a bowl. Dip the prepared zucchini sticks in the egg mixture then place them in the Crock Pot. Put the cooker's lid on and set the cooking time to 2 hours on High settings. Spread the cheese over the zucchini sticks evenly. Put the cooker's lid on and set the cooking time to 2 hours on High settings. Serve.

Cheesy Chili Pepper Dip

Ingredients: Servings: 8   Cooking Time: 9 Hours

4 chili pepper, sliced and deseeded
7 oz. Monterey cheese
3 tbsp. cream cheese
1 tbsp. onion powder
3 tbsp. dried dill
3 oz. butter
1 tbsp. cornstarch
1 tbsp. flour
¼ tsp. salt

Directions:

Add chili peppers to a blender and add salt, butter, onion powder, and dill. Blend the chili peppers well then transfer to the Crock Pot. Stir in flour, cornstarch, cream cheese, and Monterey cheese. Put the cooker's lid on and set the cooking time to 6 hours on Low settings. Serve.

Spinach Dip(2)

Ingredients: Servings: 2   Cooking Time: 1 Hour

2 tbsp. heavy cream
½ C. Greek yogurt
½ lb. baby spinach
2 garlic cloves, minced
Salt and black pepper to the taste

Directions:

In your Crock Pot, mix the spinach with the cream and the other ingredients, toss, put the lid on and cook on High for 1 hour. Blend using an immersion blender, divide into bowls and serve as a party dip.

Wild Rice Pilaf

Ingredients: Servings: 8 (6.8 oz. Per Serving)   Cooking Time: 3 Hours And 10 Minutes

2 green onion, chopped
2 C. long grain wild rice
1 C. whole tomatoes, sliced
1 tsp. seasonings, thyme, basil, rosemary
4 C. water
1 lemon rind, finely grated
4 tbsp. olive oil
Sea salt and fresh cracked pepper to taste

Directions:

Place all the ingredients in Crock-Pot except the seasonings and lemon rind, and give it a good stir. Close the lid and cook on HIGH for 1 ½ hours or on LOW for 3 hours. After done cooking add seasoning to taste. Sprinkle with lemon rind and serve hot.

Jalapeno Poppers

Ingredients: Servings: 4   Cooking Time: 3 Hours

½ lb. chorizo, chopped
10 jalapenos, tops cut off and deseeded
1 small white onion, chopped
½ lb. beef, ground
¼ tsp. garlic powder
1 tbsp. maple syrup
1 tbsp. mustard
1/3 C. water

Directions:

In a bowl, mix beef with chorizo, garlic powder and onion and stir. Stuff your jalapenos with the mix, place them in your Crock Pot, add the water, cover and cook on High for 3 hours. Transfer jalapeno poppers to a lined baking sheet. In a bowl, mix maple syrup with mustard, whisk well, brush poppers with this mix, arrange on a platter and serve.

Tomato And Mushroom Salsa

Ingredients: Servings: 2   Cooking Time: 4 Hours

1 C. cherry tomatoes, halved	12 oz. tomato sauce
1 C. mushrooms, sliced	¼ C. cream cheese, cubed
1 small yellow onion, chopped	1 tbsp. chives, chopped
1 garlic clove, minced	Salt and black pepper to the taste

Directions:

In your Crock Pot, mix the tomatoes with the mushrooms and the other ingredients, toss, put the lid on and cook on Low for 4 hours. Divide into bowls and serve as a party salsa

Almond, Zucchini, Parmesan Snack

Ingredients: Servings: 6 (5.1 oz. Per Serving) Cooking Time: 1 Hour And 40 Minutes

3 eggs, organic	Salt and pepper to taste
2 zucchinis, thinly sliced	Olive oil
1 C. almonds, ground	1 tsp. oregano
1 C. Parmesan cheese, grated	1 C. almond flour

Directions:

Wash, clean, and slice the zucchini. Salt and set aside on a paper towel. On a plate, combine Parmesan cheese, almonds, oregano, salt, and pepper and set aside. On another shallow plate, spread the almond flour. In a bowl, beat eggs with salt and pepper. Start by dipping zucchini rounds in flour, dip in the eggs, then dredge in almond mixture, pressing on them to coat. Pour olive oil in Crock-Pot and add the zucchini slices; cover and cook for 1 ½ hours on HIGH. Serve hot.

Chicken Bites

Ingredients: Servings: 4 Cooking Time: 7 Hours

1 tbsp. ginger, grated	1 lb. chicken thighs, boneless and skinless
1 yellow onion, sliced	
1 tbsp. garlic, minced	2 tbsp. lemon juice
2 tsp. cumin, ground	½ C. green olives, pitted and roughly chopped
1 tsp. cinnamon powder	
2 tbsp. sweet paprika	Salt to the taste
1 and ½ C. chicken stock	3 tbsp. olive oil
	5 pita breads, cut in quarters and heated in the oven

Directions:

Heat up a pan with the olive oil over medium-high heat, add onions, garlic, ginger, salt and pepper, stir and cook for 2 minutes. Add cumin and cinnamon, stir well and take off heat. Put chicken pieces in your Crock Pot, add onions mix, lemon juice, olives and stock, stir, cover and cook on Low for 7 hours. Shred meat, stir the whole mixture again, divide it on pita chips and serve as a snack.

Fajita Dip

Ingredients: Servings: 6 Cooking Time: 4 Hours

3 chicken breasts, skinless and boneless	8 oz. cream cheese
	16 oz. sour cream

8 oz. root beer	2 fajita seasoning mix packets
3 red bell peppers, chopped	
1 yellow onion, chopped	1 tbsp. olive oil
	Salt and black pepper to the taste
8 oz. pepper jack cheese, shredded	

Directions:

In your Crock Pot, mix chicken with root beer, bell peppers, onion, cream cheese, pepper jack cheese, sour cream, fajita seasoning, oil, salt and pepper, stir, cover and cook on High for 4 hours. Shred meat using2 forks, divide into bowls and serve.

Fava Bean Onion Dip

Ingredients: Servings: 6 Cooking Time: 5 Hours

1 lb. fava bean, rinsed	¼ C. olive oil
1 C. yellow onion, chopped	1 garlic clove, minced
4 and ½ C. of water	2 tbsp. lemon juice
1 bay leaf	Salt to the taste

Directions:

Add 4 C. water, bay leaf, salt, and fava beans to the Crock Pot. Put the cooker's lid on and set the cooking time to 3 hours on low settings. Drain the Crock Pot beans and discard the bay leaf. Return the cooked beans to the cooker and add onion, garlic, and ½ C. water. Put the cooker's lid on and set the cooking time to 2 hours on Low settings. Blend the slow-cooked beans with lemon juice and olive oil. Serve.

Potato Onion Salsa

Ingredients: Servings: 6 Cooking Time: 8 Hours

1 sweet onion, chopped	1 and ½ lbs. gold potatoes, cut into medium cubes
¼ C. white vinegar	
2 tbsp. mustard	
Salt and black pepper to the taste	¼ C. dill, chopped
	1 C. celery, chopped
	Cooking spray

Directions:

Grease the base of the Crock Pot with cooking spray. Add onion, potatoes and all other ingredients to the cooker. Put the cooker's lid on and set the cooking time to 8 hours on Low settings. Mix well and serve.

Cauliflower Dip

Ingredients: Servings: 2 Cooking Time: 5 Hours

1 C. cauliflower florets	2 tbsp. lemon juice
½ C. heavy cream	1 tbsp. basil, chopped
1 tbsp. tahini paste	1 tsp. rosemary, dried
½ C. white mushrooms, chopped	A pinch of salt and black pepper
2 garlic cloves, minced	

Directions:

In your Crock Pot, mix the cauliflower with the cream, tahini paste and the other ingredients, toss, put the lid on and cook on

Low for 5 hours.   Transfer to a blender, pulse well, divide into bowls and serve as a party dip.

Chickpeas Salsa

Ingredients: Servings: 2   Cooking Time: 6 Hours

1 C. canned chickpeas, drained
½ C. black olives, pitted and halved
1 small yellow onion, chopped
¼ tbsp. ginger, grated
4 garlic cloves, minced

1 C. veggie stock
¼ tbsp. coriander, ground
¼ tbsp. red chili powder
¼ tbsp. garam masala
1 tbsp. lemon juice

Directions:

In your Crock Pot, mix the chickpeas with the stock, olives and the other ingredients, toss, put the lid on and cook on Low for 6 hours.   Divide into bowls and serve as an appetizer.

Thyme Pepper Shrimp

Ingredients: Servings: 5   Cooking Time: 25 Minutes

1 tsp. sage
1 tbsp. Piri Piri sauce
1 tsp. thyme
1 tbsp. cayenne pepper

2 tbsp. heavy cream
1 tsp. salt
¼ C. butter
1 lb. shrimp, peeled
½ C. fresh parsley

Directions:

Blend butter with Piri Piri, thyme, sage, cayenne pepper, salt, and cream in a blender until smooth.   Add this buttercream mixture to the Crock Pot.   Put the cooker's lid on and set the cooking time to 10 minutes on High settings.   Now add the shrimp to the Crock Pot and cover again to cook for another 15 minutes.   Serve warm.

Stuffed Peppers Platter

Ingredients: Servings: 2   Cooking Time: 4 Hours

1 red onion, chopped
½ tsp. sweet paprika
½ tbsp. chili powder
1 garlic clove, minced
1 C. white rice, cooked

1 tsp. olive oil
½ C. corn
A pinch of salt and black pepper
2 colored bell peppers, tops and insides scooped out
½ C. tomato sauce

Directions:

In a bowl, mix the onion with the oil, paprika and the other ingredients except the peppers and tomato sauce, stir well and stuff the peppers the with this mix.   Put the peppers in the Crock Pot, add the sauce, put the lid on and cook on Low for 4 hours. Transfer the peppers on a platter and serve as an appetizer.

Spinach And Walnuts Dip

Ingredients: Servings: 2   Cooking Time: 2 Hours

½ C. heavy cream
½ C. walnuts, chopped
1 garlic clove, chopped

1 C. baby spinach
1 tbsp. mayonnaise
Salt and black pepper to the taste

Directions:

In your Crock Pot, mix the spinach with the walnuts and the other ingredients, toss, put the lid on and cook on High for 2 hours.   Blend using an immersion blender, divide into bowls and serve as a party dip.

Onion Dip(3)

Ingredients: Servings: 2   Cooking Time: 8 Hours

2 C. yellow onions, chopped
A pinch of salt and black pepper
½ C. heavy cream

1 tbsp. olive oil
2 tbsp. mayonnaise

Directions:

In your Crock Pot, mix the onions with the cream and the other ingredients, whisk, put the lid on and cook on Low for 8 hours. Divide into bowls and serve as a party dip.

Creamy Mushroom Spread

Ingredients: Servings: 2   Cooking Time: 4 Hours

1 lb. mushrooms, sliced
3 garlic cloves, minced
2 tsp. smoked paprika

1 C. heavy cream
Salt and black pepper to the taste
2 tbsp. parsley, chopped

Directions:

In your Crock Pot, mix the mushrooms with the garlic and the other ingredients, whisk, put the lid on and cook on Low for 4 hours.   Whisk, divide into bowls and serve as a party spread.

Apple Dip

Ingredients: Servings: 8   Cooking Time: 1 Hour And 30 Minutes

5 apples, peeled and chopped
½ tsp. cinnamon powder

12 oz. jarred caramel sauce
A pinch of nutmeg, ground

Directions:

In your Crock Pot, mix apples with cinnamon, caramel sauce and nutmeg, stir, cover and cook on High for 1 hour and 30 minutes. Divide into bowls and serve.

Corn Dip(1)

Ingredients: Servings: 12   Cooking Time: 3 Hours

9 C. corn, rice and wheat cereal
1 C. cheerios
2 C. pretzels
6 tbsp. hot, melted butter

1 C. peanuts
1 tbsp. salt
¼ C. Worcestershire sauce
1 tsp. garlic powder

Directions:

In your Crock Pot, mix cereal with cheerios, pretzels, peanuts, butter, salt, Worcestershire sauce and garlic powder, toss well, cover and cook on Low for 3 hours.   Divide into bowls and serve as a snack.

Jalapeno Salsa Snack

Ingredients: Servings: 6   Cooking Time: 3 Hours

10 Roma tomatoes, chopped	3 garlic cloves, minced
2 jalapenos, chopped	1 bunch cilantro, chopped
1 sweet onion, chopped	Salt and black pepper to the taste
28 oz. canned plum tomatoes	

Directions:

Add Roma tomatoes, onion, and all other ingredients to the Crock Pot.   Put the cooker's lid on and set the cooking time to 3 hours on High settings.   Mix well and serve.

Onion Dip(2)

Ingredients: Servings: 6   Cooking Time: 4 Hours

7 C. tomatoes, chopped	¼ C. apple cider vinegar
1 yellow onion, chopped	1 tbsp. cilantro, chopped
1 red onion, chopped	1 tbsp. sage, chopped
3 jalapenos, chopped	3 tbsp. basil, chopped
1 red bell pepper, chopped	Salt to the taste
1 green bell pepper, chopped	

Directions:

In your Crock Pot, mix tomatoes with onion, jalapenos, red bell pepper, green bell pepper, vinegar, sage, cilantro and basil, stir, cover and cook on Low for 4 hours.   Transfer to your food processor, add salt, pulse well, divide into bowls and serve.

Almond Buns

Ingredients: Servings: 6 (1.9 oz. Per Serving)   Cooking Time: 20 Minutes

3 C. almond flour	5 tbsp. butter
1 ½ tsp. sweetener of your choice (optional)	2 eggs
	1 ½ tsp. baking powder

Directions:

In a mixing bowl, combine the dry ingredients.   In another bowl, whisk the eggs.   Add melted butter to mixture and mix well.   Divide almond mixture equally into 6 parts.   Grease the bottom of Crock-Pot and place in 6 almond buns.   Cover and cook on HIGH for 2 to 2 ½ hours or LOW for 4 to 4 ½ hours.   Serve hot.

Peanut Butter Chicken

Ingredients: Servings: 7   Cooking Time: 6 Hours

3 tbsp. peanut butter, melted	1 tsp. paprika
1 lb. chicken breast, boneless, cut into strips	1 tsp. salt
	1 tsp. olive oil
	2 tbsp. almond flour
	1 tsp. cayenne pepper

Directions:

Mix the chicken strips with cayenne pepper, salt, and paprika.   Dust these with almond flour to coat.   Add olive oil and coated chicken strips to the Crock Pot.   Put the cooker's lid on and set the cooking time to 4 hours on High settings.   Flip the cooked chicken strips and cook for another 2 hours on the LOW setting.   Serve.

Peas Dip

Ingredients: Servings: 4   Cooking Time: 5 Hours

1 and ½ C. black-eyed peas	½ tsp. jalapeno powder
3 C. water	Salt and black pepper to the taste
1 tsp. Cajun seasoning	¼ tsp. liquid smoke
½ C. pecans, toasted	½ tsp. Tabasco sauce
½ tsp. garlic powder	

Directions:

In your Crock Pot, mix black-eyed pea with Cajun seasoning, salt, pepper and water, stir, cover and cook on High for 5 hours.   Drain, transfer to a blender, add pecans, garlic powder, jalapeno powder, Tabasco sauce, liquid smoke, more salt and pepper, pulse well and serve.

Mushroom Salsa

Ingredients: Servings: 4   Cooking Time: 5 Hours

2 C. white mushrooms, sliced	½ tsp. oregano, dried
1 C. cherry tomatoes halved	½ C. black olives, pitted and sliced
1 C. spring onions, chopped	3 garlic cloves, minced
½ tsp. chili powder	1 C. mild salsa
½ tsp. rosemary, dried	Salt and black pepper to the taste

Directions:

In your Crock Pot, mix the mushrooms with the cherry tomatoes and the other ingredients, toss, put the lid on and cook on Low for 5 hours.   Divide into bowls and serve as a snack.

Crispy Sweet Potatoes With Paprika

Ingredients: Servings: 4 (3.2 oz. Per Serving)   Cooking Time: 4 Hours And 45 Minutes

2 medium sweet potatoes	2 tbsp. olive oil
1 tbsp. nutritional yeast, optional	1 tsp. Cayenne pepper, optional
	Sea salt

Directions:

Wash and peel the sweet potatoes.   Slice them into wedges.   In a bowl, mix the potatoes with the other ingredients.   Grease the bottom of Crock-Pot and place the sweet potato wedges in it. Cover and cook on LOW for 4- 4 ½ hours. Serve hot.

Potato Cups

Ingredients: Servings: 8   Cooking Time: 8 Hours

5 tbsp. mashed potato	1 tsp. minced garlic
1 carrot, boiled, cubed	7 oz. puff pastry
3 tbsp. green peas	1 egg yolk, beaten
1 tsp. paprika	4 oz. Parmesan, shredded
3 tbsp. sour cream	

Directions:

Mix mashed potato with carrot cubes in a bowl. Stir in sour cream, paprika, green peas, and garlic, then mix well. Spread the puff pastry and slice it into 2x2 inches squares. Place the puff pastry square in the muffin C. of the muffin tray. Press the puff pastry and in the muffin C. and brush it with egg yolk. Divide the potatoes mixture into the muffin C.   Place the muffin tray in the Crock Pot.   Put the cooker's lid on and set the cooking time to 8 hours on Low settings.   Serve.

Paprika Cod Sticks

Ingredients: Servings: 2   Cooking Time: 2 Hours

1 eggs whisked	½ C. almond flour
½ lb. cod fillets, cut into medium strips	½ tsp. turmeric powder
½ tsp. cumin, ground	A pinch of salt and black pepper
½ tsp. coriander, ground	¼ tsp. sweet paprika
	Cooking spray

Directions:

In a bowl, mix the flour with cumin, coriander and the other ingredients except the fish, eggs and cooking spray.   Put the egg in another bowl and whisk it.   Dip the fish sticks in the egg and then dredge them in the flour mix.   Grease the Crock Pot with cooking spray, add fish sticks, put the lid on, cook on High for 2 hours, arrange on a platter and serve.

Nuts Bowls

Ingredients: Servings: 2   Cooking Time: 2 Hours

2 tbsp. almonds, toasted	½ C. coconut cream
2 tbsp. pecans, halved and toasted	2 tbsp. butter, melted
2 tbsp. hazelnuts, toasted and peeled	A pinch of cinnamon powder
2 tbsp. sugar	A pinch of cayenne pepper

Directions:

In your Crock Pot, mix the nuts with the sugar and the other ingredients, toss, put the lid on, cook on Low for 2 hours, divide into bowls and serve as a snack.

Beer And Cheese Dip

Ingredients: Servings: 10   Cooking Time: 1 Hour

12 oz. cream cheese	6 oz. beer
4 C. cheddar cheese, shredded	1 tbsp. chives, chopped

Directions:

In your Crock Pot, mix cream cheese with beer and cheddar, stir, cover and cook on Low for 1 hour.   Stir your dip, add chives, divide into bowls and serve.

Sausage Cream Dip

Ingredients: Servings: 8   Cooking Time: 5 Hours

8 oz. sausage, cooked, chopped	½ C. cream cheese
4 tbsp. sour cream	3 tbsp. chives
2 tbsp. Tabasco sauce	5 oz. salsa
	4 oz. Monterey Cheese

Directions:

Mix chopped sausages with sour cream in the Crock Pot.   Stir in Tabasco sauce, cream cheese, salsa, chives, and Monterey cheese. Put the cooker's lid on and set the cooking time to 5 hours on Low settings.   Continue mixing the dip after every 30 minutes of cooking.   Serve.

Peanut Bombs

Ingredients: Servings: 9   Cooking Time: 6 Hours

1 C. peanut	1 tsp. salt
½ C. flour	1 tsp. turmeric
1 egg	4 tbsp. milk
1 tsp. butter, melted	¼ tsp. nutmeg

Directions:

First, blend the peanuts in a blender then stir in flour.   Beat egg with milk, nutmeg, turmeric, and salt in a bowl.   Stir in the peanut-flour mixture and mix well to form a dough.   Grease the base of the Crock Pot with melted butter.   Divide the dough into golf ball-sized balls and place them the cooker.   Put the cooker's lid on and set the cooking time to 6 hours on Low settings. Serve.

Eggplant Dip

Ingredients: Servings: 4   Cooking Time: 4 Hours And 10 Minutes

1 eggplant	1 celery stick, chopped
1 zucchini, chopped	1 tomato, chopped
2 tbsp. olive oil	2 tbsp. tomato paste
2 tbsp. balsamic vinegar	1 and ½ tsp. garlic, minced
1 tbsp. parsley, chopped	A pinch of sea salt
1 yellow onion, chopped	Black pepper to the taste

Directions:

Brush eggplant with the oil, place on preheated grill and cook over medium-high heat for 5 minutes on each side.   Leave aside to cool down, chop it and put in your Crock Pot.   Also add, zucchini, vinegar, onion, celery, tomato, parsley, tomato paste, garlic, salt and pepper and stir everything.   Cover and cook on

High for 4 hours.   Stir your spread again very well, divide into bowls and serve.

Lentils Rolls

Ingredients: Servings: 4   Cooking Time: 8 Hours

1 C. brown lentils, cooked
1 green cabbage head, leaves separated
½ C. onion, chopped
1 C. brown rice, already cooked
2 oz. white mushrooms, chopped
¼ C. pine nuts, toasted
¼ C. raisins

2 garlic cloves, minced
2 tbsp. dill, chopped
1 tbsp. olive oil
25 oz. marinara sauce
A pinch of salt and black pepper
¼ C. water

Directions:

In a bowl, mix lentils with onion, rice, mushrooms, pine nuts, raisins, garlic, dill, salt and pepper and whisk well.   Arrange cabbage leaves on a working surface, divide lentils mix and wrap them well.   Add marinara sauce and water to your Crock Pot and stir.   Add cabbage rolls, cover and cook on Low for 8 hours. Arrange cabbage rolls on a platter and serve.

Cauliflower Bites

Ingredients: Servings: 2   Cooking Time: 4 Hours

2 C. cauliflower florets
1 tbsp. Italian seasoning
1 tbsp. sweet paprika
¼ C. veggie stock

2 tbsp. tomato sauce
1 tsp. sweet paprika
1 tbsp. olive oil

Directions:

In your Crock Pot, mix the cauliflower florets with the Italian seasoning and the other ingredients, toss, put the lid on and cook on Low for 4 hours.   Divide into bowls and serve as a snack.

Beef And Chipotle Dip

Ingredients: Servings: 10   Cooking Time: 2 Hours

8 oz. cream cheese, soft
2 tbsp. yellow onion, chopped
2 tbsp. mayonnaise
¼ tsp. garlic powder

2 oz. hot pepper Monterey Jack cheese, shredded
2 chipotle chilies in adobo sauce, chopped
2 oz. dried beef, chopped
¼ C. pecans, chopped

Directions:

In your Crock Pot, mix cream cheese with onion, mayo, Monterey Jack cheese, garlic powder, chilies and dried beef, stir, cover and cook on Low for 2 hours.   Add pecans, stir, divide into bowls and serve.

Spicy Dip

Ingredients: Servings: 10   Cooking Time: 3 Hours

1 lb. spicy sausage, chopped
8 oz. cream cheese, soft

8 oz. sour cream
20 oz. canned tomatoes and green chilies, chopped

Directions:

In your Crock Pot, mix sausage with cream cheese, sour cream and tomatoes and chilies, stir, cover and cook on Low for 3 hours. Divide into bowls and serve as a snack.

Mozzarella Basil Tomatoes

Ingredients: Servings: 8   Cooking Time: 30 Minutes

3 tbsp. fresh basil
5 oz. Mozzarella, sliced
4 large tomatoes, sliced

1 tsp. chili flakes
1 tbsp. olive oil
1 tsp. minced garlic
½ tsp. onion powder
½ tsp. cilantro

Directions:

Whisk olive oil with onion powder, cilantro, garlic, and chili flakes in a bowl.   Rub all the tomato slices with this cilantro mixture.   Top each tomato slice with cheese slice and then place another tomato slice on top to make a sandwich.   Insert a toothpick into each tomato sandwich to seal it.   Place them in the base of the Crock Pot.   Put the cooker's lid on and set the cooking time to 20 minutes on High settings.   Garnish with basil.   Enjoy.

Apple Chutney

Ingredients: Servings: 10   Cooking Time: 9 Hours

1 C. wine vinegar
4 oz. brown sugar
2 lbs. apples, chopped
4 oz. onion, chopped

1 jalapeno pepper
1 tsp. ground cardamom
½ tsp. ground cinnamon
1 tsp. chili flakes

Directions:

Mix brown sugar with wine vinegar in the Crock Pot.   Put the cooker's lid on and set the cooking time to 1 hour on High settings.   Add chopped apples and all other ingredients to the cooker.   Put the cooker's lid on and set the cooking time to 8 hours on Low settings.   Mix well and mash the mixture with a fork.   Serve.

Fajita Chicken Dip

Ingredients: Servings: 6   Cooking Time: 4 Hours

3 chicken breasts, skinless and boneless
8 oz. root beer
3 red bell peppers, chopped
1 yellow onion, chopped
8 oz. cream cheese

8 oz. pepper jack cheese, shredded
16 oz. sour cream
2 fajita seasoning mix packets
1 tbsp. olive oil
Salt and black pepper to the taste

Directions:

Add root beer, chicken and all other ingredients to the Crock Pot. Put the cooker's lid on and set the cooking time to 4 hours on High settings. Shred the slow-cooked chicken with the help of two forks. Mix well with its sauce and serve.

Pork Stuffed Tamales

Ingredients: Servings: 24   Cooking Time: 8 Hrs 30 Minutes

8 oz. dried corn husks, soaked for 1 day and drained	1 tbsp. chipotle chili powder
4 C. of water	2 tbsp. chili powder
3 lbs. pork shoulder, boneless and chopped	Salt and black pepper to the taste
1 yellow onion, chopped	1 tsp. cumin, ground
2 garlic cloves, crushed	4 C. masa harina
	¼ C. of corn oil
	¼ C. shortening
	1 tsp. baking powder

Directions:

Add 2 C. water, onion, black pepper, salt, garlic, chili powder, pork, cumin, and chipotle powder to the Crock Pot. Put the cooker's lid on and set the cooking time to 7 hours on Low settings. Shred the slow-cooked meat using 2 forks then mix it with 1 tbsp. cooking liquid, black pepper, and salt. Mix masa harina with baking powder, oil, shortening, black pepper, and salt in a mixer. Add the cooking liquid from the cooker and blend well until smooth. Spread the corn husks on the working surface and add ¼ C. harina mixture to the top of each husk. Add 1 tbsp. shredded pork to each husk and fold it from the top, bottom, and sideways to make a roll. Place these tamales in the Crock Pot and pour in the remaining water. Put the cooker's lid on and set the cooking time to 1.5 hours on High settings. Serve.

Sauerkraut Dip

Ingredients: Servings: 12   Cooking Time: 2 Hours

15 oz. canned sauerkraut, drained	4 oz. corned beef, chopped
8 oz. sour cream	8 oz. Swiss cheese, shredded
4 oz. cream cheese	

Directions:

In your Crock Pot, mix sauerkraut with sour cream, cream cheese, beef and Swiss cheese, stir, cover and cook on Low for 2 hours. Divide into bowls and serve.

APPETIZERS RECIPES

Sweet Corn Jalapeno Dip

Ingredients: Servings: 10   Cooking Time: 2 1/4 Hours

4 bacon slices, chopped	1 C. grated Cheddar cheese
3 cans sweet corn, drained	1/2 C. cream cheese
4 jalapenos, seeded and chopped	1 pinch nutmeg
1 C. sour cream	2 tbsp. chopped cilantro

Directions:

Combine the corn, jalapenos, sour cream, Cheddar, cream cheese and nutmeg in a Crock Pot. Cook on high settings for 2 hours. When done, stir in the cilantro and serve the dip warm. Store it in an airtight container in the fridge for up to 2 days. Re-heat it when need it.

Creamy Spinach Dip

Ingredients: Servings: 30   Cooking Time: 2 1/4 Hours

1 can crab meat, drained	1 C. sour cream
1 lb. fresh spinach, chopped	1 C. cream cheese
2 shallots, chopped	1 C. grated Cheddar cheese
2 jalapeno peppers, chopped	1 tbsp. sherry vinegar
1 C. grated Parmesan	2 garlic cloves, chopped
1/2 C. whole milk	

Directions:

Combine all the ingredients in your Crock Pot. Cover with its lid and cook on high settings for 2 hours. Serve the spinach dip warm or chilled with vegetable stick or your favorite salty snacks.

Five-spiced Chicken Wings

Ingredients: Servings: 8   Cooking Time: 7 1/4 Hours

1/2 C. plum sauce	1 tsp. salt
1/2 C. BBQ sauce	1/2 tsp. chili powder
2 tbsp. butter	4 lb. chicken wings
1 tbsp. five-spice powder	

Directions:

Combine the plum sauce and BBQ sauce, as well as butter, five-spice, salt and chili powder in a crock pot. Add the chicken wings and mix well until well coated. Cover and cook on low settings fir 7 hours. Serve warm or chilled.

Baba Ganoush

Ingredients: Servings: 4   Cooking Time: 4 1/4 Hours

1 large eggplant, halved	1 tbsp. lemon juice
2 garlic cloves, minced	1 tbsp. chopped parsley
2 tbsp. olive oil	Salt and pepper to taste
1 tbsp. tahini paste	

Directions:

Spread the garlic over each half of eggplant. Season them with salt and pepper and drizzle with olive oil. Place the eggplant halves in your Crock Pot and cook on low settings for 4 hours. When done, scoop out the eggplant flesh and place it in a bowl. Mash it with a fork. Stir in the tahini paste, lemon juice and parsley and mix well. Serve the dip fresh.

Bacon Baked Potatoes

Ingredients: Servings: 8   Cooking Time: 3 1/4 Hours

3 lb. new potatoes, halved	1 tsp. dried rosemary
8 slices bacon,	Salt and pepper to taste

chopped
1/4 C. chicken stock

Directions:

Heat a skillet over medium flame and stir in the bacon. Cook until crisp. Place the potatoes in a Crock Pot. Add the bacon bits and its fat, as well as rosemary, salt and pepper and mix until evenly distributed. Pour in the stock and cook on high heat for 3 hours. Serve the potatoes warm.

Creamy Chicken Dip

Ingredients: Servings: 6   Cooking Time: 3 1/4 Hours

1 C. cream cheese	1/4 tsp. cumin
1 1/2 C. cooked and	powder
diced chicken	2 garlic cloves,
2 C. shredded	chopped
Monterey Jack cheese	Salt and pepper to
1/4 C. white wine	taste
1 lime, juiced	

Directions:

Combine all the ingredients in your Crock Pot. Add salt and pepper to taste and cook on low settings for 3 hours. The dip is best served warm with tortilla chips or bread sticks.

Marinara Turkey Meatballs

Ingredients: Servings: 8   Cooking Time: 6 1/2 Hours

2 lb. ground turkey	4 basil leaves,
1 carrot, grated	chopped
1 potato, grated	1/2 tsp. dried mint
1 shallot, chopped	1 egg
1 tbsp. chopped	1/4 C. breadcrumbs
parsley	Salt and pepper to
1 tbsp. chopped	taste
cilantro	2 C. marinara sauce

Directions:

Mix the turkey, carrot, potato, shallot, parsley, cilantro, basil, mint, egg and breadcrumbs in a bowl. Add salt and pepper to taste and mix well. Pour the marinara sauce in your Crock Pot then form meatballs and drop them in the sauce. Cover the pot with its lid and cook on low settings for 6 hours. Serve the meatballs warm or chilled.

Bourbon Glazed Sausages

Ingredients: Servings: 10   Cooking Time: 4 1/4 Hours

3 lb. small sausage	1/2 C. apricot
links	preserves
1/4 C. maple syrup	2 tbsp. Bourbon

Directions:

Combine all the ingredients in your Crock Pot. Cover with its lid and cook on low settings for 4 hours. Serve the glazed sausages warm or chilled, preferably with cocktail sticks.

Spicy Chicken Taquitos

Ingredients: Servings: 8   Cooking Time: 6 1/2 Hours

4 chicken breasts,	1 C. cream cheese
cooked and diced	4 garlic cloves,
2 jalapeno peppers,	minced

chopped
1/2 C. canned sweet
corn, drained
1/2 tsp. cumin
powder

16 taco-sized flour
tortillas
2 C. grated Cheddar
cheese

Directions:

In a bowl, mix the chicken, cream cheese, garlic, cumin, poblano peppers and corn. Stir in the cheese as well. Place your tortillas on your working surface and top each tortilla with the cheese mixture. Roll the tortillas tightly to form an even roll. Place the rolls in your Crock Pot. Cook on low settings for 6 hours. Serve warm.

Sweet Corn Crab Dip

Ingredients: Servings: 20   Cooking Time: 2 1/4 Hours

2 tbsp. butter	1 C. sour cream
1 C. canned sweet	1 can crab meat,
corn, drained	drained
2 red bell peppers,	1 tsp. Worcestershire
cored and diced	sauce
2 garlic cloves,	1 tsp. hot sauce
chopped	1 C. grated Cheddar
2 poblano peppers,	cheese
chopped	

Directions:

Mix all the ingredients in your Crock Pot. Cover the pot with its lid and cook on low settings for 2 hours. Serve the dip warm or chilled.

Cheese And Beer Fondue

Ingredients: Servings: 10   Cooking Time: 2 1/4 Hours

4 tbsp. butter	1 shallot, chopped
2 garlic cloves,	1 C. milk
minced	1 C. light beer
2 tbsp. all-purpose	2 C. grated Cheddar
flour	1/2 tsp. chili powder
2 poblano peppers,	
chopped	

Directions:

Melt the butter in a saucepan and stir in the shallot and garlic. Sauté for 2 minutes then add the flour and cook for 2 additional minutes. Stir in the milk and cook until thickened, about 5 minutes. Pour the mixture in your Crock Pot and stir in the remaining ingredients. Cook on high settings for 2 hours and serve the fondue warm with biscuits or other salty snacks.

Mixed Olive Dip

Ingredients: Servings: 10   Cooking Time: 1 3/4 Hours

1 lb. ground chicken	1/2 C. Kalamata
2 tbsp. olive oil	olives, pitted and
1 green bell pepper,	chopped
cored and diced	1 C. green salsa
1/2 C. green olives,	1/2 C. chicken stock
chopped	1 C. grated Cheddar
1/2 C. black olives,	cheese
pitted and chopped	1/2 C. shredded
	mozzarella

Directions:

Combine all the ingredients in your Crock Pot. Cover with its lid and cook on high settings for 1 1/2 hours. The dip is best served warm.

Chipotle Bbq Meatballs

Ingredients: Servings: 10   Cooking Time: 7 1/2 Hours

3 lb. ground pork	Salt and pepper to
2 garlic cloves, minced	taste
2 shallots, chopped	2 C. BBQ sauce
2 chipotle peppers, chopped	1/4 C. cranberry sauce
	1 bay leaf

Directions:

Mix the ground pork, garlic, shallots, chipotle peppers, salt and pepper in a bowl. Combine the BBQ sauce, cranberry sauce, bay leaf, salt and pepper in your Crock Pot. Form small meatballs and drop them in the sauce. Cover the pot with its lid and cook on low settings for 7 hours. Serve the meatballs warm or chilled with cocktail skewers or toothpicks.

Pizza Dip

Ingredients: Servings: 20   Cooking Time: 6 1/4 Hours

1 lb. spicy sausages, sliced	1 onion, chopped
1/2 lb. salami, diced	2 C. tomato sauce
1 red bell pepper, cored and diced	1/2 C. grated Parmesan
1 yellow bell pepper, cored and sliced	1 C. shredded mozzarella
2 garlic cloves, minced	1/2 tsp. dried basil
	1/2 tsp. dried oregano

Directions:

Layer all the ingredients in your Crock Pot. Cook on low settings for 6 hours, mixing once during the cooking time to ensure an even distribution of ingredients. Serve the dip warm.

Cheesy Mushroom Dip

Ingredients: Servings: 16   Cooking Time: 4 1/4 Hours

1 can condensed cream of mushroom soup	1/2 tsp. chili powder
	1 C. grated Cheddar cheese
1 lb. mushrooms, chopped	1 C. grated Swiss cheese
1 tsp. Worcestershire sauce	
1/4 C. evaporated milk	

Directions:

Mix the cream of mushroom soup, mushrooms, Worcestershire sauce, evaporated milk and chili powder in your Crock Pot. Top with grated cheese and cook on low settings for 4 hours. Serve the dip warm or re-heated.

Cranberry Baked Brie

Ingredients: Servings: 6   Cooking Time: 2 1/4 Hours

1 wheel of Brie	1/2 tsp. dried thyme
1/2 C. cranberry sauce	

Directions:

Spoon the cranberry sauce in your Crock Pot. Sprinkle with thyme and top with the Brie cheese. Cover with a lid and cook on low settings for 2 hours. The cheese is best served warm with bread sticks or tortilla chips.

Turkey Meatloaf

Ingredients: Servings: 8   Cooking Time: 6 1/4 Hours

1 1/2 lb. ground turkey	1/4 tsp. chili powder
1 carrot, grated	Salt and pepper to taste
1 sweet potato, grated	1 C. shredded mozzarella
1 egg	
1/4 C. breadcrumbs	

Directions:

Mix all the ingredients in a bowl and season with salt and pepper as needed. Give it a good mix then transfer the mixture in your Crock Pot. Level the mixture well and cover with the pot's lid. Cook on low settings for 6 hours. Serve the meatloaf warm or chilled.

White Bean Hummus

Ingredients: Servings: 8   Cooking Time: 8 1/4 Hours

1 lb. dried white beans, rinsed	1 thyme sprig
2 C. water	Salt and pepper to taste
2 C. chicken stock	2 tbsp. canola oil
1 bay leaf	2 large sweet onions, sliced
4 garlic cloves, minced	

Directions:

Combine the white beans, water, stock, bay leaf and thyme in your Crock Pot. Add salt and pepper to taste and cook the beans on low settings for 8 hours. When done, drain the beans well (but reserve 1/4 C. of the liquid) and discard the bay leaf and thyme. Transfer the bean in a food processor. Add the reserved liquid and pulse until smooth. Season with salt and pepper and transfer in a bowl. Heat the canola oil in a skillet and add the onions. Cook for 10 minutes over medium flame until the onions begin to caramelize. Top the hummus with caramelized onions and serve.

Mediterranean Dip

Ingredients: Servings: 20   Cooking Time: 6 1/4 Hours

2 tbsp. canola oil	1/2 C. black olives, pitted and chopped
1 lb. ground beef	
2 shallots, chopped	1/2 tsp. dried oregano
2 garlic cloves, chopped	1 tsp. dried basil
	1/4 C. white wine
4 ripe tomatoes, peeled and diced	1/2 C. tomato sauce
1/2 C. Kalamata olives, pitted and chopped	Salt and pepper to taste

Directions:

Heat the oil in a skillet and stir in the beef. Cook for 5 minutes then add the shallots and garlic and cook for 5 additional minutes. Transfer the mixture in your Crock Pot and add the remaining ingredients. Season with salt and pepper and cook on low settings for 6 hours. Serve the dip warm or chilled.

Spicy Enchilada Dip

Ingredients: Servings: 8   Cooking Time: 6 1/4 Hours

1 lb. ground chicken	1 shallot, chopped
1/2 tsp. chili powder	2 tomatoes, diced
2 garlic cloves, chopped	1 C. tomato sauce
1 red bell pepper, cored and diced	Salt and pepper to taste
	1 1/2 C. grated Cheddar cheese

Directions:

Combine the ground chicken with chili powder, shallot and garlic in your Crock Pot. Add the remaining ingredients and cook on low settings for 6 hours. Serve the dip warm with tortilla chips.

Boiled Peanuts With Skin On

Ingredients: Servings: 8   Cooking Time: 7 1/4 Hours

2 lb. uncooked, whole peanuts	1/2 C. salt
	4 C. water

Directions:

Combine all the ingredients in your Crock Pot. Cover and cook on low settings for 7 hours. Drain and allow to cool down before servings.

Bacon Crab Dip

Ingredients: Servings: 20   Cooking Time: 2 1/4 Hours

1 lb. bacon, diced	1 tsp. Dijon mustard
1 C. cream cheese	1 can crab meat, drained and shredded
1/2 C. grated Parmesan cheese	1 tsp. hot sauce
1 tsp. Worcestershire sauce	

Directions:

Heat a skillet over medium flame and add the bacon. Sauté for 5 minutes until fat begins to drain out. Transfer the bacon in a Crock Pot. Stir in the remaining ingredients and cook on high settings for 2 hours. Serve the dip warm or chilled.

Roasted Bell Peppers Dip

Ingredients: Servings: 8   Cooking Time: 2 1/4 Hours

4 roasted red bell peppers, drained	1 shallot, chopped
2 cans chickpeas, drained	Salt and pepper to taste
1/2 C. water	2 tbsp. lemon juice
4 garlic cloves, minced	2 tbsp. olive oil

Directions:

Combine the bell peppers, chickpeas, water, shallot and garlic in a Crock Pot. Add salt and pepper as needed and cook on high settings for 2 hours. When done, puree the dip in a blender, adding the lemon juice and olive oil as well. Serve the dip fresh or store it in the fridge in an airtight container for up to 2 days.

Hoisin Chicken Wings

Ingredients: Servings: 8   Cooking Time: 7 1/4 Hours

4 lb. chicken wings	1 tsp. sesame oil
2/3 C. hoisin sauce	1 tbsp. molasses
4 garlic cloves, minced	1 tsp. hot sauce
1 tsp. grated ginger	1/4 tsp. ground black pepper
	1/2 tsp. salt

Directions:

Mix the hoisin sauce, garlic, ginger, sesame oil, molasses, hot sauce, black pepper and salt in your Crock Pot. Add the chicken wings and toss them around until evenly coated. Cover with a lid and cook on low settings for 7 hours. Serve the wings warm or chilled.

Asian Marinated Mushrooms

Ingredients: Servings: 8   Cooking Time: 8 1/4 Hours

2 lb. mushrooms	1/4 C. rice vinegar
1 C. soy sauce	1/2 tsp. chili powder
1 C. water	
1/2 C. brown sugar	

Directions:

Combine all the ingredients in your Crock Pot. Cover the crock pot and cook on low settings for 8 hours. Allow to cool in the pot before serving.

Balsamico Pulled Pork

Ingredients: Servings: 6   Cooking Time: 8 1/4 Hours

2 lb. boneless pork shoulder	1/4 C. hoisin sauce
2 tbsp. honey	1/4 C. chicken stock
1/4 C. balsamic vinegar	2 garlic cloves, minced
1 tbsp. Dijon mustard	2 shallots, sliced
	2 tbsp. soy sauce

Directions:

Combine the honey, vinegar, hoisin sauce, mustard, stock, garlic, shallots and soy sauce in your Crock Pot. Add the pork shoulder and roll it in the mixture until evenly coated. Cover the Crock Pot and cook on low settings for 8 hours. When done, shred the meat into fine pieces and serve warm or chilled.

Cheeseburger Dip

Ingredients: Servings: 20   Cooking Time: 6 1/4 Hours

2 lb. ground beef	1 tbsp. Dijon mustard
1 tbsp. canola oil	2 tbsp. pickle relish
2 sweet onions, chopped	1 C. shredded processed cheese
4 garlic cloves, chopped	1 C. grated Cheddar
1/2 C. tomato sauce	

Directions:

Heat the canola oil in a skillet and stir in the ground beef. Sauté for 5 minutes then add the meat in your Crock Pot. Stir in the remaining ingredients and cover with the pot's lid. Cook on low settings for 6 hours. The dip is best served warm.

Three Cheese Artichoke Sauce

Ingredients: Servings: 16   Cooking Time: 4 1/4 Hours

1 jar artichoke hearts, drained and chopped	1 C. grated Swiss cheese
1 shallot, chopped	1/2 tsp. dried thyme
2 C. shredded mozzarella	1/4 tsp. chili powder
1 C. grated Parmesan	

Directions:
Combine all the ingredients in your Crock Pot. Cover the pot with its lid and cook on low setting for 4 hours. The sauce is great served warm with vegetable sticks or biscuits or even small pretzels.

Spicy Glazed Pecans

Ingredients: Servings: 10   Cooking Time: 3 1/4 Hours

1/2 C. butter, melted	2 lb. pecans
1 tsp. chili powder	1 tsp. dried thyme
1 tsp. smoked paprika	1/4 tsp. cayenne pepper
1 tsp. dried basil	1/2 tsp. garlic powder
	2 tbsp. honey

Directions:
Combine all the ingredients in your Crock Pot. Mix well until all the ingredients are well distributed and the pecans are evenly glazed. Cook on high settings for 3 hours. Allow them to cool before serving.

Chili Chicken Wings

Ingredients: Servings: 8   Cooking Time: 7 1/4 Hours

4 lb. chicken wings	1/4 C. maple syrup
1 tsp. garlic powder	1 tbsp. Dijon mustard
1 tsp. chili powder	1 tsp. Worcestershire sauce
2 tbsp. balsamic vinegar	1/2 C. tomato sauce
	1 tsp. salt

Directions:
Combine the chicken wings and the remaining ingredients in a Crock Pot. Toss around until evenly coated and cook on low settings for 7 hours. Serve the chicken wings warm or chilled.

Tropical Meatballs

Ingredients: Servings: 20   Cooking Time: 7 1/2 Hours

1 can pineapple chunks (keep the juices)	1/4 C. brown sugar
2 poblano peppers, chopped	2 lb. ground pork
	1 lb. ground beef
2 tbsp. soy sauce	4 garlic clove, minced
2 tbsp. cornstarch	1 tsp. dried basil
1 tbsp. lemon juice	1 egg
	1/4 C. breadcrumbs
	Salt and pepper to taste

Directions:
Mix the pineapple, poblano peppers, brown sugar, soy sauce, cornstarch and lemon juice in a Crock Pot. Combine the ground meat, garlic, basil, egg and breadcrumbs in a bowl. Add salt and pepper to taste and mix well. Form small meatballs and place them in the sauce. Cover and cook on low settings for 7 hours. Serve the meatballs warm or chilled.

Eggplant Caviar

Ingredients: Servings: 6   Cooking Time: 3 1/4 Hours

2 large eggplants, peeled and cubed	1 tsp. dried oregano
4 tbsp. olive oil	2 garlic cloves, minced
1 tsp. dried basil	Salt and pepper to taste
1 lemon, juiced	

Directions:
Combine the eggplant cubes, olive oil, basil and oregano in a Crock Pot. Add salt and pepper to taste and cook on high settings for 3 hours. When done, stir in the lemon juice, garlic, salt and pepper and mash the mix well with a potato masher. Serve the dip chilled.

Marmalade Glazed Meatballs

Ingredients: Servings: 8   Cooking Time: 7 1/2 Hours

2 lb. ground pork	1 C. orange marmalade
1 shallot, chopped	2 C. BBQ sauce
4 garlic cloves, minced	1 bay leaf
1 carrot, grated	1 tsp. Worcestershire sauce
1 egg	Salt and pepper to taste
Salt and pepper to taste	

Directions:
Mix the ground pork, shallot, garlic, carrot, egg, salt and pepper in a bowl. Form small meatballs and place them on your working surface. For the sauce, mix the orange marmalade, sauce, bay leaf, Worcestershire sauce, salt and pepper in your Crock Pot. Place the meatballs in the sauce. Cover with its lid and cook on low settings for 7 hours. Serve the meatballs warm.

Stuffed Artichokes

Ingredients: Servings: 6   Cooking Time: 6 1/2 Hours

6 fresh artichokes	1 C. breadcrumbs
6 anchovy fillets, chopped	1 tbsp. chopped parsley
4 garlic cloves, minced	Salt and pepper to taste
2 tbsp. olive oil	1/4 C. white wine

Directions:
Cut the stem of each artichoke so that it sits flat on your chopping board then cut the top off and trim the outer leaves, cleaning the center as well. In a bowl, mix the anchovy fillets, garlic, olive oil, breadcrumbs and parsley. Add salt and pepper to taste. Top each artichoke with breadcrumb mixture and rub it well into the leaves. Place the artichokes in your Crock Pot and pour in the white wine. Cook on low settings for 6 hours. Serve the artichokes warm or chilled.

Pretzel Party Mix

Ingredients: Servings: 10   Cooking Time: 2 1/4 Hours

4 C. pretzels
1 C. peanuts
1 C. crispy rice cereals
1/4 C. butter, melted

1 C. pecans
1 tsp. Worcestershire sauce
1 tsp. salt
1 tsp. garlic powder

Directions:

Combine the pretzels, peanuts, pecans and rice cereals in your Crock Pot.   Drizzle with melted butter and Worcestershire sauce and mix well then sprinkle with salt and garlic powder. Cover and cook on high settings for 2 hours, mixing once during cooking.   Allow to cool before serving.

Sausage Dip

Ingredients: Servings: 8   Cooking Time: 6 1/4 Hours

1 lb. fresh pork sausages
1 lb. spicy pork sausages

1 C. cream cheese
1 can diced tomatoes
2 poblano peppers, chopped

Directions:

Combine all the ingredients in a crock pot.   Cook on low settings for 6 hours.   Serve warm or chilled.

Zesty Lamb Meatballs

Ingredients: Servings: 10   Cooking Time: 7 1/4 Hours

3 lb. ground lamb
1 shallot, chopped
2 garlic cloves, minced
1 tbsp. lemon zest
1/4 tsp. five-spice powder
1/2 tsp. cumin powder
1/4 tsp. cumin powder

1/4 tsp. chili powder
1/2 C. raisins, chopped
1 tsp. dried mint
Salt and pepper to taste
2 C. tomato sauce
1 lemon, juiced
1 bay leaf
1 thyme sprig
1 red chili, chopped

Directions:

Mix the tomato sauce, lemon juice, bay leaf, thyme sprig and red chili in your Crock Pot.   Combine the remaining ingredients in a bowl and mix well. Season with salt and pepper and give it a good mix.   Form small balls and place them in the sauce. Cover with its lid and cook on low settings for 7 hours.   Serve the meatballs warm or chilled.

Green Vegetable Dip

Ingredients: Servings: 12   Cooking Time: 2 1/4 Hours

10 oz. frozen spinach, thawed and drained
1 jar artichoke hearts, drained
1 C. chopped parsley
1 C. cream cheese
1 C. sour cream

1/2 C. grated Parmesan cheese
1/2 C. feta cheese, crumbled
1/2 tsp. onion powder
1/4 tsp. garlic powder

Directions:

Combine all the ingredients in your Crock Pot and mix gently. Cover with its lid and cook on high settings for 2 hours.   Serve the dip warm or chilled with crusty bread, biscuits or other salty snacks or even vegetable sticks.

Teriyaki Chicken Wings

Ingredients: Servings: 6   Cooking Time: 6 1/4 Hours

2 tbsp. brown sugar
1 tbsp. molasses
1/2 tsp. garlic powder
1/2 tsp. ground ginger
1/2 C. soy sauce

1/2 C. pineapple juice
1/4 C. water
2 tbsp. canola oil
3 lb. chicken wings

Directions:

Combine all the ingredients in a Crock Pot and mix until evenly coated.   Cover the pot with its lid and cook on low settings for 6 hours.   Serve the chicken wings warm or chilled.

Cheesy Beef Dip

Ingredients: Servings: 8   Cooking Time: 3 1/4 Hours

2 lb. ground beef
1 lb. grated Cheddar
1/2 C. cream cheese

1/2 C. white wine
1 poblano pepper, chopped

Directions:

Combine all the ingredients in a crock pot.   Cook on high settings for 3 hours.   Serve preferably warm.

Carne Asada Nachos

Ingredients: Servings: 8   Cooking Time: 10 1/2 Hours

2 lb. flanks steak
1 tsp. smoked paprika
1/2 tsp. chili powder
2 tbsp. brown sugar
1 tsp. cumin powder
1 tsp. garlic powder
2 tbsp. canola oil

1 tsp. salt
1 C. dark beer
8 oz. tortillas chips
1 C. red salsa
1 can sweet corn, drained
2 C. grated Monterey jack cheese
Sour cream for serving
Chopped cilantro for serving

Directions:

Mix the salt, paprika, chili powder, sugar, cumin powder and garlic powder in a bowl. Spread this mix over the steak and rub it well into the meat.   Heat the oil in a skillet and add the steak in the hot oil. Cook on all sides for 4-5 minutes just to sear it. Transfer the meat in your Crock Pot and pour the beer over. Cook on low settings for 8 hours.   When done, remove from the pot and cut the flank steak into thin slices.   Clean the pot then place the tortilla chips on the bottom.   Cover the tortilla chips with red salsa, followed by flank steak, corn and cheese.   Cook on low settings for 2 additional hours.   Serve right away.

Blue Cheese Chicken Wings

Ingredients: Servings: 8   Cooking Time: 7 1/4 Hours

4 lb. chicken wings
1/2 C. spicy tomato

1/2 C. buffalo sauce
1 tbsp.

sauce
1 tbsp. tomato paste
2 tbsp. apple cider vinegar

Worcestershire sauce
1 C. sour cream
2 oz. blue cheese, crumbled
1 thyme sprig

Directions:

Combine the buffalo sauce, tomato sauce, vinegar, Worcestershire sauce, sour cream, blue cheese and thyme in a Crock Pot. Add the chicken wings and toss them until evenly coated. Cook on low settings for 7 hours. Serve the chicken wings preferably warm.

Candied Kielbasa

Ingredients: Servings: 8   Cooking Time: 6 1/4 Hours

2 lb. kielbasa sausages
1/2 C. brown sugar
1 tsp. prepared horseradish

1 C. BBQ sauce
1/2 tsp. black pepper
1/4 tsp. cumin powder

Directions:

Combine all the ingredients in a Crock Pot, adding salt if needed. Cook on low settings for 6 hours. Serve the kielbasa warm or chilled.

Parmesan Zucchini Frittata

Ingredients: Servings: 8   Cooking Time: 6 1/4 Hours

2 zucchinis, finely sliced
2 garlic cloves, minced
1 tsp. dried mint
1 tsp. dried oregano
6 eggs

2 tbsp. plain yogurt
1 tbsp. chopped parsley
1/2 C. grated Parmesan
Salt and pepper to taste

Directions:

Mix the zucchinis, garlic, dried mint and oregano in a Crock Pot. Add salt and pepper to taste. In a bowl, mix the eggs, yogurt, parsley and Parmesan. Pour the egg mixture over the zucchinis and cover the pot with its lid. Cook on low settings for 6 hours. Serve the frittata sliced, warm or chilled.

Bacon Wrapped Dates

Ingredients: Servings: 8   Cooking Time: 1 3/4 Hours

16 dates, pitted
16 almonds

16 slices bacon

Directions:

Stuff each date with an almond. Wrap each date in bacon and place the wrapped dates in your Crock Pot. Cover with its lid and cook on high settings for 1 1/4 hours. Serve warm or chilled.

Curried Chicken Wings

Ingredients: Servings: 10   Cooking Time: 7 1/4 Hours

4 lb. chicken wings
1 C. tomato sauce
1/4 C. red curry paste
1/2 C. coconut milk

2 shallots, chopped
1/2 tsp. dried basil
Salt and pepper to taste

Directions:

Combine all the ingredients in a Crock Pot and toss around until evenly coated. Adjust the taste with salt and pepper and cook on low settings for 7 hours. Serve the chicken wings warm or chilled.

Cheesy Bacon Dip

Ingredients: Servings: 20   Cooking Time: 4 1/4 Hours

1 sweet onions, chopped
1 tsp. Worcestershire sauce
1 tsp. Dijon mustard
1 C. cream cheese

10 bacon slices, chopped
1 C. grated Gruyere
1/2 C. whole milk
Salt and pepper to taste

Directions:

Combine all the ingredients in a Crock Pot. Adjust the taste with salt and pepper and cover with its lid. Cook on low settings for 4 hours. Serve the dip warm or chilled with vegetable sticks, biscuits or other salty snacks.

Spiced Buffalo Wings

Ingredients: Servings: 8   Cooking Time: 8 1/4 Hours

4 lb. chicken wings
1 C. BBQ sauce
1/4 C. butter, melted
1 tbsp. Worcestershire sauce
1 tsp. dried oregano
1 tsp. dried basil

1 tsp. onion powder
1 tsp. garlic powder
1/2 tsp. cumin powder
1/2 tsp. cinnamon powder
1 tsp. hot sauce
1 tsp. salt

Directions:

Combine all the ingredients in a Crock Pot. Mix until the wings are evenly coated. Cook on low settings for 8 hours. Serve warm or chilled.

Wild Mushroom Dip

Ingredients: Servings: 20   Cooking Time: 4 1/4 Hours

1 lb. wild mushrooms, chopped
1 can condensed cream of mushroom soup
1 C. white wine
1 C. cream cheese
1 C. heavy cream
1/2 C. grated Parmesan

1 tsp. dried tarragon
1/2 tsp. dried oregano
1/2 tsp. ground black pepper
Salt and pepper to taste

Directions:

Combine all the ingredients in your Crock Pot. Adjust the taste with salt and pepper and cook on low settings for 4 hours. Serve the dip warm or chilled.

Mozzarella Stuffed Meatballs

Ingredients: Servings: 8   Cooking Time: 6 1/2 Hours

2 lb. ground chicken
1 tsp. dried basil

1/2 C. breadcrumbs
Salt and pepper to

1/2 tsp. dried
oregano

1 egg

taste
Mini-mozzarella balls
as needed
1/2 C. chicken stock

Directions:

Mix the ground chicken, basil, oregano, egg, breadcrumbs, salt and pepper in a bowl. Take small pieces of the meat mixture and flatten it in your palm. Place a mozzarella ball in the center and gather the meat around the mozzarella. Shape the meatballs, making sure they are well sealed and place them in a Crock Pot. Add the chicken stock and cook on low settings for 6 hours. Serve the meatballs warm or chilled.

Southwestern Nacho Dip

Ingredients: Servings: 10   Cooking Time: 6 1/4 Hours

1 lb. ground pork
1 C. apple juice
4 garlic cloves,
chopped
2 C. BBQ sauce
2 tbsp. brown sugar
Salt and pepper to
taste
1 1/2 C. sweet corn

1 can black beans,
drained
1 C. diced tomatoes
2 jalapeno peppers,
chopped
2 tbsp. chopped
cilantro
2 C. grated Cheddar
1 lime, juiced
Nachos for serving

Directions:

Heat a skillet over medium flame and add the pork. Cook for a few minutes, stirring often. Transfer the pork in your Crock Pot and add the apple juice, garlic, BBQ sauce, brown sugar, salt and pepper. Cook on high settings for 2 hours. After 2 hours, add the remaining ingredients and continue cooking for 4 hours on low settings. Serve the dip warm with nachos.

Charred Tomato Salsa

Ingredients: Servings: 8   Cooking Time: 3 Hours

4 ripe tomatoes,
sliced
2 tbsp. olive oil
1 tsp. dried basil
1/2 tsp. dried mint
2 shallots, chopped

1 jalapeno pepper,
chopped
1 can black beans,
drained
1/4 C. chicken stock
1 bay leaf
Salt and pepper to
taste

Directions:

Place the tomato slices in a baking tray and sprinkle with salt, pepper, basil and mint. Drizzle with olive oil and cook in the preheated oven at 350F for 35-40 minutes until the slices begin to caramelize. Transfer the tomatoes in a Crock Pot and add the remaining ingredients. Cook on high settings for 2 hours and serve the salsa warm or chilled.

Spicy Asian Style Mushroom

Ingredients: Servings: 8   Cooking Time: 2 1/4 Hours

1/4 C. hoisin sauce
1/4 C. soy sauce
2 garlic cloves,
minced

1/2 tsp. red pepper
flakes
2 lb. fresh
mushrooms, cleaned

Directions:

Mix the hoisin sauce, soy sauce, garlic and red pepper flakes in a bowl. Place the mushrooms in your Crock Pot and drizzle them with the sauce. Cook on high settings for 2 hours. Allow the mushrooms to cool in the pot before serving.

Caramelized Onion Dip

Ingredients: Servings: 12   Cooking Time: 4 1/2 Hours

4 red onions, sliced
2 tbsp. butter
1 tbsp. canola oil
1 C. beef stock
1 tsp. dried thyme
1/2 C. white wine

2 garlic cloves,
chopped
2 C. grated Swiss
cheese
1 tbsp. cornstarch
Salt and pepper to
taste

Directions:

Heat the butter and oil in a skillet. Add the onions and cook over medium flame until the onions begin to caramelize. Transfer the onions in your Crock Pot and add the remaining ingredients. Season with salt and pepper and cook on low settings for 4 hours. Serve the dip warm with vegetable sticks or your favorite crunchy snacks.

Bacon Chicken Sliders

Ingredients: Servings: 8   Cooking Time: 4 1/2 Hours

2 lb. ground chicken
1 egg
1/2 C. breadcrumbs

1 shallot, chopped
Salt and pepper to
taste
8 bacon slices

Directions:

Mix the chicken, egg, breadcrumbs and shallot in a bowl. Add salt and pepper to taste and give it a good mix. Form small sliders then wrap each slider in a bacon slice. Place the sliders in a Crock Pot. Cover with its lid and cook on high settings for 4 hours, making sure to flip them over once during cooking. Serve them warm.

Bacon Black Bean Dip

Ingredients: Servings: 6   Cooking Time: 6 1/4 Hours

6 bacon slices
2 cans black beans,
drained
2 shallots, sliced
1 garlic cloves,
chopped
1 C. red salsa
1 tbsp. brown sugar

1/2 C. beef stock
1 tbsp. molasses
1/2 tsp. chili powder
1 tbsp. apple cider
vinegar
2 tbsp. Bourbon
Salt and pepper to
taste

Directions:

Heat a skillet over medium flame and add the bacon. Cook until crisp then transfer the bacon and its fat in your Crock Pot. Stir in the remaining ingredients and cook on low settings for 6 hours. When done, partially mash the beans and serve the dip right away.

Artichoke Bread Pudding

Ingredients: Servings: 10   Cooking Time: 6 1/2 Hours

6 C. bread cubes
6 artichoke hearts, drained and chopped
1/2 C. grated Parmesan
4 eggs
1/2 C. sour cream
1 C. milk
4 oz. spinach, chopped
1 tbsp. chopped parsley
2 tbsp. olive oil
Salt and pepper to taste
1/2 tsp. dried oregano
1/2 tsp. dried basil

Directions:
Combine the bread cubes, artichoke hearts and Parmesan in your Crock Pot. Add the spinach and parsley as well. In a bowl, mix the eggs, sour cream, milk, oregano and basil, as well as salt and pepper. Pour this mixture over the bread and press the bread slightly to make sure it soaks up all the liquid. Cover the pot with its lid and cook on low settings for 6 hours. The bread can be served both warm and chilled.

Mexican Chili Dip

Ingredients: Servings: 20   Cooking Time: 2 1/4 Hours

1 can black beans, drained
1 can red beans, drained
1 can diced tomatoes
1/2 tsp. cumin powder
1/2 tsp. chili powder
1/2 C. beef stock
Salt and pepper to taste
1 1/2 C. grated Cheddar

Directions:
Combine the beans, tomatoes, cumin powder, chili and stock in your Crock Pot. Add salt and pepper to taste and top with grated cheese. Cook on high settings for 2 hours. The dip is best served warm.

Pepperoni Pizza Dip

Ingredients: Servings: 10   Cooking Time: 3 1/4 Hours

1 1/2 C. pizza sauce
4 peperoni, sliced
2 red bell peppers, diced
1/2 C. black olives, pitted and chopped
2 shallots, chopped
1 C. cream cheese
1 C. shredded mozzarella
1/2 tsp. dried basil

Directions:
Combine the pizza sauce and the rest of the ingredients in your Crock Pot. Cover the pot with its lid and cook on low settings for 3 hours. The dip is best served warm with bread sticks or tortilla chips.

Bean Queso

Ingredients: Servings: 10   Cooking Time: 6 1/4 Hours

1 can black beans, drained
1 C. chopped green chiles
1/2 C. red salsa
1 tsp. dried oregano
1/2 tsp. cumin powder
1 C. light beer
1 1/2 C. grated Cheddar
Salt and pepper to taste

Directions:
Combine the beans, chiles, oregano, cumin, salsa, beer and cheese in your Crock Pot. Add salt and pepper as needed and cook on low settings for 6 hours. Serve the bean queso warm.

Honey Glazed Chicken Drumsticks

Ingredients: Servings: 8   Cooking Time: 7 1/4 Hours

3 lb. chicken drumsticks
1/4 C. soy sauce
1/4 C. honey
1 tsp. rice vinegar
1/2 tsp. sesame oil
2 tbsp. tomato paste
1/2 tsp. dried Thai basil

Directions:
Combine all the ingredients in your Crock Pot and toss them around until the drumsticks are evenly coated. Cover the pot with its lid and cook on low settings for 7 hours. Serve the chicken drumsticks warm or chilled.

Spanish Chorizo Dip

Ingredients: Servings: 8   Cooking Time: 6 1/4 Hours

8 chorizo links, diced
1 can diced tomatoes
1 chili pepper, chopped
1 C. cream cheese
2 C. grated Cheddar cheese
1/4 C. white wine

Directions:
Combine all the ingredients in your Crock Pot. Cook the dip on low settings for 6 hours. Serve the dip warm.

Molasses Lime Meatballs

Ingredients: Servings: 10   Cooking Time: 8 1/4 Hours

3 lb. ground beef
2 garlic cloves, minced
1 shallot, chopped
1/2 C. oat flour
1/2 tsp. cumin powder
1/2 tsp. chili powder
1 egg
Salt and pepper to taste
1/2 C. molasses
1/4 C. soy sauce
2 tbsp. lime juice
1/2 C. beef stock
1 tbsp. Worcestershire sauce

Directions:
Combine the molasses, soy sauce, lime juice, stock and Worcestershire sauce in your Crock Pot. In a bowl, mix the ground beef, garlic, shallot, oat flour, cumin powder, chili powder, egg, salt and pepper and mix well. Form small balls and place them in the sauce. Cover the pot and cook on low settings for 8 hours. Serve the meatballs warm or chilled.

Creamy Potatoes

Ingredients: Servings: 6   Cooking Time: 6 1/4 Hours

3 lb. small new potatoes, washed
4 bacon slices, chopped
1 tsp. dried oregano
1 shallot, chopped
2 tbsp. olive oil
2 garlic cloves, chopped
Salt and pepper to taste
1 C. sour cream
2 green onions, chopped

2 tbsp. chopped
parsley

Directions:

Combine the potatoes, bacon, oregano, shallot, olive oil and garlic in a Crock Pot. Add salt and pepper and mix until the ingredients are well distributed. Cover the pot with its lid and cook on low settings for 6 hours. When done, mix the cooked potatoes with sour cream, onions and parsley and serve right away.

Quick Layered Appetizer

Ingredients: Servings: 10   Cooking Time: 7 1/2 Hours

4 chicken breasts, cooked and diced	1 C. cream cheese
1 tsp. dried basil	Salt and pepper to taste
1 tsp. dried oregano	4 tomatoes, sliced
1/4 tsp. chili powder	4 large tortillas
	2 C. shredded mozzarella

Directions:

Mix the chicken, basil, oregano, cream cheese, chili powder, salt and pepper in a bowl. Begin layering the chicken mixture, tomatoes, tortillas and mozzarella in your Crock Pot. Cover and cook on low settings for 7 hours. Allow to cool then slice and serve.

Cranberry Sauce Meatballs

Ingredients: Servings: 12   Cooking Time: 7 1/2 Hours

3 lb. ground pork	Salt and pepper to taste
1 lb. ground turkey	
1 egg	2 C. cranberry sauce
1/2 C. breadcrumbs	1 C. BBQ sauce
1 shallot, chopped	1 tsp. hot sauce
1/2 tsp. ground cloves	1 thyme sprig

Directions:

Mix the ground pork, turkey, egg, breadcrumbs, shallot, ground cloves, salt and pepper and mix well. In the meantime, combine the cranberry sauce, BBQ sauce, hot sauce and thyme sprig in your Crock Pot. Form small meatballs and drop them in the sauce. Cook on low settings for 7 hours. Serve the meatballs warm or chilled.

Bacon New Potatoes

Ingredients: Servings: 6   Cooking Time: 3 1/4 Hours

3 lb. new potatoes, washed and halved	2 tbsp. white wine
12 slices bacon, chopped	Salt and pepper to taste
	1 rosemary sprig

Directions:

Place the potatoes, wine and rosemary in your Crock Pot. Add salt and pepper to taste and top with chopped bacon. Cook on high settings for 3 hours. Serve the potatoes warm.

Goat Cheese Stuffed Mushrooms

Ingredients: Servings: 6   Cooking Time: 4 1/4 Hours

12 medium size mushrooms	1 poblano pepper, chopped
6 oz. goat cheese	1 tsp. dried oregano
1 egg	
1/2 C. breadcrumbs	

Directions:

Mix the goat cheese, egg, breadcrumbs, pepper and oregano in a bowl. Stuff each mushroom with the goat cheese mixture and place them all in a Crock Pot. Cover the pot and cook on low settings for 4 hours. Serve the mushrooms warm or chilled.

Sausage And Pepper Appetizer

Ingredients: Servings: 8   Cooking Time: 6 1/4 Hours

2 tbsp. olive oil	6 fresh pork sausages, skins removed
1 can fire roasted tomatoes	
4 roasted bell peppers, chopped	1 shallot, chopped
1 poblano pepper, chopped	1 C. grated Provolone cheese
	Salt and pepper to taste

Directions:

Heat the oil in a skillet and stir in the sausage meat. Cook for 5 minutes, stirring often. Transfer the meat in your Crock Pot and add the remaining ingredients. Season with salt and pepper and cook on low settings for 6 hours. Serve the dish warm or chilled.

Ham And Swiss Cheese Dip

Ingredients: Servings: 6   Cooking Time: 4 1/4 Hours

1 lb. ham, diced	1 C. cream cheese
1 can condensed cream of mushroom soup	2 C. grated Swiss cheese
1 can condensed onion soup	1/2 tsp. chili powder

Directions:

Combine all the ingredients in a Crock Pot. Cook on low settings for 4 hours. Serve the dip preferably warm.

Swiss Cheese Fondue

Ingredients: Servings: 10   Cooking Time: 4 1/4 Hours

1 garlic cloves	1 C. grated Cheddar
2 C. dry white wine	2 tbsp. cornstarch
2 C. grated Swiss cheese	1 pinch nutmeg

Directions:

Rub the inside of your Crock Pot with a garlic clove. Discard the clove once done. Add the remaining ingredients and cook on low heat for 4 hours. Serve the fondue warm with vegetable sticks, croutons or pretzels.

Chipotle Bbq Sausage Bites

Ingredients: Servings: 10   Cooking Time: 2 1/4 Hours

3 lb. small smoked sausages	1 tbsp. tomato paste
	1/4 C. white wine

1 C. BBQ sauce
2 chipotle peppers in adobo sauce
Salt and pepper to taste

Directions:
Combine all the ingredients in your Crock Pot. Add salt and pepper if needed and cover with a lid. Cook on high settings for 2 hours. Serve the sausage bites warm or chilled.

Quick Parmesan Bread

Ingredients: Servings: 8   Cooking Time: 1 1/4 Hours

4 C. all-purpose flour
1/2 tsp. salt
1/2 C. grated Parmesan cheese
1 tsp. baking soda
2 C. buttermilk
2 tbsp. olive oil

Directions:
Mix the flour, salt, parmesan cheese and baking soda in a bowl. Stir in the buttermilk and olive oil and mix well with a fork. Shape the dough into a loaf and place it in your Crock Pot. Cover with its lid and cook on high heat for 1 hour. Serve the bread warm or chilled.

Taco Dip

Ingredients: Servings: 20   Cooking Time: 6 1/2 Hours

2 lb. ground beef
2 tbsp. canola oil
1 can black beans, drained
1/2 C. beef stock
1 C. tomato sauce
1 tbsp. taco seasoning
2 C. Velveeta cheese, shredded

Directions:
Heat the oil in a skillet and add the beef. Cook for 10 minutes, stirring often. Transfer the beef in your Crock Pot. Add the remaining ingredients and cook on low settings for 6 hours. Serve the dip warm.

Cheeseburger Meatballs

Ingredients: Servings: 8   Cooking Time: 6 14 Hours

2 lb. ground pork
1 shallot, chopped
2 tbsp. beef stock
1 egg
1 tsp. Cajun seasoning
14 C. breadcrumbs
12 tsp. dried basil
Salt and pepper to taste
2 C. shredded processed cheese

Directions:
Mix the pork, shallot, beef stock, egg, breadcrumbs, Cajun seasoning and basil in a bowl. Add salt and pepper to taste and mix well. Form small meatballs and place them in the Crock Pot. Top with shredded cheese and cook on low settings for 6 hours. Serve the meatballs warm.

Beer Bbq Meatballs

Ingredients: Servings: 10   Cooking Time: 7 1/2 Hours

2 lb. ground pork
1 lb. ground beef
1 carrot, grated
2 shallots, chopped
1 egg
1/2 C. breadcrumbs
1 C. dark beer
1 C. BBQ sauce
1 bay leaf
1/2 tsp. chili powder

1/2 tsp. cumin powder
Salt and pepper to taste
1 tsp. apple cider vinegar

Directions:
Mix the ground pork and beef in a bowl. Add the carrot, shallots, egg, breadcrumbs, cumin, salt and pepper and mix well. Form small meatballs and place them on your chopping board. For the beer sauce, combine the beer, BBQ sauce, bay leaf, chili powder and vinegar in a Crock Pot. Place the meatballs in the pot and cover with its lid. Cook on low settings for 7 hours. Serve the meatballs warm or chilled.

Queso Verde Dip

Ingredients: Servings: 12   Cooking Time: 4 1/4 Hours

1 lb. ground chicken
2 shallots, chopped
2 tbsp. olive oil
2 C. salsa verde
1 C. cream cheese
2 poblano peppers, chopped
2 C. grated Cheddar
1 tbsp. Worcestershire sauce
4 garlic cloves, minced
1/4 C. chopped cilantro
Salt and pepper to taste

Directions:
Combine all the ingredients in your Crock Pot. Add salt and pepper to taste and cook on low heat for 4 hours. The dip is best served warm.

Oriental Chicken Bites

Ingredients: Servings: 10   Cooking Time: 7 1/4 Hours

4 chicken breasts, cubed
2 sweet onions, sliced
1 tsp. grated ginger
4 garlic cloves, minced
1/2 tsp. cinnamon powder
1 tsp. smoked paprika
1 tsp. cumin powder
1 C. chicken stock
1/2 lemon, juiced
2 tbsp. olive oil
Salt and pepper to taste

Directions:
Combine all the ingredients in your Crock Pot. Add salt and pepper to taste and mix well until the ingredients are evenly distributed. Cover and cook on low settings for 7 hours. Serve the chicken bites warm or chilled.

Cocktail Meatballs

Ingredients: Servings: 10   Cooking Time: 6 1/2 Hours

2 lb. ground pork
1 lb. ground beef
4 garlic cloves, minced
1 shallot, chopped
1 egg
1/4 C. breadcrumbs
2 tbsp. chopped parsley
1 tbsp. chopped cilantro
1/2 tsp. chili powder
2 tbsp. cranberry sauce
1 C. BBQ sauce
1/2 C. tomato sauce
1 tsp. red wine vinegar
1 bay leaf
Salt and pepper to taste

Directions:

Combine the cranberry sauce, BBQ sauce, tomato sauce and vinegar, as well as bay leaf, salt and pepper in your Crock Pot. In a bowl, mix the two types of meat, garlic, shallot, egg, breadcrumbs, parsley, cilantro and chili powder. Add salt and pepper to taste. Form small meatballs and place them all in the sauce in the Crock Pot. Cover and cook on low settings for 6 hours. Serve the meatballs warm or chilled with cocktail skewers.

Artichoke Dip

Ingredients: Servings: 20   Cooking Time: 6 1/4 Hours

2 sweet onions, chopped	1 red chili, chopped
2 garlic cloves, chopped	1 C. cream cheese
1 jar artichoke hearts, drained and chopped	1 C. heavy cream
	2 oz. blue cheese, crumbled
	2 tbsp. chopped cilantro

Directions:

Mix the onions, chili, garlic, artichoke hearts, cream cheese, heavy cream and blue cheese in a Crock Pot. Cook on low settings for 6 hours. When done, stir in the cilantro and serve the dip warm or chilled.

VEGETABLE & VEGETARIAN RECIPES

Soft Sweet Potato Halves

Ingredients: Servings: 4   Cooking Time: 5 Hours

4 sweet potatoes, halved	1 tsp. dried thyme
4 tsp. coconut oil	½ tsp. dried oregano
1 tsp. salt	¼ C. of water

Directions:

Pour water in the Crock Pot. Then rub the sweet potato halves with dried thyme, oregano, and salt. Put the sweet potato halves in the Crock Pot. Top every sweet potato halves with coconut oil and close the lid. Cook the sweet potato halves for 5 hours on Low.

Onion Balls

Ingredients: Servings: 4   Cooking Time: 2 Hours

½ C. red lentils, cooked	¼ C. flax meal
½ C. onion, minced	1 tsp. cornflour
1 tsp. ground black pepper	½ tsp. salt
	½ C. of water
	½ C. ketchup

Directions:

In the mixing bowl mix red lentils with minced onion, ground black pepper, flax meal, cornflour, and salt. Make the balls from the onion mixture and freeze them in the freezer for 20 minutes. After this, mix water and ketchup in the Crock Pot.

Add frozen balls and close the lid. Cook the meal on High for 2 hours.

Eggplant Parmesan Casserole

Ingredients: Servings: 3   Cooking Time: 3 Hours

1 medium eggplant, sliced	1 large egg
Salt and pepper to taste	1 C. almond flour
	1 C. parmesan cheese

Directions:

Place the eggplant slices in the crockpot. Pour in the eggs and season with salt and pepper. Stir in the almond flour and sprinkle with parmesan cheese. Stir to combine everything. Close the lid and cook on low for 3 hours or on high for 2 hours.

Beet And Capers Salad

Ingredients: Servings: 4   Cooking Time: 4 Hours

2 tsp. capers	1 tbsp. sunflower oil
1 C. lettuce, chopped	1 tsp. flax seeds
2 oz. walnuts, chopped	3 C. of water
1 tbsp. lemon juice	2 C. beets, peeled

Directions:

Pour water in the Crock Pot and add beets. Cook them on High for 4 hours. Then drain water, cool the beets and chop. Put the chopped beets in the salad bowl. Add capers, lettuce, walnuts, lemon juice, sunflower oil, and flax seeds. Carefully mix the salad.

Zucchini Spinach Lasagne

Ingredients: Servings: 7   Cooking Time: 5 Hours

1 lb. green zucchini, sliced	1 tbsp. minced garlic
7 tbsp. tomato sauce	1 onion, chopped
½ C. fresh parsley, chopped	4 tbsp. ricotta cheese
1 tbsp. fresh dill, chopped	5 oz. mozzarella, shredded
7 oz. Parmesan, shredded	2 eggs
	½ C. baby spinach
	1 tsp. olive oil

Directions:

Grease the base of your Crock Pot with olive oil. Spread 3 zucchini slices at the bottom of the cooker. Whisk tomato sauce with garlic, onion, dill, ricotta cheese, parsley, and spinach. Stir in shredded parmesan, mozzarella, and eggs, then mix well. Add a layer of this tomato-cheese mixture over the zucchini layer. Again, place the zucchini slices over this tomato mixture layer. Continue adding alternating layers of zucchini and tomato sauce Put the cooker's lid on and set the cooking time to 5 hours on High settings. Slice and serve warm.

Lazy Minestrone Soup

Ingredients: Servings: 4   Cooking Time: 3 Hours

1 C. zucchini, sliced	2 C. chicken broth
1 package diced vegetables of your choice	2 tbsp. basil, chopped
	½ C. diced celery

Directions:

Place all ingredients in the crockpot. Season with salt and pepper to taste. Close the lid and cook on low for 3 hours or on high for 1 hour.

Rice Cauliflower Casserole

Ingredients: Servings: 6   Cooking Time: 8 Hrs 10 Minutes

1 C. white rice
5 oz. broccoli, chopped
4 oz. cauliflower, chopped
1 C. Greek Yogurt
6 oz. Cheddar cheese, shredded

1 C. chicken stock
1 tsp. onion powder
2 yellow onions, chopped
1 tsp. paprika
1 tbsp. salt
2 C. of water
1 tsp. butter

Directions:

Add cauliflower, broccoli, water, chicken stock, salt, paprika, rice, and onion powder to the Crock Pot. Top the broccoli-cauliflower mixture with onion slices. Put the cooker's lid on and set the cooking time to 8 hours on Low settings. Add butter and cheese on top of the casserole. Put the cooker's lid on and set the cooking time to 10 minutes on High settings. Serve warm.

Curry Couscous

Ingredients: Servings: 4   Cooking Time: 20 Minutes

1 C. of water
1 C. couscous

½ C. coconut cream
1 tsp. salt

Directions:

Put all ingredients in the Crock Pot and close the lid. Cook the couscous on High for 20 minutes.

Curried Vegetable Stew

Ingredients: Servings: 10   Cooking Time: 3 Hours

1 tsp. olive oil
2 tbsp. curry powder
1 tbsp. grated ginger
3 cloves of garlic, minced
1/8 tsp. cayenne pepper
1 C. tomatoes, crushed

1 onion, diced
1 bag baby spinach
1 yellow bell pepper, chopped
1 red bell pepper, chopped
2 C. vegetable broth
1 C. coconut milk
Salt and pepper to taste

Directions:

Place all ingredients in the CrockPot. Give a good stir. Close the lid and cook on high for 2 hours or on low for 3 hours.

Eggplant Casserole

Ingredients: Servings: 4   Cooking Time: 6 Hours

1 tsp. minced garlic
2 C. eggplants, chopped
2 tbsp. sunflower oil

1 tsp. salt
½ C. potato, diced
1 C. of water
1 C. vegan Cheddar cheese, shredded

Directions:

Brush the Crock Pot bottom with sunflower oil. The mix eggplants with minced garlic and salt. Put the vegetables in the Crock Pot. Add potatoes and water. After this, top the vegetables with vegan Cheddar cheese and close the lid. Cook the casserole on Low for 6 hours.

Light Chana Masala

Ingredients: Servings: 4   Cooking Time: 8 Hours

1 tsp. ginger, peeled, minced
1 tsp. minced garlic
¼ C. fresh cilantro, chopped

1 jalapeno, chopped
1 C. tomatoes, pureed
1 C. chickpeas
4 C. of water

Directions:

Put all ingredients in the Crock Pot and close the lid. Cook the meal on Low for 8 hours.

Cauliflower Stuffing

Ingredients: Servings: 4   Cooking Time: 5 Hours

1-lb. cauliflower, chopped
½ C. panko breadcrumbs
1 C. Mozzarella, shredded

1 C. of coconut milk
2 tbsp. sour cream
1 tsp. onion powder

Directions:

Put all ingredients in the Crock Pot and carefully mix. Then close the lid and cook the stuffing on low for 5 hours. Cool the stuffing for 10-15 minutes and transfer in the bowls.

Apples Sauté

Ingredients: Servings: 4   Cooking Time: 2 Hours

4 C. apples, chopped
1 C. of water

1 tsp. ground cinnamon
1 tsp. sugar

Directions:

Put all ingredients in the Crock Pot. Cook the apple sauté for 2 hours on High. When the meal is cooked, let it cool until warm.

Cauliflower Mac And Cheese

Ingredients: Servings: 6   Cooking Time: 4 Hours

1 large cauliflower, cut into small florets
2 tbsp. butter
1 C. heavy cream
2 oz. grass-fed cream cheese
1 ½ tsp. Dijon mustard

1 ½ C. organic sharp cheddar cheese
1 tbsp. garlic powder
½ C. nutritional yeast
Salt and pepper to taste

Directions:

Place all ingredients in the CrockPot. Give a good stir. Close the lid and cook on high for 3 hours or on low for 4 hours.

Minestrone Zucchini Soup

Ingredients: Servings: 8   Cooking Time: 4 Hours

2 zucchinis, chopped	3 carrots, chopped
1 yellow onion, chopped	1 lb. lentils, cooked
1 C. green beans, halved	4 C. veggie stock
3 celery stalks, chopped	28 oz. canned tomatoes, chopped
4 garlic cloves, minced	1 tsp. curry powder
10 oz. canned garbanzo beans	½ tsp. garam masala
	½ tsp. cumin, ground
	Salt and black pepper to the taste

Directions:

Add carrots, zucchinis, and all other ingredients to the Crock Pot. Put the cooker's lid on and set the cooking time to 4 hours on High settings.   Serve warm.

Spinach With Halloumi Cheese Casserole

Ingredients: Servings: 4   Cooking Time: 2 Hours

1 package spinach, rinsed	1 tbsp. balsamic vinegar
½ C. walnuts, chopped	1 ½ C. halloumi cheese, grated
Salt and pepper to taste	

Directions:

Place spinach and walnuts in the crockpot.   Season with salt and pepper. Drizzle with balsamic vinegar.   Top with halloumi cheese and cook on low for 2 hours or on high for 30 minutes

Dill Brussel Sprouts

Ingredients: Servings: 4   Cooking Time: 2 Hours

4 C. Brussel sprouts, halved	1 tbsp. dried dill
2 tbsp. avocado oil	1 tbsp. vegan butter
½ tsp. salt	2 C. of water

Directions:

Pour water in the Crock Pot. Add Brussel sprouts.   Then close the lid and cook the vegetables on high for 2 hours.   After this, drain water and transfer the vegetables in the hot skillet. Sprinkle them with avocado oil, dried dill, salt, and vegan butter. Roast Brussel sprouts for 3-4 minutes on high heat.

Zucchini Soup With Rosemary And Parmesan

Ingredients: Servings: 6   Cooking Time: 3 Hours

2 tbsp. olive oil	1 onion, chopped
1 tbsp. butter	2 lb. zucchini, chopped
1 tsp. minced garlic	8 C. vegetable stock
1 tsp. Italian seasoning	Salt and pepper to taste
4 tsp. rosemary, chopped	1 C. grated parmesan cheese

Directions:

Place all ingredients except for the parmesan cheese in the CrockPot.   Give a good stir.   Close the lid and cook on high for 3 hours or on low for 4 hours   Place inside a blender and pulse until smooth.   Serve with parmesan cheese on top.

Fragrant Jackfruit

Ingredients: Servings: 4   Cooking Time: 2 Hours

1-lb. jackfruit, canned, chopped	1 tsp. taco seasoning
1 tsp. tomato paste	½ C. coconut cream
1 onion, diced	1 tsp. chili powder

Directions:

In the mixing bowl mix taco seasoning, chili powder, tomato paste, and coconut cream.   Put the jackfruit and diced onion in the Crock Pot.   Pour the tomato mixture over the vegetables and gently mix them.   Close the lid and cook the meal on High for 2 hours.

Beet Salad

Ingredients: Servings: 4   Cooking Time: 5 Hours

2 C. beet, peeled, chopped	1 tbsp. olive oil
3 oz. goat cheese, crumbled	1 tsp. liquid honey
4 C. of water	3 pecans, chopped

Directions:

Put beets in the Crock Pot.   Add water and cook them on high for 5 hours.   The drain water and transfer the cooked beets in the bowl.   Add olive oil, honey, and pecans. Shake the vegetables well and transfer them to the serving plates.   Top every serving with crumbled goat cheese.

Coconut Cauliflower Florets

Ingredients: Servings: 4   Cooking Time: 4 Hours

2 C. cauliflower, florets	1 C. of coconut milk
1 tbsp. coconut flakes	1 tsp. salt
	1 tsp. ground turmeric

Directions:

Sprinkle the cauliflower florets with ground turmeric and salt, and transfer in the Crock Pot.   Add coconut flakes and coconut milk.   Close the lid and cook the meal on Low for 4 hours. Carefully mix the cauliflower before serving.

Tofu Kebabs

Ingredients: Servings: 4   Cooking Time: 2 Hours

2 tbsp. lemon juice	1 tsp. chili powder
1 tsp. ground turmeric	¼ C. of water
2 tbsp. coconut cream	1 tsp. avocado oil
	1-lb. tofu, cubed

Directions:

Pour water in the Crock Pot.   After this, in the mixing bowl mix lemon juice, ground turmeric, coconut cream, chili powder, and avocado oil.   Coat every tofu cube in the coconut cream mixture and string on the wooden skewers. Place them in the Crock Pot. Cook the tofu kebabs on Low for 2 hours.

Thyme Fennel Bulb

Ingredients: Servings: 4   Cooking Time: 3 Hours

16 oz. fennel bulb	1 tsp. salt
1 tbsp. thyme	1 tsp. peppercorns
1 C. of water	

Directions:

Chop the fennel bulb roughly and put it in the Crock Pot. Add thyme, water, salt, and peppercorns. Cook the fennel on High for 3 hours. Then drain water, remove peppercorns, and transfer the fennel in the serving plates.

Pinto Beans With Rice

Ingredients: Servings: 6   Cooking Time: 3 Hours

1 lb. pinto beans, dried	½ tsp. cumin, ground
1/3 C. hot sauce	1 tbsp. chili powder
Salt and black pepper to the taste	3 bay leaves
1 tbsp. garlic, minced	½ tsp. oregano, dried
1 tsp. garlic powder	1 C. white rice, cooked

Directions:

Add pinto beans along with the rest of the ingredients to your Crock Pot. Put the cooker's lid on and set the cooking time to 3 hours on High settings. Serve warm on top of rice.

Quinoa Avocado Salad(1)

Ingredients: Servings: 6   Cooking Time: 7 Hours

½ lemon, juiced	1 tsp. canola oil
1 avocado, pitted, peeled and diced	½ C. fresh dill
1 red onion, diced	1 C. green peas, frozen
1 C. white quinoa	1 tsp. garlic powder
1 C. of water	

Directions:

Add quinoa, green peas and water to the Crock Pot. Put the cooker's lid on and set the cooking time to 7 hours on Low settings. Transfer the cooked quinoa and peas to a salad bowl. Stir in the remaining ingredients for the salad and toss well. Serve fresh.

Wild Rice Peppers

Ingredients: Servings: 5   Cooking Time: 7.5 Hours

1 tomato, chopped	1 tsp. turmeric
1 C. wild rice, cooked	1 tsp. curry powder
4 oz. ground chicken	1 C. chicken stock
2 oz. mushroom, sliced	2 tsp. tomato paste
½ onion, sliced	1 oz. black olives
1 tsp. salt	5 red sweet pepper, cut the top off and seeds removed

Directions:

Toss rice with salt, turmeric, olives, tomato, onion, chicken, mushrooms, curry powder in a bowl. Pour tomato paste and chicken stock into the Crock Pot. Stuff the sweet peppers with chicken mixture. Place the stuffed peppers in the cooker. Put the cooker's lid on and set the cooking time to 7 hours 30 minutes on Low settings. Serve warm with tomato gravy.

Brussel Sprouts

Ingredients: Servings: 4   Cooking Time: 2.5 Hours

1-lb. Brussel sprouts	1 tsp. cayenne pepper
2 oz. tofu, chopped, cooked	1 tbsp. vegan butter
2 C. of water	

Directions:

Pour water in the Crock Pot. Add Brussel sprouts and cayenne pepper. Cook the vegetables on high for 2.5 hours. Then drain water and mix Brussel sprouts with butter and tofu. Shake the vegetables gently.

Asian Broccoli Sauté

Ingredients: Servings: 4   Cooking Time: 3 Hours

1 tbsp. coconut oil	1 tsp. ginger, grated
1 head broccoli, cut into florets	Salt and pepper to taste
1 tbsp. coconut aminos or soy sauce	

Directions:

Place the ingredients in the crockpot. Toss everything to combine. Close the lid and cook on low for 3 hours or on high for an hour. Once cooked, sprinkle with sesame seeds or sesame oil.

Potato Bake

Ingredients: Servings: 3   Cooking Time: 7 Hours

2 C. potatoes, peeled, halved	1 tbsp. vegan butter, softened
4 oz. vegan Provolone cheese, grated	½ C. vegetable stock
1 tsp. dried dill	1 carrot, diced

Directions:

Grease the Crock Pot bottom with butter and put the halved potato inside. Sprinkle it with dried dill and carrot. Then add vegetable stock and Provolone cheese. Cook the potato bake on low for 7 hours.

Rice Stuffed Apple Cups

Ingredients: Servings: 4   Cooking Time: 6 Hours

4 red apples	7 tbsp. water
1 C. white rice	1 tsp. salt
3 tbsp. raisins	1 tsp. curry powder
1 onion, diced	4 tsp. sour cream

Directions:

Remove the seeds and half of the flesh from the center of the apples to make apple cups. Toss onion with white rice, curry powder, salt, and raisin in a separate bowl. Divide this rice-raisins mixture into the apple cups. Pour water into the Crock

Pot and place the stuffed C. in it. Top the apples with sour cream. Put the cooker's lid on and set the cooking time to 6 hours on Low settings. Serve.

Cauliflower Hash

Ingredients: Servings: 4   Cooking Time: 2.5 Hours

3 C. cauliflower, roughly chopped	½ C. potato, chopped
3 oz. Provolone, grated	1 C. milk
2 tbsp. chives, chopped	½ C. of water
	1 tsp. chili powder

Directions:
Pour water and milk in the Crock Pot. Add cauliflower, potato, chives, and chili powder. Close the lid and cook the mixture on high for 2 hours. Then sprinkle the hash with provolone cheese and cook the meal on High for 30 minutes.

Rice Stuffed Eggplants

Ingredients: Servings: 4   Cooking Time: 8 Hours

4 medium eggplants	1 tsp. paprika
1 C. rice, half-cooked	½ C. fresh cilantro
½ C. chicken stock	3 tbsp. tomato sauce
1 tsp. salt	1 tsp. olive oil

Directions:
Slice the eggplants in half and scoop 2/3 of the flesh from the center to make boats. Mix rice with tomato sauce, paprika, salt, and cilantro in a bowl. Now divide this rice mixture into the eggplant boats. Pour stock and oil into the Crock Pot and place the eggplants in it. Put the cooker's lid on and set the cooking time to 8 hours on Low settings. Serve warm.

Corn Salad

Ingredients: Servings: 4   Cooking Time: 1.5 Hours

2 C. corn kernels	1 C. of water
1 tsp. vegan butter	1 tsp. chili flakes
1 C. lettuce, chopped	1 tsp. salt
1 C. tomatoes, chopped	1 tbsp. sunflower oil

Directions:
Pour water in the Crock Pot, add corn kernels and cook them on high for 5 hours. Then drain water and transfer the corn kernels in the salad bowl. Add lettuce, tomatoes, chili flakes, salt, and sunflower oil. Shake the salad gently.

Turmeric Parsnip

Ingredients: Servings: 2   Cooking Time: 7 Hours

10 oz. parsnip, chopped	½ tsp. onion powder
1 tsp. ground turmeric	½ tsp. salt
1 tsp. chili flakes	1 C. of water
	1 tsp. vegan butter

Directions:

Put parsnip in the Crock Pot, Add chili flakes and ground turmeric. Then add onion powder, salt, water, and butter. Close the lid and cook the meal on Low for 7 hours.

Broccoli Fritters

Ingredients: Servings: 4   Cooking Time: 40 Minutes

2 C. broccoli, shredded	1 egg, beaten
1 tsp. chili flakes	1 tbsp. cornflour
1 tsp. salt	1 tbsp. sunflower oil
2 tbsp. semolina	¼ C. coconut cream

Directions:
In the mixing bowl mix shredded broccoli, chili flakes, salt, semolina, egg, and cornflour. Make the small fritters from the broccoli mixture. Then pour sunflower in the Crock Pot. Out the fritters in the Crock Pot in one layer. Add coconut cream. Cook the fritters on High for 40 minutes.

Mushroom Saute

Ingredients: Servings: 4   Cooking Time: 2.5 Hours

2 C. cremini mushrooms, sliced	1 tsp. ground black pepper
1 white onion, sliced	¼ C. vegan Cheddar cheese, shredded
½ C. fresh dill, chopped	1 tbsp. coconut oil
1 C. coconut cream	

Directions:
Toss the coconut oil in the skillet and melt it. Add mushrooms and onion. Roast the vegetables on medium heat for 5 minutes. Then transfer them in the Crock Pot. Add all remaining ingredients and carefully mix. Cook the mushroom saute on High for 2.5 hours.

Creamy White Mushrooms

Ingredients: Servings: 4   Cooking Time: 8 Hours

1-lb. white mushrooms, chopped	1 tsp. ground black pepper
1 C. cream	1 tbsp. dried parsley
1 tsp. chili flakes	

Directions:
Put all ingredients in the Crock Pot. Cook the mushrooms on low for 8 hours. When the mushrooms are cooked, transfer them in the serving bowls and cool for 10-15 minutes.

Yam Fritters

Ingredients: Servings: 1   Cooking Time: 4 Hours

1 yam, grated, boiled	1 egg, beaten
1 tsp. dried parsley	1 tsp. flour
¼ tsp. chili powder	5 tbsp. coconut cream
¼ tsp. salt	Cooking spray

Directions:
In the mixing bowl mix grated yams, dried parsley, chili powder, salt, egg, and flour. Make the fritters from the yam mixture. After this, spray the Crock Pot bottom with cooking spray. Put the fritters inside in one layer. Add coconut cream and cook the meal on Low for 4 hours.

Sweet Onions

Ingredients: Servings: 4   Cooking Time: 4 Hours

2 C. white onion,
sliced
½ C. vegan butter
1 tsp. ground black
pepper

¼ C. of water
1 tbsp. maple syrup
1 tsp. lemon juice

Directions:
Put all ingredients in the Crock Pot.   Close the lid and cook the
onions on low for 4 hours.

Walnut Kale

Ingredients: Servings: 4   Cooking Time: 5 Hours

5 C. kale, chopped
2 oz. walnuts,
chopped
1 tsp. vegan butter

1 C. of coconut milk
1 C. of water
1 oz. vegan Parmesan,
grated

Directions:
Put all ingredients in the Crock Pot and gently stir.   Then close
the lid and cook the kale on Low for 5 hours.

Marinated Jalapeno Rings

Ingredients: Servings: 4   Cooking Time: 1 Hour

1 C. of water
¼ C. apple cider
vinegar
1 tsp. peppercorns

1 garlic clove, crushed
3 tbsp. sunflower oil
5 oz. jalapeno, sliced

Directions:
Put the sliced jalapeno in the plastic vessel (layer by layer).
Then put peppercorns in the Crock Pot.   Add the garlic clove,
sunflower oil, and apple cider vinegar.   Close the lid and cook
the liquid on High for 1 hour.   After this, cool the liquid to the
room temperature and pour it over the jalapenos.   Close the
plastic vessel and leave it in the fridge for 30-40 minutes before
serving.

Mushroom Steaks

Ingredients: Servings: 4   Cooking Time: 2 Hours

4 Portobello
mushrooms
1 tbsp. avocado oil
1 tbsp. lemon juice

2 tbsp. coconut cream
½ tsp. ground black
pepper

Directions:
Slice Portobello mushrooms into steaks and sprinkle with
avocado oil, lemon juice, coconut cream, and ground black
pepper.   Then arrange the mushroom steaks in the Crock Pot in
one layer (you will need to cook all mushroom steaks by 2 times).
Cook the meal on High for 1 hour.

Aromatic Artichokes

Ingredients: Servings: 2   Cooking Time: 3 Hours

4 artichokes,
trimmed

4 tsp. olive oil
1 tsp. dried rosemary
1 C. of water

2 tbsp. lemon juice
1 tsp. minced garlic

Directions:
Mix lemon juice with olive oil, minced garlic, and dried rosemary.
Then rub every artichoke with oil mixture and arrange it in the
Crock Pot.   Add water and close the lid.   Cook the artichoke on
High for 3 hours.

Saag Aloo

Ingredients: Servings: 6   Cooking Time: 6 Hours

1 yellow onion,
chopped
1 C. potatoes,
chopped
3 garlic cloves, diced
1 chili pepper,
chopped
2 C. of water

1 tsp. ground cumin
1 tsp. garam masala
1 C. tomatoes,
chopped
1 C. spinach, chopped

Directions:
Put onion, potatoes, and chili pepper in the Crock Pot.   Add
tomatoes and spinach.   After this, add sprinkle the ingredients
with garam masala, ground cumin, and garlic.   Add water and
close the lid.   Cook the meal on Low for 6 hours.

Oat Fritters

Ingredients: Servings: 4   Cooking Time: 2 Hours

1 C. rolled oats
¼ tsp. ground
paprika
2 sweet potatoes,
peeled, boiled

1 tsp. salt
1 tbsp. coconut oil
2 tbsp. coconut cream

Directions:
In the mixing bowl mix rolled oats, ground paprika, salt, and
potatoes.   When the mixture is homogenous, make the fritters
and transfer them in the Crock Pot.   Add coconut cream and
coconut oil.   Cook the fritters in High for 1 hour.   Then flip the
fritters on another side and cook them for 1 hour more.

Broccoli And Cheese Casserole

Ingredients: Servings: 4   Cooking Time: 4 Hours

¾ C. almond flour
1 head of broccoli, cut
into florets
2 large eggs, beaten

Salt and pepper to
taste
½ C. mozzarella
cheese

Directions:
Place the almond flour and broccoli in the crockpot.   Stir in the
eggs and season with salt and pepper to taste.   Sprinkle with
mozzarella cheese.   Close the lid and cook on low for 4 hours or
on high for 2 hours.

Okra Curry

Ingredients: Servings: 4   Cooking Time: 2.5 Hours

1 C. potatoes,
chopped
1 C. okra, chopped

1 tsp. curry powder
1 tsp. dried dill

| 1 C. tomatoes, chopped | 1 C. coconut cream |
| | 1 C. of water |

Directions:

Pour water in the Crock Pot. Add coconut cream, potatoes, tomatoes, curry powder, and dried dill. Cook the ingredients on High for 2 hours. Then add okra and carefully mix the meal. Cook it for 30 minutes on High.

Cauliflower Curry

Ingredients: Servings: 4   Cooking Time: 2 Hours

| 4 C. cauliflower | 2 C. of coconut milk |
| 1 tbsp. curry paste | |

Directions:

In the mixing bowl mix coconut milk with curry paste until smooth. Put cauliflower in the Crock Pot. Pour the curry liquid over the cauliflower and close the lid. Cook the meal on High for 2 hours.

Spicy Okra

Ingredients: Servings: 2   Cooking Time: 1.5 Hours

2 C. okra, sliced	1 tsp. chili flakes
½ C. vegetable stock	1 tsp. dried oregano
1 tsp. chili powder	1 tbsp. butter
½ tsp. ground turmeric	

Directions:

Put okra in the Crock Pot. Add vegetable stock, chili powder, ground turmeric, chili flakes, and dried oregano. Cook the okra on High for 1.5 hours. Then add butter and stir the cooked okra well.

Marinated Poached Aubergines

Ingredients: Servings: 6   Cooking Time: 4 Hours

½ C. apple cider vinegar	¼ C. avocado oil
1-lb. eggplants, chopped	3 garlic cloves, diced
1 C. of water	1 tsp. salt
	1 tsp. sugar

Directions:

Put all ingredients in the Crock Pot. Cook the meal on Low for 4 hours. Cool the cooked aubergines well.

Masala Eggplants

Ingredients: Servings: 2   Cooking Time: 2 Hours

½ C. coconut cream	½ C. of water
1 tsp. garam masala	2 eggplants, chopped
	1 tsp. salt

Directions:

Sprinkle the eggplants with salt and leave for 10 minutes. Then drain eggplant juice and transfer the vegetables in the Crock Pot. Add garam masala, water, and coconut cream. Cook the meal on High for 2 hours.

Braised Swiss Chard

Ingredients: Servings: 4   Cooking Time: 30 Minutes

1-lb. swiss chard, chopped	1 tbsp. sunflower oil
1 lemon	1 tsp. salt
1 tsp. garlic, diced	2 C. of water

Directions:

Put the swiss chard in the Crock Pot. Cut the lemon into halves and squeeze it over the swiss chard. After this, sprinkle the greens with diced garlic, sunflower oil, salt, and water. Mix the mixture gently with the help of the spoon and close the lid. Cook the greens on High for 30 minutes.

Arugula And Halloumi Salad

Ingredients: Servings: 4   Cooking Time: 30 Minutes

1 tbsp. coconut oil	½ tsp. garlic powder
1 tsp. smoked paprika	2 C. arugula, chopped
½ tsp. ground turmeric	1 tbsp. olive oil
1 C. cherry tomatoes	6 oz. halloumi

Directions:

Slice the halloumi and sprinkle with melted coconut oil. Put the cheese in the Crock Pot in one layer and cook on high for 15 minutes per side. Meanwhile, mix arugula with cherry tomatoes in the salad bowl. Add cooked halloumi, smoked paprika, ground turmeric, garlic powder, and olive oil. Shake the salad gently.

Cauliflower Rice

Ingredients: Servings: 6   Cooking Time: 2 Hours

4 C. cauliflower, shredded	1 tbsp. cream cheese
1 C. vegetable stock	1 tsp. dried oregano
1 C. of water	

Directions:

Put all ingredients in the Crock Pot. Close the lid and cook the cauliflower rice on High for 2 hours.

Sesame Asparagus

Ingredients: Servings: 4   Cooking Time: 3 Hours

1-lb. asparagus	½ C. vegetable stock
½ C. of soy sauce	1 tbsp. vegan butter
1 tsp. sesame seeds	

Directions:

Trim the asparagus and put it in the Crock Pot. Add soy sauce and vegetable stock. Then add sesame seeds and butter. Close the lid and cook the meal on High for 3 hours.

Butter Asparagus

Ingredients: Servings: 4   Cooking Time: 5 Hours

| 1-lb. asparagus | 1 tsp. ground black pepper |
| 2 tbsp. vegan butter | 1 C. vegetable stock |

Directions:

Pour the vegetable stock in the Crock Pot. Chop the asparagus roughly and add in the Crock Pot. Close the lid and cook the asparagus for 5 hours on Low. Then drain water and transfer the asparagus in the bowl. Sprinkle it with ground black pepper and butter.

Shallot Saute

Ingredients: Servings: 2   Cooking Time: 2.5 Hours

½ C. carrot, grated	½ tsp. salt
1 C. shallot, sliced	1 tsp. garlic, diced
1 tsp. ground turmeric	½ C. milk

Directions:

Put all ingredients in the Crock Pot. Close the lid and cook the saute on High for 2 hours. Then leave the cooked meal for 30 minutes to rest.

Garlic Eggplant Rings

Ingredients: Servings: 6   Cooking Time: 40 Minutes

4 eggplants, sliced	1 tsp. salt
2 tsp. garlic, minced	2 tbsp. coconut oil
3 tbsp. mayonnaise	½ C. of water

Directions:

Mix the eggplants with salt and leave for 10 minutes. Then melt the coconut oil in the skillet. Put the sliced eggplants in the hot coconut oil and roast them for 2 minutes per side. Then transfer the eggplants in the Crock Pot. Add water and cook on High for 30 minutes. Transfer the cooked eggplant rings in the plate and sprinkle with mayonnaise and minced garlic.

Sweet Pineapple Tofu

Ingredients: Servings: 2   Cooking Time: 15 Minutes

1/3 C. pineapple juice	¼ tsp. ground cardamom
1 tsp. brown sugar	7 oz. firm tofu, chopped
1 tsp. ground cinnamon	1 tsp. olive oil

Directions:

Put tofu in the mixing bowl. Then sprinkle it with pineapple juice, brown sugar, ground cinnamon, cardamom, and olive oil. Carefully mix the tofu and leave it for 10-15 minutes. Then transfer the tofu mixture in the Crock Pot and close the lid. Cook it on High for 15 minutes.

Sweet Potato And Lentils Pate

Ingredients: Servings: 4   Cooking Time: 6 Hours

1 C. sweet potato, chopped	1 tbsp. soy milk
½ C. red lentils	1 tsp. cayenne pepper
2.5 C. water	½ tsp. salt

Directions:

Put all ingredients in the Crock Pot. Close the lid and cook the mixture on low for 6 hours. When the ingredients are cooked, transfer them in the blender and blend until smooth. Put the cooked pate in the bowl and store it in the fridge for up to 4 days.

Fragrant Appetizer Peppers

Ingredients: Servings: 2   Cooking Time: 1.5 Hours

4 sweet peppers, seeded	1 red onion, sliced
¼ C. apple cider vinegar	½ tsp. sugar
1 tsp. peppercorns	¼ C. of water
	1 tbsp. olive oil

Directions:

Slice the sweet peppers roughly and put in the Crock Pot. Add all remaining ingredients and close the lid. Cook the peppers on high for 1.5 hours. Then cool the peppers well and store them in the fridge for up to 6 days.

Zucchini Caviar

Ingredients: Servings: 4   Cooking Time: 5 Hours

4 C. zucchini, grated	1 tsp. salt
2 onions, diced	1 tsp. ground black pepper
2 tbsp. tomato paste	1 C. of water
	1 tsp. olive oil

Directions:

Put all ingredients in the Crock Pot. Close the lid and cook the meal on Low for 5 hours. Then carefully stir the caviar and cool it to the room temperature.

Spaghetti Cheese Casserole

Ingredients: Servings: 8   Cooking Time: 7 Hours

1 lb. cottage cheese	3 tbsp. white sugar
7 oz. spaghetti, cooked	1 tsp. vanilla extract
5 eggs	1 tsp. marjoram
1 C. heavy cream	1 tsp. lemon zest
5 tbsp. semolina	1 tsp. butter

Directions:

Start by blending cottage cheese in a blender jug for 1 minute. Add eggs to the cottage cheese and blend again for 3 minutes. Stir in semolina, cream, sugar, marjoram, vanilla extract, butter and lemon zest. Blend again for 1 minute and keep the cheese-cream mixture aside. Spread the chopped spaghetti layer in the Crock Pot. Top the spaghetti with 3 tbsp. with the cheese-cream mixture. Add another layer of spaghetti over the mixture. Continue adding alternate layers in this manner until all ingredients are used. Put the cooker's lid on and set the cooking time to 7 hours on Low settings. Slice and serve.

Chili Okra

Ingredients: Servings: 6   Cooking Time: 7 Hours

6 C. okra, chopped	½ tsp. cayenne pepper
1 C. tomato juice	
1 tsp. salt	1 tbsp. olive oil
½ tsp. chili powder	1 C. vegetable stock

Directions:

Put all ingredients from the list above in the Crock Pot. Mix them gently and cook on Low for 7 hours.

Vegan Kofte

Ingredients: Servings: 4   Cooking Time: 4 Hours

2 eggplants, peeled, boiled	½ C. chickpeas, canned
1 tsp. minced garlic	3 tbsp. breadcrumbs
1 tsp. ground cumin	1/3 C. water
¼ tsp. minced ginger	1 tbsp. coconut oil

Directions:

Blend the eggplants until smooth. Add minced garlic, ground cumin, minced ginger, chickpeas, and blend the mixture until smooth. Transfer it in the mixing bowl. Add breadcrumbs. Make the small koftes and put them in the Crock Pot. Add coconut oil and close the lid. Cook the meal on Low for 4 hours.

Herbed Mushrooms

Ingredients: Servings: 4   Cooking Time: 4.5 Hours

1-lb. cremini mushrooms	1 tsp. fennel seeds
1 tsp. cumin seeds	3 tbsp. sesame oil
1 tsp. coriander seeds	1 tsp. salt
2 C. of water	3 tbsp. lime juice

Directions:

Pour water in the Crock Pot. Add mushrooms. Close the lid and cook them on High for 4.5 hours. Then drain water and transfer mushrooms in the big bowl. Sprinkle them with cumin seeds, coriander seeds, fennel seeds, sesame oil, salt, and lime juice. Carefully mix the mushrooms and leave them to marinate for 30 minutes.

Tofu And Cauliflower Bowl

Ingredients: Servings: 3   Cooking Time: 2.15 Hours

5 oz. firm tofu, chopped	¼ C. of coconut milk
1 tsp. curry paste	1 tbsp. sunflower oil
1 tsp. dried basil	2 C. cauliflower, chopped
	1 C. of water

Directions:

Put cauliflower in the Crock Pot. Add water and cook it on High for 2 hours. Meanwhile, mix curry paste with coconut milk, dried basil, and sunflower oil. Then add tofu and carefully mix the mixture. Leave it for 30 minutes. When the cauliflower is cooked, drain water. Add tofu mixture and shake the meal well. Cook it on High for 15 minutes.

Sweet Potato Puree

Ingredients: Servings: 2   Cooking Time: 4 Hours

2 C. sweet potato, chopped	1 oz. scallions, chopped
1 C. of water	1 tsp. salt
¼ C. half and half	

Directions:

Put sweet potatoes in the Crock Pot. Add water and salt. Cook them on High for 4 hours. The drain water and transfer the sweet potatoes in the food processor. Add half and half and

blend until smooth. Transfer the puree in the bowl, and scallions, and mix carefully.

Crockpot Vindaloo Vegetables

Ingredients: Servings: 6   Cooking Time: 4 Hours

3 cloves of garlic, minced	½ tsp. cardamom
1 tbsp. ginger, chopped	½ tsp. turmeric powder
1 ½ tsp. coriander powder	1 onion, chopped
1 ¼ tsp. ground cumin	4 C. cauliflower florets
½ tsp. dry mustard	1 red bell peppers, chopped
½ tsp. cayenne pepper	1 green bell peppers, chopped
	Salt and pepper to taste

Directions:

Place all ingredients in the Crock Pot. Give a good stir. Close the lid and cook on high for 3 hours or on low for 4 hours.

Buffalo Cremini Mushrooms

Ingredients: Servings: 4   Cooking Time: 6 Hours

3 C. cremini mushrooms, trimmed	½ C. of water
2 oz. buffalo sauce	2 tbsp. coconut oil

Directions:

Pour water in the Crock Pot. Melt the coconut oil in the skillet. Add mushrooms and roast them for 3-4 minutes per side. Transfer the roasted mushrooms in the Crock Pot. Cook them on Low for 4 hours. Then add buffalo sauce and carefully mix. Cook the mushrooms for 2 hours on low.

Sauteed Spinach

Ingredients: Servings: 3   Cooking Time: 1 Hour

3 C. spinach	2 oz. Parmesan, grated
1 tbsp. vegan butter, softened	1 tsp. pine nuts, crushed
2 C. of water	

Directions:

Chop the spinach and put it in the Crock Pot. Add water and close the lid. Cook the spinach on High for 1 hour. Then drain water and put the cooked spinach in the bowl. Add pine nuts, Parmesan, and butter. Carefully mix the spinach.

Crockpot Cumin-roasted Vegetables

Ingredients: Servings: 2   Cooking Time: 4 Hours

1 red bell pepper, chopped	6 C. kale leaves, chopped
1 yellow bell pepper, chopped	4 tbsp. olive oil
1 green bell pepper, chopped	1 tsp. cumin
½ C. cherry tomatoes	1 tsp. dried oregano
¼ C. pepita seeds	¼ tsp. salt

Directions:

Place all ingredients in a mixing bowl. Toss to coat everything with oil. Line the bottom of the CrockPot with foil. Place the vegetables inside. Close the lid and cook on low for 4 hours or on high for 6 hours until the vegetables are a bit brown on the edges.

Info Calories per serving:380; Carbohydrates: 13.8g; Protein: 8.6g; Fat:35.8g; Sugar:1.7 g; Sodium: 512mg; Fiber: 6.6g

Braised Sesame Spinach

Ingredients: Servings: 4   Cooking Time: 35 Minutes

1 tbsp. sesame seeds	¼ C. of soy sauce
2 tbsp. sesame oil	4 C. spinach, chopped
	1 C. of water

Directions:

Pour water in the Crock Pot. Add spinach and cook it on High for 35 minutes. After this, drain water and transfer the spinach in the big bowl. Add soy sauce, sesame oil, and sesame seeds. Carefully mix the spinach and transfer in the serving plates/bowls.

Cinnamon Banana Sandwiches

Ingredients: Servings: 4   Cooking Time: 2 Hours

2 bananas, peeled and sliced	¼ tsp. ground cinnamon
8 oz. French toast slices, frozen	5 oz. Cheddar cheese, sliced
1 tbsp. peanut butter	¼ tsp. turmeric

Directions:

Layer half of the French toast slices with peanut butter. Whisk cinnamon with turmeric and drizzle over the peanut butter layer. Place the banana slice and cheese slices over the toasts. Now place the remaining French toast slices on top. Place these banana sandwiches in the Crock Pot. Put the cooker's lid on and set the cooking time to 2 hours on High settings. Serve.

Quinoa Casserole

Ingredients: Servings: 6   Cooking Time: 3 Hours

1 tsp. nutritional yeast	1 C. broccoli florets, chopped
1 C. quinoa	1 C. cashew cream
1 C. bell pepper, chopped	1 tsp. chili flakes
1 tsp. smoked paprika	3 C. of water

Directions:

Mix quinoa with nutritional yeast and put in the Crock Pot. Add bell pepper, smoked paprika, broccoli florets, and chili flakes. Add cashew cream and water. Close the lid and cook the casserole for 3 hours on high.

Mung Beans Salad

Ingredients: Servings: 4   Cooking Time: 3 Hours

½ avocado, chopped	3 C. of water
1 C. cherry tomatoes, halved	1 tbsp. lemon juice
	1 tbsp. avocado oil
½ C. corn kernels, cooked	
1 C. mung beans	

Directions:

Put mung beans in the Crock Pot. Add water and cook them on High for 3 hours. Then drain water and transfer the mung beans in the salad bowl. Add avocado, cherry tomatoes, corn kernels, and shake well. Then sprinkle the salad with avocado oil and lemon juice.

Curry Paneer

Ingredients: Servings: 2   Cooking Time: 2 Hours

6 oz. paneer, cubed	½ C. coconut cream
1 tsp. garam masala	1 tsp. olive oil
1 chili pepper, chopped	½ onion, diced
	1 tsp. garlic paste

Directions:

In the mixing bowl mix diced onion, garlic paste, olive oil, chili pepper, coconut cream, and garam masala. Then mix the mixture with cubed paneer and put in the Crock Pot. Cook it on Low for 2 hours.

Creamy Garlic Potatoes

Ingredients: Servings: 6   Cooking Time: 7 Hours

2 lb. potatoes	½ tsp. salt
1 C. heavy cream	1 tbsp. fresh dill
1 tbsp. minced garlic	1 tsp. butter
1 tsp. garlic powder	

Directions:

Liberally rub the potatoes with butter and place them in the Crock Pot. Whisk cream with garlic powder, minced garlic fill, and salt in a bowl. Add cream mixture to the potatoes. Put the cooker's lid on and set the cooking time to 7 hours on Low settings. Serve warm.

Vanilla Applesauce

Ingredients: Servings: 4   Cooking Time: 6 Hours

4 C. apples, chopped, peeled	½ tsp. ground cardamom
1 tsp. vanilla extract	1 tbsp. lemon juice
1 C. of water	2 tbsp. sugar

Directions:

Put all ingredients in the Crock Pot. Close the lid and cook them on Low for 6 hours. Then blend the mixture with the help of the immersion blender. Transfer the smooth applesauce in the glass cans.

Potato Balls

Ingredients: Servings: 6   Cooking Time: 1.5 Hours

2 C. mashed potato	1 tsp. dried dill
1 tbsp. coconut cream	2 oz. scallions, diced
3 tbsp. breadcrumbs	1 egg, beaten
	2 tbsp. flour
	½ C. of coconut milk

Directions:

In the mixing bowl mix mashed potato with coconut cream, breadcrumbs, dried dill, scallions, egg, and flour. Make the potato balls and put them in the Crock Pot. Add coconut milk and cook the meal on High for 1.5 hours.

Green Peas Puree

Ingredients: Servings: 2   Cooking Time: 1 Hour

2 C. green peas, frozen	1 tsp. smoked paprika
1 tbsp. coconut oil	1 C. vegetable stock

Directions:

Put green peas, smoked paprika, and vegetable stock in the Crock Pot. Cook the ingredients in high for 1 hour. Then drain the liquid and mash the green peas with the help of the potato masher. Add coconut oil and carefully stir the cooked puree.

Mushroom Bourguignon

Ingredients: Servings: 3   Cooking Time: 7 Hours

½ C. mushrooms, chopped	¼ C. carrot, diced
¼ C. onion, chopped	1 tsp. salt
½ C. green peas, frozen	2 tbsp. tomato paste
1 tsp. dried thyme	3 C. vegetable stock

Directions:

Mix vegetable stock with tomato paste and pour liquid in the Crock Pot. Add all remaining ingredients and close the lid. Cook the meal on Low for 7 hours.

Paprika Baby Carrot

Ingredients: Servings: 2   Cooking Time: 2.5 Hours

1 tbsp. ground paprika	2 C. baby carrot
1 tsp. cumin seeds	1 C. of water
	1 tsp. vegan butter

Directions:

Pour water in the Crock Pot. Add baby carrot, cumin seeds, and ground paprika. Close the lid and cook the carrot on High for 2.5 hours. Then drain water, add butter, and shake the vegetables.

Beans Bake

Ingredients: Servings: 4   Cooking Time: 5 Hours

1-lb. green beans	1 tsp. salt
1 tbsp. olive oil	2 tbsp. breadcrumbs
½ tsp. ground black pepper	4 eggs, beaten

Directions:

Chop the green beans roughly and sprinkle them with salt and ground black pepper. Then put them in the Crock Pot. Sprinkle the vegetables with breadcrumbs and eggs. Close the lid and cook the beans bake on Low for 5 hours.

Braised Root Vegetables

Ingredients: Servings: 4   Cooking Time: 8 Hours

1 C. beets, chopped	1 tsp. raisins
1 C. carrot, chopped	1 tsp. salt
2 C. vegetable stock	1 tsp. onion powder

Directions:

Put all ingredients in the Crock Pot. Close the lid and cook them on Low for 8 hours.

Corn Pudding

Ingredients: Servings: 4   Cooking Time: 5 Hours

3 C. corn kernels	2 C. heavy cream
3 tbsp. muffin mix	1 oz. Parmesan, grated

Directions:

Mix heavy cream with muffin mix and pour the liquid in the Crock Pot. Add corn kernels and Parmesan. Stir the mixture well. Close the lid and cook the pudding on Low for 5 hours.

Egg Cauliflower

Ingredients: Servings: 2   Cooking Time: 4 Hours

2 C. cauliflower, shredded	1 tbsp. vegan butter
4 eggs, beaten	½ tsp. salt

Directions:

Mix eggs with salt. Put the shredded cauliflower in the Crock Pot. Add eggs and vegan butter. Gently mix the mixture. Close the lid and cook the meal on low for 4 hours. Stir the cauliflower with the help of the fork every 1 hour.

Baked Onions

Ingredients: Servings: 4   Cooking Time: 2 Hours

4 onions, peeled	1 tsp. brown sugar
1 tbsp. coconut oil	1 C. coconut cream
1 tsp. salt	

Directions:

Put coconut oil in the Crock Pot. Then make the small cuts in the onions with the help of the knife and put in the Crock Pot in one layer. Sprinkle the vegetables with salt, and brown sugar. Add coconut cream and close the lid. Cook the onions on High for 2 hours.

Rainbow Carrots

Ingredients: Servings: 4   Cooking Time: 3.5 Hours

2-lb. rainbow carrots, sliced	1 onion, sliced
1 C. vegetable stock	1 tsp. salt
1 C. bell pepper, chopped	1 tsp. chili powder

Directions:

Put all ingredients in the Crock Pot. Close the lid and cook the meal on High for 3.5 hours. Then cool the cooked carrots for 5-10 minutes and transfer in the serving bowls.

Sugar Yams

Ingredients: Servings: 4   Cooking Time: 2 Hours

4 yams, peeled   2 tbsp. vegan butter

1 C. of water

1 tbsp. sugar

Directions:

Cut the yams into halves and put them in the Crock Pot.   Add water and cook for 2 hours on high.   Then melt the butter in the skillet.   Add sugar and heat it until sugar is melted.   Then drain water from the yams.   Put the yams in the sugar butter and roast for 2 minutes per side.

Recipe index

C

M

N

Printed in the USA
CPSIA information can be obtained
at www.ICGtesting.com
LVHW060243280823
756471LV00007B/86